Th

The Impact of Hospitals

John Henderson, Peregrine Horden, and Alessandro Pastore (eds)

The Impact of Hospitals

300-2000

PETER LANG

Oxford · Bern · Berlin · Bruxelles · Frankfurt am Main · New York · Wien

Bibliographic information published by Die Deutsche Bibliothek
Die Deutsche Bibliothek lists this publication in the Deutsche
Nationalbibliografie; detailed bibliographic data is available on
the Internet at ‹http://dnb.ddb.de›.

British Library and Library of Congress Cataloguing-in-Publication Data:
A catalogue record for this book is available from *The British Library,*
Great Britain, and from *The Library of Congress,* USA

Cover image: Prospect of St Thomas's Hospital, London, as published
in John Strype's 1720 edition of John Stow's *Survey of London*
(photo: Wellcome Library, London).

ISBN 978-3-03911-001-8

© Peter Lang AG, International Academic Publishers, Bern 2007
Hochfeldstrasse 32, Postfach 746, CH-3000 Bern 9, Switzerland
info@peterlang.com, www.peterlang.com, www.peterlang.net

Printed in Germany

Contents

Part Two: The Visual Impact

Part Three: The Impact on Rural Landscape

Part Four: The Impact on the Patient

Preface

The chapters of this collection derive principally from papers read to the second conference of the International Network for the History of Hospitals, 'Hospitals and Health: The Balance Sheet', held at Verona in April 2001. The volume also includes authors who contributed to the Network's inaugural conference, 'From Liturgy to Therapy', held at Norwich in November 1999. The two conferences were organised respectively by Alessandro Pastore and Carole Rawcliffe. The editors' thanks go to those who administered these gatherings: for Verona, Marina Garbellotti of Trento University; for Norwich, Becky Fitt of the University of East Anglia. The editors are heavily indebted to the contributors for their patience, and their willingness to recast their papers extensively for publication. They wish to thank the Wellcome Trust for its long-standing and generous support of the International Network's ventures, and the sponsors of the Verona conference: the Università degli Studi di Verona and the Fondazione Cassa di Risparmio di Verona Vicenza Belluno e Ancona. Humaira Erfan Ahmed prepared camera-ready copy with her customary speed, skill and good humour. We offer her our warmest thanks.

The chapters that follow interlock in a number of ways. The editors have grouped them under five main headings to bring out just some of their recurrent themes. No volume of manageable length could fully reflect the scholarship now being lavished on hospital history. We hope, however, that this collection of studies, especially when read in conjunction with the global history of hospitals and the survey of recent writing contained in the Introduction, will alert not only historians of medicine, but historians of all kinds to the value and interest of institutions that were and remain, in Carole Rawcliffe's memorable phrase, 'a mirror to society'.

JH

PH

AP

List of Figures

JOHN HENDERSON, PEREGRINE HORDEN and ALESSANDRO PASTORE

Introduction. The World of the Hospital: Comparisons and Continuities

> The whole earth is our hospital
> Endowed by the ruined millionaire
> T.S. Eliot, *Four Quartets*, 'East Coker', IV

I   A Cross-Roads of Hospital History?

Vienna around the year 1780.[1] Anyone with a time machine and a desire to gain some vantage point on the long-term history of hospitals, but allowed just one period and place to visit, could make a far worse choice of venue. In this city with a population of over a quarter of a million people, some 1,000 hospital beds were available for the care of the sick and needy. They were distributed across a range of institutions that varied greatly in size and services. But most exemplified a tradition of Catholic charity that would have been instantly recognisable back in the Middle Ages. Under the Church's aegis, though subsidised – inadequately – by the government, they offered shelter and nursing to poor immigrants, the homeless, the elderly, and the needy sick. There was the Bürgerspital, the oldest in the city, with 200 beds, founded in the thirteenth century. There was the Bäckenhäusel, which had been established as a lazaretto or plague house in 1656, a year in which the Viennese suffered very badly from plague. And there was the Great Poorhouse dating from 1693. Reports of high institutional mortality, in these and a few other lesser establishments, did nothing to diminish their reputations as gateways to death. By the 1780s one-third of hospital patients were reckoned to have contracted the *morbus Viennensis*, the 'Viennese disease' of pulmonary tuberculosis.

At the more salubrious end of the spectrum, a few private institutions such as the seventy-bed Spanish hospital could attract paying middle-class patients and a monastic hospital in the city even set aside rooms for the nobility. Nor was learned medicine lacking. Formal clinical medical instruction was already several decades old in Vienna in 1780. It had been formally instituted in 1753 by Gerard van Swieten, the Empress Maria Theresa's personal physician and a disciple of Hermann Boerhaave, whose ward round was observed by his students in Leyden's municipal hospital from the gallery of a special ward.[2] This ward was the *collegium medico-practicum* in which lay six male and six female patients each selected for some exemplary pathological condition. In Vienna another Boerhaave student, Anton de Haen, carried out what has been famed (mistakenly) as the first such bedside teaching.[3] It took place in two rooms of six beds each in the Bürgerspital, by the eighteenth century metamorphosed into a retirement home for the elderly. This contribution to university teaching was financed by the emperor, and was part of a sweeping curricular reform designed to produce a corps of well-trained professionals who would oversee, police-like, the public health and medical needs of the Austrian masses. Though a follower of Hippocrates, and thus guided by two thousand years of tradition in his clinical observations, de Haen also developed an interest in thermometry, and many of his colleagues were engaged in research that would, within decades, contribute to the dissolution of the Hippocratic paradigm.

In 1784, not only the teaching but the whole configuration of Vienna's hospital regime changed. Having seen the fire-ravaged and decrepit Hôtel-Dieu in Paris while visiting his sister Marie Antoinette in 1777, Joseph II decided to centralise hospital care and to confine it to the sick, emulating (as he hoped) the best and avoiding the worst of the French model.[4] Poor relief was clumsily devolved to parishes and fraternities. Foreign beggars were expelled. The assets of twelve existing Viennese hospitals were 'nationalised'. The massive old almshouse was turned into the 2,000-bed *Allgemeines Krankenhaus* or General Hospital, although it still sheltered the poor as well as providing medicine for the sick.

In accordance with Enlightenment rationalism, the general hospital was neatly divided into four medical and two surgical sections, one venereal section, and one for contagious diseases. There was a lying-in facility, a tower for the insane, and an establishment for foundlings. Some space in private rooms was reserved for patients with means. The emphasis lay on using secular medicine to help the sick recover. The hospital had a staff of some fifteen university-educated physicians, an equal number of surgeons, and 140 lay attendants. Yet even though no altars were to be seen, two resident Catholic priests toured the wards daily, administering the sacraments. By 1800, after some vicissitudes, the hospital had added its own medical library. Stables were converted into isolation wards. A surgical amphitheatre was constructed so that operations would no longer be performed on the wards; and there was a new mortuary in which physicians and senior students dissected their own deceased patients. Since 1785, there had also been a subordinate military hospital, the *Josephinum*.

Some of these reforms and developments were attributable to Johann Peter Frank, author of the *System of a Complete Medical Police.*[5] His totalitarian ambitions for the health of the masses appealed to Joseph II's 'enlightened despotism'. The emperor's successor but one, Francis II, appointed Frank director of the General Hospital in 1795, his mission being in part to combat the enormous risk of cross-infection run by patients in such a large establishment.

What first strikes the time traveller about the hospitals of late Enlightenment Vienna is their sheer variety and the range of functions that they performed, even when rationalised by despotic emperors and medical 'policemen'. The poor – whether indigenous or immigrant – the aged, the pregnant, the insane, the syphilitic are all embraced by them, alongside the acutely and chronically sick. The environment in which some attempt is made to meet their needs is an 'over-determined' one (the Freudian analogy surely permissible in this of all cities.) That is, it is subject to pressures from every conceivable direction – demographic, financial, governmental, and ideological as well as medical. It has to be interpreted within the widest context of Viennese history.

Aspects of this hospital scene apparently point to the future. In the general hospital there is a clear shift from almshouse to house of the sick: the new purpose is to promote recovery rather than to offer palliative care. This hospital is no longer primarily an agent of poor relief. University-trained physicians are present, if not in proportionally very large numbers. There is a degree of secularisation: in the absence of altars the liturgical round becomes far less prominent than the ward round.

'Fast forward' only a few decades and it is in the maternity wards of the same general hospital that, in 1848, Ignaz Semmelweiss will make the observations and deductions that herald modern – biologically effective – antisepsis. Such antisepsis is one of the essential preconditions of the hospital as we have known it in the later twentieth and early twenty-first centuries: the hospital that is accepted, and indeed preferred, as the place of treatment for serious conditions by all socio-economic groups, not only the poor. In Enlightenment Vienna, there were already better-off patients paying for privacy and superior medical attention, and their history, as we shall see, is a good deal older than that. Frank was combating the cross-infections that would keep many away from hospital wards.

Also pointing to what we take to be modernity is the use of the wards and the autopsy room by physicians or surgeons for medical education and enquiry. We are at an early chapter – though by no means the first, as Boerhaave shows, without even looking back to the real beginnings in the Renaissance – in a story that will lead to the conception of the hospital as situated at the 'cutting edge' of medical technology and research.[6] In such a hospital, so its critics have contended, patients almost cease to be persons and become more like specimens. Removed from their normal surroundings they can be treated in ways that ignore those surroundings precisely because the physician is now focusing on disease entities, undistracted by the 'whole person'. That reductionism, which only in relatively recent times has shown any sign of being reversed in favour of paying attention to patient 'narratives', originates in clinical education and its conceptual or physical alignment of cases that are medically, rather than socially, similar.

Such education was centuries old in Joseph II's Vienna, and is one respect in which the example of the city's hospital seems to point us back in time as well as forwards. Another respect is the emperor's desire for centralisation under governmental control. This is really a phenomenon that historians label 'early modern' or even 'Renaissance' rather than 'Enlightenment'.[7] In many ways it was old-fashioned in France when Joseph visited his sister and inspected the massive and not very salubrious Hôtel-Dieu. Large hospitals had long been seen by reformers to generate at least as much disease as they cured. In France, where the general hospitals were most numerous and prominent, their mission to house and discipline the disorderly poor actually had the effect of enhancing the medical, curative function of other smaller hospitals, to whom they passed suitable cases.

The old hospitals still functioning in Joseph II's time not surprisingly take us deepest into the past of hospital history. Here was exemplified a tradition of Catholic charity that, if a millennium younger than the Hippocratic medicine with which it could be associated, was still of considerable antiquity. The earliest of Vienna's surviving hospitals had been a part of a great wave of foundations that spread right across western Europe in the 'high' Middle Ages of the twelfth to thirteenth centuries. The lack of 'true' medical attention, the low discharge rate and the corresponding patient mortality were always likely to be exaggerated by later 'reformers' of the sixteenth to eighteenth centuries, blackening the objects of their reform to an extent that later historians can easily accept too uncritically. The least we can say, by way of counter-argument, is that there were notable havens in which the best and most expensive of contemporary medicine was available free to patients. And it was not only in Protestant northern Europe that an emphasis on ensuring the patient a safe passage to the other world was counterbalanced by a this-worldly concern to get a sick or injured labourer quickly back to work. That aim had for example been demonstrated much earlier in some of the hospitals of Italian Renaissance cities. Still, surveying European hospitals over several centuries preceding the reign of Joseph II makes three conclusions unavoidable. First, hospitals were essentially institutions of charity in which the primary criteria of admission were as likely to be economic and social as they were to be medical. Second, secular medicine was almost always subordinate to the therapy of the sacraments in Catholic countries, or the ethical imperatives of a godly community in Protestant ones. Finally, those who could afford to stay at home for treatment or poor relief nearly always did so. It was only when hospitals, under financial pressure, took in better-off pensioners offering life-time security in return for benefactions that the choice between hospital and home became more evenly balanced.

II   A View of the Long-Term in Hospital History

Taking Vienna *c.* 1780 as a 'moment' in hospital history alerts us to many components in the generally accepted outlines of the subject.[8] We shall now retrace those outlines, adding some minor modifications of our own without, we hope, distorting the received view, and giving proportionate space to the medieval and early modern period instead of cantering briskly through them as mere warm-up to 'modernity'. More substantial reservations and additions will be set out in the next section.

Hospitals were originally Christian charitable foundations for the overnight care of transients or immigrants, the local poor also lacking in the support networks that transients would have left behind, and the sick who could not pay for treatment.[9] They had, as we shall see later, a few forerunners in pagan antiquity, but they were essentially an architectural expression of the Christian charitable imperative. They began to be founded by rulers, leading churchmen, and wealthy pious individuals with the 'establishment' of the Christian Church by Constantine in the early fourth century. These *xenodocheia* (houses for strangers as they were originally called) spread rapidly across the Byzantine empire and, more slowly, around the Mediterranean, to France, Italy, and Spain. Some, especially in major pilgrimage centres, were quite large. Some, again in the largest cities, were highly 'medicalised' in that they had wards for specific diseases or conditions, and physicians and surgeons on their staff. Others specialised in the care of the poor, the elderly, the blind, and so on.

In general, early medieval hospitals increase in size and complexity, and probably also in numbers, as one transverses Eurasia in an easterly direction. Thus western European hospitals were, on the whole, more hospice-like, offering the ultimate therapy of the sacraments, less intent on returning patients to the community than in easing chronic need and the effects of aging – or of leprosy. The biggest Byzantine hospitals displayed a more obvious emphasis on secular medicine. When the 'hospital idea' was exported from Byzantium to Islam, through the intermediary of Christian communities in Islamic lands, in the ninth and tenth centuries, hospitals attained what it is tempting to conceive as a new stage in their development. Islamic hospitals were not so overwhelmingly charitable, catering more prominently for well-to-do patients. They offered medical treatment by court physicians. They were, indeed, centres of medical learning and teaching. And many of them introduced a relatively novel element: they housed the insane – treating them perhaps harshly, but in a medical manner, as sick rather than possessed.

The hospital spread eastwards, across Asia, principally with Islam (as did Islamic medicine) rather than with Christian missionaries. Thus one major chapter in hospital history is the story of Islamic foundations, a story that stretches with few interruptions from tenth-century Baghdad to parts of India and Sri Lanka in the present day. But the next major phase of European hospital history begins in the twelfth century.[10] In Byzantine Constantinople, medicalisation seemingly reached its apogee in the Pantocrator hospital (attached to a monastery) in which there were almost more physicians and support staff than patients. In the Crusader states the Knights Hospitaller's hospital of St John in Jerusalem stands out as, by western standards, a medically intensive establishment, and as one which showed its charitable ethos in a pronounced and individual way, by proclaiming the 'Lordship of the Poor' – whom the Knights of St John were to serve as if the poor underlings were really their 'feudal' superiors.[11] More generally, across the crusaders' home territories in western Europe, hospitals were founded for the poor and, among the sick, especially for the leprous. Yet this was not because paupers and lepers were becoming proportionately more numerous, but because the prayers of such unfortunates were increasingly recognised as a sure means of helping donors' souls through purgatorial fire. The Catholic doctrine of purgatory may not have solidified until the thirteenth century, but its ingredients were already clearly recognised long before.

In parts of northern Europe, the wave of foundations that began in the twelfth century lost impetus by the time of the Black Death. Fewer hospitals were founded. In England, for example, the alms-house, with its distinct if conjoined dwellings for the respectable elderly, became the favoured type of foundation. Many existing hospitals also mutated into retirement homes, or into chantries (offering liturgy rather than charity) or into colleges of priests.

Naturally there were exceptions to this general picture, mostly to be found in the larger cities. Paris, with its Hôtel-Dieu, is one of them. No medieval English hospital could measure up to its size or the number of its medical personnel. The main contrast to the northern pattern is, however, to be found in southern Europe, to some extent in Spain,[12] but especially in the Italian city-states of the later Middle Ages and Renaissance. The hospitals of Renaissance Florence in the fifteenth and sixteenth centuries were, for example, widely admired and often the objects of emulation, as in the case of Santa Maria Nuova, which became the model for the Savoy Hospital in London, the subject of Eric Gruber von Arni's chapter in this volume. In their combination of a continuing religious ethos – altars in view of the patients, the literal centrality of the sacraments to daily life – with lay, sometimes civic, control, they show how difficult it is to carve hospital history up into periods. For they straddle the end of the Middle Ages and the beginnings of the early modern period. And, right back in the fourteenth century, they already anticipate what are usually taken to be early modern features of hospitals in major cities: lay control, centralisation, learned physicians in attendance, pharmacies attached, rapid turnover of patients (no gateways to death here, al-though women patients did stay for longer than men). It is in Italy too that we encounter the first specialised hospitals in Europe to have been founded in any numbers since the *leprosaria* of the twelfth and thir-teenth centuries: large foundling hospitals like the famous Innocenti in Florence and, later, hospitals for victims of the era's two greatest scourges, plague and the Great Pox.[13]

A degree of continuity across the supposed medieval/early modern divide is evident not only in Catholic Europe but even in England. The dissolution of almost all hospitals at the Henrician Reformation, as well as monasteries, obviously marked a break in hospital history. But many hospitals were quite rapidly refounded and new ones added – not just in London (as is commonly said), but in provincial cities such as Norwich.[14] These hospitals of the later sixteenth century broke with English traditions only in one respect, which aligns them more with their continental coevals. They, or the bigger ones at least, had attendant physicians; they were attuned to ideas about the potential of hospitals that had been aired in Italy over two centuries previously.

As we move closer in time to the Viennese example with which we began, we return to developments already sketched. The French model has usually been taken as defining the next distinct phase. In this, a division arose. On the one hand, there were the general hospitals that provided some medical care, but served primarily as catch-all establishments for the supposed work-shy, vagrants, gypsies, religious dissidents, prostitutes, beggars, the disabled, and the insane. On the other hand, there were the older *hôtels-Dieu* that, with the aforementioned social groups interned elsewhere, could concentrate more on acute and curable sickness.[15] But it should be remembered that the *hôpital général* was not peculiar to France. It was in some respects an elaboration of that English sixteenth-century invention and export, the workhouse. Further, the apparently clear distinction between it and the Hôtel-Dieu is muddied by all the other kinds of hospital that continued to develop alongside them, in France and elsewhere in Europe. These included lying-in hospitals, hostels for vagabonds, houses for the reform of prostitutes, 'conservatories' for the moral education of orphans, and, not least, the military hospital, 'a kind of laboratory for experimentation in medical services within a hospital setting'.[16]

At the opposite extreme from the governmental schemes manifested in large general hospitals, we find the 'voluntary hospitals'. These establishments began to appear in England in the 1720s and are often treated as another distinct chapter in hospital history. They are projected against a background from which hospitals had mostly disappeared, which makes them seem a novel departure. And they are presented as peculiarly English when they in fact had continental counterparts or imitations, in Germany, Switzerland and elsewhere. Seen in the *longue durée* of hospital history their peculiarity is less in the fact that they were, at least to begin with, controlled by their leading (financially most beneficent) 'voluntary' subscribers than in the particular way in which this control was exercised. Hospital benefactors had been determining the nature of institutions to which they lent their support since the earliest Christian foundations of the fourth century. They had set the criteria of admission in generic terms and doubtless exercised influence over the selection of individual patients on occasion. What was new in the eighteenth century was the regularisation of this connection between patron and patient, such that the purchase of a subscription at a particular level brought corresponding privileges in the nomination of inmates.[17]

Power to the patrons is one strident theme in hospital history of the eighteenth century – and many preceding centuries. The equivalent for the nineteenth century and since is conventionally: power to the physicians, and to the surgeons; and then power to the professional administrators. The centuries do not divide neatly, of course; and developments since the late eighteenth century are so many and various that they defeat all brief generalisation. The two largest and clearest phenomena of the nineteenth and early twentieth centuries are these. First, the enormous expansion of patient demand for hospital services (crudely estimated as a tenfold increase across the nineteenth century in Britain)[18] and concomitant increase in the number of hospital beds (over four-fold in England and Wales between 1861 and 1938).[19] Second, the growing status of hospital medicine and surgery, such that by about 1920 they had achieved the dominance that we take to be the defining feature of the modern hospital. General hospitals consumed more resources and offered a greater range of services than any other type of health care provider. So it was *c.*1800–*c.*1920, so it has been ever since.[20]

To elaborate only on the second phenomenon: from the later eighteenth century, doctors on the whole supplanted governors in the determination of hospital admissions, staff appointments, and overall policy. For the first time in history, hospital medicine was different in kind from non-hospital medicine, and not just a simplified, cheaper, version of a medical 'vernacular'. New techniques and instruments – the electro-cardiograph in the nineteenth century, the iron lung and dialysis machine in the twentieth – were either developed in hospitals or were used in them as nowhere else. The medicine with which they were involved was based conceptually in pathological anatomy – as revealed in the post mortem and refined in the hospital laboratory. With effective antisepsis and anaesthesia the hospital became by the early twentieth century the almost exclusive locus of surgery too. The criteria for admission were now chiefly medical rather than socio-economic. In England, as the Poor Law hospitals of the later nine-teenth century removed pauper patients from the voluntary hospitals, so the latter became far more acceptable to paying patients than they had ever been before – either middle-class fee payers or the working poor who contributed to some insurance scheme. Design was chang-ing too – the pavilion style advocated by Florence Nightingale being adopted in response to concerns about the hospital environment and the need for fresh air and cleanliness. (Such concerns were hardly new and clearly affected hospital architecture in, for instance, Renaissance Florence, but on the basis of a very different – humoral – medical theory.) Mention of Nightingale is a reminder, if any were needed, to add to the overall picture the changing image of the hospital nurse be-tween 1830 and *c.*1918 – from *relatively* unskilled carer to respectable educated professional – even though the image does a serious injustice to the longer-term background of women in nursing orders who pro-vided hospital food and basic medication and surgery in eighteenth-century France,[21] not to mention earlier generations of women who had been dispensing remedies in hospitals since the Middle Ages.[22]

Enhanced specialisation is the final major feature of nineteenth to twentieth century hospitals to be noted: hospitals for teaching; eye, skin, and fever hospitals; and above all that characteristically nineteenth-century phenomenon, the lunatic asylum. The insane had a long, if patchy history of being admitted to general hospitals in Europe since the later Middle Ages (earlier in some places, especially in Islamic lands, but even in the late antique Mediterranean world).[23] Small private asylums proliferated in the second half of the eighteenth century, but the large, dedicated asylum and the whole social and legal culture of 'asylumdom' is a nineteenth-century development lasting until the decarceration movement of the 1960s. By the mid-nineteenth century, in parallel to the centrality of the hospital to general medicine, 'the asylum was endorsed as the sole, officially approved response to the problems posed by mental illness'.[24]

Perhaps the most recent phase to date in hospital history should be assigned a beginning in the 1960s. What distinguishes the twentieth century may prove to be less the formation of the British National Health Service, or national or individual insurance schemes in other countries, but the sharply rising costs of the capital- and technology-intensive hospital medicine, of which such schemes are only particular expressions. The critique of hospitals that emerged in the 1960s and that has continued to be voiced in the twenty-first century seemingly marks the end of a relatively brief, quite positive, phase in hospital history. There had been 'anti-hospital' movements before, in later medieval England perhaps, as patrons favoured other types of foundation, and at the close of the late eighteenth century for example;[25] and the hospital had often (although not nearly as often as modern historians used to maintain) been stigmatised as a locus of pauperism, infection, and death. Yet it has experienced no downturn in its general reputation quite as dramatic as that registered by the biomedical 'high-tech' hospital in the later twentieth century. After many decades of growing popularity, hospitals are now a focus of those anxieties about bureaucratic, corporate modern medicine, its costs and allegedly skewed priorities, and the infections that it passes to those whom it should be curing – anxieties that enhance the attraction of alternative therapies. Hospitals are likely victims of further cost-reducing decentralisation: the devolving of services to outpatient clinics and primary health care providers. It is not hard to foresee a time when the power and cheapness of computer-run medical technology could nullify the economies of scale and concentration that have been the rationale for hospitals' existence since the time of Joseph II, if not from the very beginning. As the late Roy Porter wrote in one of his last books:

> Whether, for its part, the general medicine of the future needs, or can afford, the ever-expanding hospital complex remains unclear. Today's huge general

hospitals may soon seem medicine's dinosaurs. Will they go the way of the lunatic asylums?[26]

III Minding the Gaps

Such is one possible view of the long term in hospital history, from the fourth century to the twenty-first. It adds a few local twists and comments of its own, but essentially is meant to convey a broadly uncontroversial narrative. It is, of course, nevertheless seriously deficient, and not just in the ways that inevitably attend summaries of over 1,500 years history in a few paragraphs.

Some of the deficiencies are glaring. First, the story has been mainly European. We have not so far mentioned hospitals in North America.[27] The earliest such hospital is the Pennsylvania Hospital (1751), followed by the New York Hospital (1791), and then, after a gap, the Massachusetts General (1821). These were modelled on the English voluntary hospitals, and, in outline, the story of American hospitals is that of European hospitals – telescoped in the initial stages, varied in subsequent ones, but still overall clearly recognisable. The wealthy physicians who specialised in diseases of the rich nonetheless used poor patients to burnish their expertise, and these patients lay in the hospitals philanthropically financed by the physicians' rich patients.

The multiplication of institutions that in Europe began in the twelfth century came late to North America even when allowance is made for its having started only in 1751. A survey of 1873 revealed no more than 120 general hospitals in the entire country. The Civil War, with its one million hospital cases in the North alone, seemingly produced no major lasting changes to hospital provision. At the end of the war the military hospitals were closed and most of the soldiers still needing treatment were packed off to their families. It required the unprecedented immigration, urbanisation and industrialisation of the century's closing decades to produce a significant expansion of hospital establishment. By 1909 there were over 4,300 hospitals with

420,000 beds, but it had been only relatively recently (after *c.* 1880) that middle-class patients could be enticed to occupy any of them.

There is obviously much more to American hospital history – and not only since 1900. In keeping with the Eurocentricity of most hospital history written in English, America is only North America, and only since 1751. Yet there is wider history, both earlier and contemporary, that remains to be written in detail: colonial hospitals, exported from Old Spain to New Spain, for instance, as instruments of attempted control, conversion, acculturation, the containment of epidemics – and even medical experimentation.[28] There was a hospital on the Spanish Caribbean island of Santo Domingo from the very early sixteenth century, and one opened in what would become Mexico City soon after the subjugation of the Aztecs. It was followed in the 1530s by the first establishment exclusively for indigenous people. By the beginning of the seventeenth century there were some 128 hospitals in New Spain. Later that century, in New France, supposedly even the rich settlers availed themselves of hospital services.

This colonial hospital history of course extends to Asia and, later, Africa.[29] In Asia it again begins in the early sixteenth century. The Portuguese founded a hospital in Goa – for their own soldiers and seamen – soon after the creation of the colony in 1510. In the comparatively brief period during which Japan was open to foreigners, 1549– 1639, the Portuguese were responsible for the first western-style hospital at the other end of Asia.[30] Such a history is but one aspect of the 'globalisation' of the hospital, the earlier phases of which were outlined above. Filling out the picture in this way does not go far enough, however. The narrative presented in section 2 above was not only European. It was also Christian. It takes the beginnings of Christian hospitals in the fourth century CE as the beginnings of hospital history *tout court*. That does a small injustice to the various settings in which historians of the ancient world have, mostly without convincing result, tried to detect the pagan equivalent of the Christian hospital: in the courtyards of healing shrines in which the sick camped out for days at a time hoping for a therapeutic dream; in doctors' private clinics; and, above all, in the *valetudinaria* (literally recovery homes; seldom medicalised; and few in number) in which some sick or injured soldiers and slaves were for a short time, during the 'high' Roman Empire, nursed back to health.[31]

Beginning – as we did – with Christianity may do another, and perhaps greater, injustice to the Jewish contribution. Jewish hospitals are first clearly attested in the sixth-century CE. But both their medical development, and the extent to which they inspired or imitated Christian hospitals, remains unclear. It may be that, within synagogue complexes, a room or rooms had been set aside, hospital-like, for lodging transients a long time before the sixth century. And there was at least one first-century CE hospital-cum-guest house to cope with the great influx to the Jerusalem Temple. The history of the Jewish hospital deserves to be rescued from the margins and set alongside that of, on the one hand, the Christian hospital and, on the other, the mutation of the clearly Christian-inspired hospital idea characteristic of hospital founders in Islam.

Three religions of Abraham; three intertwined histories of hospital 'diasporas'. Even recognising that does not take us quite far enough. Hinduism, Buddhism, and Jainism each have their hospital histories – charitable in emphasis, and to that extent rather like the Judaeo-Christian type; but in the case of Jainism also producing the unusual feature (unusual in pre-modern times) of the hospital for sick animals.

This wider history of Asian hospitals brings out interesting, though presumably coincidental, similarities between East and West. It is not just that the groups to whom hospital charity is extended are similar – the sick poor, those unable to work, widows, orphans and so on. Chronological parallels are also detectable.

In the early fifth century CE, a Chinese Buddhist pilgrim touring India recorded:

> The cities and towns of this country are the greatest of all in the Middle Kingdom. The inhabitants are rich and prosperous, and vie with one another in the practice of benevolence and righteousness [...] The heads of the Vaiśya [merchant] families in them [all the kingdoms of north India] establish in the cities houses for dispensing charity and medicine. All the poor and destitute in the country, orphans, widowers, and childless men, maimed people and cripples, and all who are diseased, go to those houses, and are provided with every kind of help, and doctors examine their diseases. They get the food and

medicines which their cases require, and are made to feel at ease; and when they are better, they go away of themselves.[32]

This has been called an account of a 'civic hospital system'.[33] It may not quite be that, but it prompts interesting comparisons with the hospitals contemporaneously being founded in the Byzantine Empire.

The Middle Ages reveal other parallels. The medieval wave of foundations beginning in the twelfth century is echoed in the government-sponsored poorhouses and hospitals being set up in northern Sung China.[34] A little later, at the time this western wave was cresting, around 1200 CE Jayarvarman VII of the Cambodian kingdom of Angkor was founding or restoring 102 hospitals across his kingdom. Some details of their intended organisation can be derived from inscriptions, for instance the stele of Say-feng, close to Vientiane in Laos, and among the northernmost points of the Angkorian kingdom. To quote an authoritative summary:

> The text of this inscription mentions the persons employed by the hospital: nursing staff and servants. The hospital is open to the four castes. Two doctors are to attend to each caste; they are assisted by a man and two women 'with a right to lodging'. The personnel also includes: 'two dispensers responsible for the distribution of remedies, receiving the measures of rice. Two cooks, with a right to fuel and water, who have to tend the flowers and the lawn, and to clean the temple [...] fourteen hospital warders, entrusted with the administration of the remedies [...] two women to grind the rice.' As the hospital is a religious foundation, 'two sacrificers and one astrologer, all three pious, are to be named by the Superior of the royal monastery. Every year each of them shall be provided with the following: three coats and three lengths of cloth, fifteen pairs of garments, three pewter vases.' In addition they were to receive paddy, wax and pepper. The sick are to be fed with 'the rice forming part of the oblation to the deities [fixed] at one bushel a day' and with the remains of the sacrifices. The text next gives a long list of the medicaments placed by the king at the disposition of the sick: honey, sesame, clarified butter, a mixture of pepper, cumin and rottleria tinctoria, musk, asafoetida, camphor, sugar, 'aquatic animals,' turpentine, sandalwood, coriander, cardamum, ginger, kakola, origano, mustard seed, senna, curcumaaromatica of two kinds etc.[35]

To mention only one other, final, example: in nineteenth to twenty-first century India, hospitals dispensing either Ayurvedic medicine, or *Unani Tibb* – the 'Greek medicine' brought to India by Islam – have been erected, if not alongside, then not far from those dispensing western biomedicine.[36] Of course, the different medical systems have not remained uncontaminated by one another; in particular Ayurveda and *Unani Tibb* have accommodated aspects of their therapeutics to biomedicine. But the globalising of biomedicine has hardly produced a uniformly modern medical landscape, whether in hospitals or in medicine generally.

IV Against Grand Narrative

Hospital history is large and complicated – far more so than conventional Christocentric, Eurocentric, accounts suggest. Not surprisingly, historians who seek an Olympian view try to divide this history up into phases or stages; we have done the same ourselves in the opening sections.

Several classifications are currently on offer, all essentially similar. Back in 1936 Henry Sigerist sensibly divided hospital history into three broad stages.[37] The first saw the institutional care of the sick arising in the medical facilities incidentally offered by poor houses, guest houses and (implausible as it now seems) prisons. The second stage began in the thirteenth century where hospitals emerged as medical institutions for the indigent and dependent. The third, and so far final, stage began in the mid-nineteenth century when the 'progress of medicine and surgery' induced the emergence of the modern hospital – the hospital that we, in the 2000s, know and do not all love.

Much more recently than Sigerist, Guenter Risse, who in a very helpful monograph favours a series of case studies over a continuous narrative, none the less essays a summary typology.[38] Overall he sees hospitals as symbols of community, deliverers of social welfare, and mechanisms for coping with suffering, illness and death. The hospital is first, originally, a 'house of mercy'; then in the later Middle Ages (also the start of Sigerist's phase two) a 'house of segregation'; then in the Renaissance a 'house of rehabilitation'. In the eighteenth century the hospital becomes a 'house of care', as doctors come to dominate (in ways sketched above). From the 1880s it is a 'house of surgery', because of antisepsis, and for the first time it is used on a significant scale by the middle classes. For the last century or so, it has been a 'house of science'.

Risse's typology is elegant and memorable – and subtly qualified in all the appropriate ways. It may be preferable to proceeding by conventional historical periods (medieval, early modern, Enlightenment, and so on); as does Lindsay Granshaw, whose final division and longest section in her excellent survey article is, however, somewhat crudely, 'early modern and modern'.[39] But the problem with all these various ways of dividing up the hospital's past is not their artificiality or over-simplicity. All chronological schemes over-simplify, and are to be judged only by the heuristic value of the generalisations that result from them. The problem, rather, is in the way that the particular historiographical schemes that hospitals have attracted are all skewed towards a modernity defined by medicalisation. The background assumption is that true hospitals are medicalised – with medicalisation defined basically in terms of the presence of doctors and surgeons and, at a more sophisticated level, of the degree of authority that they wield, over the patients and over the institution as a whole. For Sigerist, that process began in the thirteenth century. For Risse, as for many others, it belongs above all to the nineteenth century and since. Whatever its particular inflection, the underlying idea is that there has been a great 'before' and 'after' in hospital history; some pivotal period in which charity gives way to medicine, care to cure, stigma to pride, the mortuary to the recovery room, the poor to the middle classes.

Why do we tend to think like this? Why do we look so persistently for the 'genesis of the modern', assessing over 1,500 years of hospital history on a yardstick calibrated for the last two centuries? The economic history of Europe since antiquity is not (or not usually) conceived solely as a search for the origins of capitalism, nor the history of transport as a frustratingly long build-up to the railway and the steamship. Yet the historiography of hospitals is more often than not written with an eye on the present, or at least on the modern. Sometimes this is an effect of the rhetoric of hospital reformers over the past two centuries: reformers have tended to exaggerate the difference of 'before' from 'after', as if they are always engaged in dragging their particular hospitals from medieval darkness into modern light.

Historians have sometimes been seduced by this rhetoric from the past. But they have also generated theories of their own. The sociologist Nicholas Jewson strikingly identified the 'disappearance of the sick man' (and woman) in hospitals around the turn of the nineteenth century. A system of hospital medicine founded in a holistic view of the individual patient and his or her environment gave way to a reductive clinical emphasis on diseased parts; the individual person was disregarded (an accusation normally reserved for, and perhaps unduly influenced by, later twentieth-century medicine).[40]

The most famous proponent of a 'big bang' theory of the origins of the modern hospital is of course Michel Foucault. His identification of the French Revolution as the brief but explosive period of 'the birth of the clinic' has proved so influential that historians have to continue rehearsing it even though few of them now accept it. Indeed, his account perhaps continues to enjoy currency precisely because it offers a clear theory to attack so that a more 'smoothed out' view of hospital medicine in the eighteenth and early nineteenth centuries can be substituted without having to arrive at some alternative conception of the period. This 'smoother' historiography finds medicalisation (when it happened at all) to have been a far more complex phenomenon than Foucauldians have alleged, yielding perhaps surprising agents of change:

> Probably the most medical process in [French] hospitals in the seventeenth century was the diffusing of nursing communities. Far from such women being – as is often simplistically alleged – the bearers of a religiously inspired anti-medicine, careful study of the contracts they passed with hospitals reveals nursing communities as a prime agent of hospital medicalization.[41]

Or again:

> to a considerable extent, we may see in military hospitals one of the prime sites in which the hospital patient qua patient was constructed over the eighteenth century, long in advance of the 'birth of the clinic' in the 1790s. Their overtly functional orientation made it more likely that their inmates were more truly sick than might be the case in civilian hospitals.[42]

The modern medicalisation of the hospital – however we define 'modernity' and 'medicalisation' – is undeniably important. But it does not have to skew the overall history of hospitals – an outline into which specialists insert their particular contributions – to quite the extent that it mostly has up to now. It may be that, for the first millennium of its history, indeed for longer than that, the modal hospital – the commonest form of hospital – was charitable, funded for the poor and offering the therapy of religion, a regulated environment and a proper diet, rather than the attentions of secular physicians. That first millennium must be viewed in its own light, rather than that cast by the period since 1900.

Alongside the modal European hospital, we must also place others that make up the rest of the global population. The modal hospital of the early Byzantine Empire was grounded in the therapy of the sacraments, even though right from the very documented beginning of Byzantine hospitals some foundations had doctors attached. The modal Islamic hospital of say the eleventh century, like the modal Cambodian hospital of the twelfth, was on the other hand highly medicalised, to judge simply by medical manpower. Considering Renaissance Florence, the highly medicalised, seemingly modern, though still essentially religious, Santa Maria Nuova may distort our overall picture. But the modal Florentine hospital of the fifteenth century remained what it had been in the twelfth – small, without medical staff, and providing overnight accommodation to pilgrims and poor travellers rather than treating large numbers of sick people.

As we move later in period so the mode becomes more elusive. We saw at the start, with the example of Josephine Vienna, and later when we returned to the Enlightenment in England and France, that towards 1800 the hospital population was still extremely diverse, old and novel elements kaleidoscopically interconnected. And the twentieth century? It might seem obvious that the modal hospital has been the one at the forefront of medical technology and intervention. But that may be true only on a circular definition – that all genuine hospitals are medicalised to that degree. If we add to the list of hospital types the hospices for palliative care of the terminally ill that have multiplied since the 1970s, and other similar institutions that would have been counted as hospitals in any period before *c*. 1800, then the mode may not be so certain. Abandon the outright privileging of western biomedicine; add in the global 'population' of famine relief centres, Ayurvedic hospitals, private hospitals owned and run by individual physicians (as in twentieth-century Japan), small temporary clinics offering only basic medication, leper sanctuaries – and the commonest form of hospital in the world since 1900 may not be the technological showcase we thought it was.

V   Hospital Historiography

Of the making of hospital histories there is no end. The modal study remains local, institutional, introspective, celebratory – a story of physicians and local activists, and above all of progress. Yet since the 1970s a 'new' hospital historiography has also developed. It is comparative (not looking at just one institution at a time) and in the broadest sense sociological or contextual. That is, it studies hospitals in their social, cultural, and religious, as well as their medical setting, recognising that there is always much more to a hospital than its doctors.

An excellent sample of this more recent approach – now not so new, of course, but still not the numerically dominant form of historical writing on the subject – is the collection edited by Lindsay Granshaw and Roy Porter, *The Hospital in History* (1989).[43] Theirs is a volume of enormous chronological scope, ranging from about 1100 to 1980. And, although six of its ten chapters deal with Britain, there are papers covering Italy, Germany, and the USA. The volume decisively breaks the traditional paradigm of hospital history written as if from the doctor's point of view. It offers a much more inclusive interpretation of the hospital in society based on an admirably broad variety of source material, not least visual evidence.[44] The functions of the hospital are shown to change over time and an unprecedentedly wide range of institutions is considered, including children's hospitals. The volume also places a new emphasis on the vital relationship between hospitals, their founders and patrons, and the wider socio-political context, thus providing a valuable tool for re-interpreting the narrow, institutional, vision of the hospital in history. The experience of patients before, during and even after hospitalisation was brought into the picture. Another advance was to produce a more nuanced conception of the relationship between hospitals and their staff of administrators and nurses.

And yet, for all its sophistication, in the background of most of the contributions to Granshaw and Porter can be detected the Foucauldian master narrative of hospital history – a narrative predicated on the centrality to hospital history of the presence or absence of doctors and focused on the question of when they appeared on the scene so as to inaugurate modernity.[45] The overall trend of identifying some great transition from care to cure was, for the contributors to this volume, contradicted only by the history of cancer hospices. They were the exception proving the rule (even though some cancer hospices prescribe not only palliative treatment but also therapy based on pain relief).[46]

Since the publication of the Granshaw-Porter volume in 1989, there has, predictably, been a cascade of studies in hospital history. The catalogue of the Wellcome Library for the History and Understanding of Medicine, to look no further, lists more than 450 publications in English alone, over half of them monographs. Many of these are substantial contributions, but they are still often chronologically restricted; others are local and introspective in scope and celebratory in tone;[47] others continue to chew over old debates.[48] Few collections in English have rivalled Granshaw and Porter in breadth.[49]

In what follows, rather than attempt to report comprehensively on this massive yet, on the whole, fragmented, literature we shall anticipate the themes of the papers below and relate them where we can to trends in recent historiography.

VI The Impact of Hospitals

In contrast to Granshaw and Porter, the present volume reflects a deliberate decision to get away from medicalisation as the leitmotiv. Instead we expand their liberating multi-disciplinary perspective still further – to convey some of the most recent and innovative approaches in the wider field of the social history of medicine, not privileging any one aspect or period, so as to arrive at a rounded view of the hospital in society. Medicine and doctors certainly appear, but as only one facet of changing varieties of therapy rather than as the defining moment in the arrival of modernity. Indeed the hospital's health-promoting role is seen within a much wider context than that of doctors, whether in relation to physicians of the soul (priests) or singers of the liturgy or the nursing staff or more broadly to the built and natural environments as stimulants to recovery.[50] Eric von Arni's discussion of the two major military hospitals for sick and maimed soldiers in seventeenth-century London, the Savoy and Ely House, serves as a good example of what conventional accounts of medicalisation so often downplay. Emphasis was placed on increasing patients' mobility with, for example, special wooden limbs being made. Ely House had a 'hot house' for sweating 'pox' patients with mercury, and sufferers were also sent to Bath for spa-water treatment. Considerable attention was paid to the environment in each hospital so that wards were frequently fumigated with burning pitch, although, as von Arni points out, patients must have suffered from inadequate ventilation.

To avoid the teleology of looking for precocious signs of modernity we consider the hospital over the *longue durée*. The chapters that follow range from what Peregrine Horden calls the 'invention' of the hospital in the late antique Mediterranean world to Annmarie Adams's discussion of the construction of Canadian hospitals in the twenty-first century. Although we thus include North America and parts of the Middle East, and have in earlier sections of this Introduction sketched a world-wide history of hospitals, our main focus has remained European and is indeed envisaged as complementary to Mark Harrison's edited collection on 'the hospital beyond the west'. This adds the much-needed African and Asian dimensions to the subject.[51]

In the present collection, as we move between early modern Italy (Bologna, Brescia, Verona), nineteenth-century Germany (Munich, Leipzig), and nineteenth- and early twentieth-century Britain (East Anglia and London), one of the recurrent themes is the range of institutions which called themselves 'hospital', whether for the sick poor or other disadvantaged groups, from pilgrims to foundlings and sick children to abandoned women or the insane. (The last of these are not considered in the chapters that follow because they have a mature historiography of their own; we shall simply note parallels with developments in adjacent fields of scholarship.)[52] Within the broad categories that recur, we find an enormous variety of function – from isolation to control, from treating the curable to comforting the incurable, from providing education[53] to the aim of returning patients to the community so that they continue to make a useful contribution to society.

A related theme, already encountered in our opening historical sketch, is specialisation, as prominent during the Middle Ages and Renaissance as it is today. A series of institutions are represented below which were established to cope with the casualties of both natural and man-made disasters. Thus Max Satchell discusses rural *leprosaria* in medieval England and Flurin Condrau looks at sanatoria for TB patients in Germany and Italy. These papers are part of a wider recent trend to examine specialised institutions, not only *leprosaria* and military establishments but isolation hospitals (*lazzaretti* for plague victims, and the new hospitals which emerged in the sixteenth century in response to that other 'new' disease, the Great Pox).[54] Hospitals set up to cope with the epidemics of more recent times, such as the isolation wards for Polio and AIDS, also belong in this tradition. Indeed each new epidemic underlines the broad continuity of society's response over the centuries, a main plank of which remains the isolation hospital, whether during the outbreak of plague in India in the mid-1990s or the SARS epidemic in 2003.

Specialisation of function relates to another theme of both this volume and recent historiography, the centralisation of resources and the development of 'systems' of care, whether (as we saw above) in

Renaissance Italy or late eighteenth-century Vienna or (as below) in the move towards municipal medicine in Britain during the 1920s and 1930s and the foundation of the National Health Service after the Second World War.[55] This topic is at the heart of two of our chapters on central and northern Italy during the Renaissance. In his discussion of the finances of Bolognese hospitals, Matthew Sneider discusses the 'rationalising' of smaller hospitals, which led to the centralisation of hospitals in Bologna, thereby helping to provide some security to the larger institutions living close to the financial edge. Marina Garbellotti demonstrates the decisive role of the government of Venice, producing, in collaboration with the citizenry and religious fraternities, a radical reorganisation of hospitals. The Veronese elite played a similar role in the life of their city's hospitals, symbolised by the communal coat of arms on the façade of the hospital of Sts Giacomo e Lazzaro. The same hospital had capital invested in the communal bank of the Monte di Pietà; any interest was distributed annually to other welfare organisations in financial difficulties, or was even given to the city administration to help them cope with emergencies, as during Venice's war against the Turks in 1686–7. This process, through which the political élite gradually took over the direction of hospitals, was common to most European cities, but was even more pronounced in sixteenth-century Italy as an outcome of the gradual exclusion of the aristocracy from the governance of the state.[56] As for France, recent analysis of the social background of hospital rectors has shown that, in the minor centres, they were drawn from groups of leading citizens, while in major cities they were nobles.[57] It would, however, be a mistake to assume too monolithic a power structure. As Kevin Robbins shows in his piece on the Hôtel-Dieu in Beaune, the administrative staff and nursing sisters mounted a spirited defence of the 'public honesty' of the hospital against the patronal family of the de Pernes, who had wanted to use their institution as a hotel.

Centralisation had its limits at the 'macro' level too. Just as Foucault's 'birth of the clinic' is no longer identifiable in the way he suggested, so it is now generally accepted that his related thesis of the early modern state's power over charitable institutions, and in particular of its 'great confinement' of the poor in the seventeenth century, is to say the least exaggerated. The mechanisms through which charities and their inmates might be controlled were far more flexible.[58] Furthermore, the charitable and religious institutions of the Counter-Reformation were – as Brian Pullan has shown – separated from the world to help to convert the sick, the poor, prostitutes and Jews to a life of salvation and virtue.[59] Indeed it has been argued that 'spiritual salvation' was the main objective in the hospitalisation of such patients – a perspective to be set against Foucault's emphasis on the dangers of poverty and the insanitary conditions of the early modern city.[60]

Moral discipline was a more subtle form of the exercise of power over the bodies and souls of patients. It represented a means of enforcing religious conformity and a moral way of life that one finds equally in the hospitals of Elizabethan London, in Friuli, and in areas under the influence of the Ottoman Empire.[61] This was the same kind of intrusive surveillance, as Nathan Wachtel has outlined, that penetrated into the cells of the prisons of the Inquisition, recording secretly and efficiently the glances, words, gestures and the actions of the inmates.[62] From the political and moral standpoint, discipline was justified by reference to the campaign against licence, vice, disorder and the desire for change that supposedly characterised the insolent masses. They were seen as contaminating, infecting and offending the dignity and decorum of the city, since they did not observe rules and laws. They represented a danger to social stability and were therefore 'la plus dangereuse peste des Etats'.[63]

Government policy, then, as in other places and times, originated in a set of more or less noble motives, ranging from a desire to protect hospitals from impoverishment to exploitation of their resources to using them as a means to control the poor and sick when they were seen as threats to public order and health. And if institutional patrons in the shape of governments had mixed motivations, so did individual patrons when seeking to establish and maintain hospitals. At the very centre of a number of the chapters below dealing with earlier periods is the theology of alms-giving, which links the provision of charity with salvation. This was clearly the case in Byzantium, where the major 'monastic multiplex' in Constantinople was founded principally for the commemoration of the soul of the emperor. Indeed, so concerned with commemoration were medieval patrons that hospital statutes frequently gave more space to the details of masses than to the treatment of inmates. Carole Rawcliffe argues that in late-medieval England the larger hospitals were transformed into liturgical spaces for the Christian departed. Kevin Robbins also shows how the founder of the great hospital of Beaune, Chancellor Rolin, made sure that he continued to control his institution from the grave. He laid down that his coats-of-arms should be visible on all the buildings as a constant reminder of his presence and patronage. As for Italy, Sneider demonstrates that a significant proportion of the expenditure of the four most affluent hospitals of Bologna was devoted to commemorative masses and other religious activities.

The role of religion in hospitals in medieval and early modern Europe went far beyond the provision of masses. The aim of the hospital was to cure the soul of the patient and not just the body. Indeed the vital role of religion in the treatment of the sick has been underlined by a series of major studies, not least the books by Carole Rawcliffe on the hospitals of late medieval Norwich and John Henderson on the Renaissance hospitals of Florence.[64] In her paper in this volume, Rawcliffe demonstrates the fundamental role of images in healing, from altarpieces to stained-glass windows and sculpture, stressing how the commissioning of major works such as Roger van der Weiden's *Last Judgement* or the *Isenheim Altarpiece* played a fundamental role not simply in commemorating the patron, but also in the hospital's everyday life.[65]

Splendid altarpieces and sculptural or fresco-cycles in hospital churches and wards as well as important collections of relics performed an essential role in promoting the profile of the hospital and thereby encouraging almsgiving. Indeed the maintenance of a constant income was vital for the flourishing of any hospital, as is brought out by two chapters in this volume which deal with British voluntary hospitals, Christine Stevenson on the eighteenth century and Andrea Tanner on the Great Ormond Hospital for Children founded in London in 1852. As we noted above, Georgian England saw a flowering of hospitals and infirmaries for the sick poor supported by voluntary subscriptions. By 1800 there were thirty general infirmaries outside London and seven in the capital. Then, in the following century, London became the centre of a hospital boom fuelled by the growth of medical schools: by 1850 there were forty-five hospitals with 26,000 beds.

Such initiatives were clearly expensive. One way to finance them adopted in eighteenth-century England was to distribute to potential subscribers prints 'proper to shew to Gentlemen': prints of, for example, St Bartholomew's rebuilding programme under James Gibbs or the elevations and plans of St George's in London. Great Ormond Street was also a voluntary hospital and its founder, the physician Charles West, mounted a significant campaign to raise cash. It is significant that at this time there were no children's hospitals in Britain, partly because the establishment opposed children's hospitals for fear of competition, and partly because physicians did not take children's ailments seriously. West therefore involved important people on the hospital's Board. They included Charles Dickens, who had done so much to raise contemporary awareness of the plight of poor children, and Queen Victoria herself, who was persuaded to become the patron. Also, following a tradition of gracious ladies distributing their bounty to the poor in hospitals (a tradition that goes back to late antiquity), West encouraged visits from society ladies and female journalists, who were to spread the good news that Great Ormond Street was a means of inculcating middle-class values into working-class families. The 'catechism' of cleanliness and godliness became a leitmotif designed to improve mothers and children. As Andrea Tanner shows, these women's role was vital in day-to-day fund-raising, including the year-round bazaars, collections and tea parties, as well as in raising subscriptions towards the hospital and in urging London female 'society' to visit the wards as part of their social round. Most significant was Queen Victoria's support; she was a regular visitor and on one occasion sent hundreds of toys from a German toy factory that she had visited.

The physical structure of the hospital is another recurrent topic in many of the following chapters, whether the vast Pantocrator of Constantinople, the smaller leprosaria of medieval England, the impressive Renaissance hospitals of central and northern Italy, the British voluntary hospitals or the nineteenth to twentieth-century hospitals of North America. The architectural history of hospitals has recently attracted an increasing amount of attention.[66] Few scholars, however, have followed the example of Thompson and Goldin's classic study of 1975, which traced the developing structure of the hospital in western Europe across the centuries.[67] Indeed a theme which emerges both from their book and from the present collection is the extent to which the physical form of the hospital was adapted to changing contexts and circumstances and yet also how far architectural models were imitated across time and space. A classic example of that imitation is provided by cruciform ward design, which became standard in some of the major Renaissance hospitals of central and northern Italy and was copied in other parts of both the Mediterranean (Spain and Portugal) and northern Europe.[68]

A common assumption of many hospital historians, questioned by Annmarie Adams, is how far form really followed function. Once we move away from the narrow vision of the 'medicalisation model', it becomes increasingly apparent that every hospital building represents a variety of interrelated motives, including those of patrons, governments and patients as well as other interest groups. As Adams reminds us, 'medical change does not necessarily inspire new architectural forms', even in recent years. Rather, hospital architecture is more culturally than medically determined. Hospitals in nineteenth-century Canada looked like Scottish castles and interwar and post-modern hospitals like luxury hotels and shopping malls, while modern hospitals tend to resemble office buildings. Christine Stevenson also demonstrates that both the exterior elevations of hospitals and their disposition of space responded not just to demands of medical science, but also to the grandiose concerns of patrons, as in the splendid example of Greenwich Hospital. And Kevin Robbins notes a telling reaction to Rolin's extraordinary creation at Beaune; visitors admired the hospital, characterising it as more like a prince's palace than a hospital for the poor.

None of this is to deny that form was ever related to function. One has to distinguish between exterior and interior. Frequently the appreciation of the literate classes, these gentlemen on their Grand Tours of Europe, was excited above all by the outward design; such observers were less concerned with the interior. It was rather the role of master masons, architects, and medical authorities to consider how space should be used. There was, for example, a long-held belief in the necessity to promote airiness for the dispersal of the noxious fumes of disease. This can be discovered just as much in writers of the Italian Renaissance, like Marsilio Ficino, as in the designers of voluntary hospitals in the eighteenth century or the pavilion style of the age of Nightingale. St Bartholomew's Hospital in London, for example, was planned with four detached wings around a square, large windows in the wards, and separate isolation facilities for contagious disease such as smallpox.

Up to this point, we have followed the lead of much of the literature in the field and examined the hospital principally as an urban phenomenon. Just as it is necessary, however, to ensure that the hospital is not detached from the wider social and political patronage networks of the city, so it is essential not to divorce it from the rural context. Indeed, in his study of English hospitals between 1100 and 1300 Max Satchell concludes that one in five of them can be defined as 'rural' (although it should be stressed that in this period England was indeed a rural 'backwater' in comparison with Italy). With the advantage of the *longue durée*, we can trace the origins of the whole hospital movement in Western Europe to the countryside. Some of the earliest Middle Eastern hospitals were attached to rural or suburban monasteries. Their medieval European successors have left visible reminders of the scale and importance of these monasteries' infirmaries, such as the vast wards of Ourscamps and Tonerre, while some of the numerous pilgrim hospices on the routes to Compostella or Rome expanded in time into substantial hospitals.

Some hospitals in the smaller urban centres and villages seem to have declined in the early modern period, partly because they were seen as centres of local solidarity and resistance to central authority. An example of this has been seen above at Beaune, but was also more generally true of France in the sixteenth to seventeenth centuries, as Daniel Hickey has shown.[69] Yet curiously, as so often in hospital history, the trend came to be reversed. The reversal happened in the nineteenth century, at least in northern Italy and southeast England, as Sergio Onger and Steve Cherry show in their respective chapters. Onger's study of health facilities in the Brescian territory reveals that there were a number of factors involved in the creation of new rural hospitals and the reduction of those in the main conglomerations.

They were established to cope with the spread of disease, both endemic pellagra, the main cause of hospitalisation until the end of the nineteenth century, and epidemic typhus and cholera. It was also believed that new hospitals lent prestige to local communities and promoted social harmony in a period when the countryside was undergoing great economic change. The Brescian example confirms our general contention that changes in hospital history can be understood only in relation to wider factors which often have little to do with medicine.[70]

Finally, under this rural heading, we should invoke an English initiative in heath care, the cottage hospital. Because of the high levels of poverty, those at the bottom of the social pile would have been unable to pay for professional medical treatment unless they were fortunate enough to belong to friendly societies and workers' clubs. Cottage hospitals were particularly significant for rural areas because they addressed local needs. These hospitals were run by GPs, who performed simple operations in them and, along with competent nursing staff, offered patients the necessary periods of recuperation that they would have been unlikely to obtain in larger city hospitals.

Whether in urban or rural contexts, the one constant of all these hospitals was the patient, the subject of Part Four of our collection. So far in our discussion he or she has remained obscure, the object of patrons, administrators, priests, doctors and nurses, rather than self-determining. Largely due to the influence of Roy Porter, much has been done to redress this longstanding imbalance in the historiography and restore the viewpoint of the patient to the historian's purview. The publication of a number of studies of patients in early modern Europe based on analysis of letter collections, diaries and trial records is part of a wider scholarly trend to explore the narratives of everyday events.[71] It is, however, rare that this type of evidence survives from the hand of the *hospital* patient. He or she normally remains silent since, before the nineteenth century, surviving documentation relating to patients tends to consist only of entry and death registers. These, as will be seen below, provide invaluable information on demographic events and social background, but little on the patient's personal experience of the hospital.

Petitions are one type of source that does allow us to come closer to understanding when and why the sick wanted to be hospitalised, as is demonstrated by Louise Gray's study of those seeking admission to a hospital in rural southern Germany in the seventeenth and eighteenth centuries. Even though the 'voice' of the poor was mediated through the hand of the scribes who actually wrote the petitions, accompanying witness statements from priests, administrators and doctors did confirm the veracity of their claims. These patients were, however, unusual in that they suffered from chronic conditions, excluded from the average general hospital. The petitions reveal that men and women applied to the hospital as a last resort, for their sickness had made it impossible for them to survive by any other means. Some of them, however, declared their willingness to work in the hospital, and they were given light tasks, such as cutting wood for the kitchen and harvesting fruit. Indeed, work was encouraged since it was seen as combating idleness and diabolical temptation; only prisoners and the bed-ridden were exempt. Emphasis on work was also an important aspect of the British treatment of TB patients in the nineteenth century. Flurin Condrau describes such treatment as 'graduated labour therapy' for the working-class; the aim was to return the patient to his profession. That this did not always happen is attested by the early twentieth-century case of the young worker Moritz Bromme, who kept an autobiography of his repeated visits to the sanatorium. Though each time he was discharged as 'cured', the necessity to support a family of four children meant that he had to return to his factory job, only to get worse again and to have to return to what his foreman described as the 'cougher's castle'. Bromme recorded a growing scepticism of the therapy offered him.

We should not generalise too readily. Sometimes the hospital was indeed a last resort, as Gray shows. On other occasions, as Sandra Cavallo's work on early modern Turin has demonstrated, it was a strategic resource of the family or individual in managing what we might call the patient's career – a resource to be drawn on in some phases of illness or economic need, and by no means necessarily the final phases.[72] This is also reflected at Great Ormond Street. Parents were not simply passive and unthinking recipients of charity. It was not unknown for them to remove their offspring early because of perceived poor treatment or the unhappiness of their children, whom they were rarely allowed to see. Thus 800 patients were removed by families between 1852 and 1899, often against medical advice. That behaviour reminds us of the power of the family to reject or accept hospital treatment, contradicting a prevalent view of the London poor as helpless and unable to evaluate the medicine provided by professionals. Such manifestations of patient power further undermine Foucault's twin conceptions of a great confinement and the power of the clinical 'gaze'.

Physicians' diagnoses and their disease terminology none the less underlay the selection of patients for some of the more specialised hospitals. Many of the chapters in this book have dealt sensitively with contemporary classifications and prompt questions of a comparative kind. Did the term 'incurable' mean the same in the sixteenth century as in the eighteenth? Did the terms 'healed' or 'cured' change over time? The two papers on Germany, for example (Gray and Condrau), suggest that the condition of 'cured' was often taken to mean that an individual was again fit to work. Through her examination of the petitions of the poor, Gray also shows that disease categories and labels could even change from day to day and according to the person who was recording them. Condrau points out that, although some sanatoria claimed high success rates, in fact 50 per cent of those who left as 'cured' died within five years from the date of discharge.

Levels of mortality have long been a major concern for hospitals: they affect their public reputation and ultimately the willingness of both private and public sponsors to continue financial support. Mortality was especially a preoccupation for anybody running a foundling home, given the general recognition throughout pre-industrial Europe that up to a third of all babies born would die in infancy. The constant tension between available finance and required services is well brought out by Alysa Levene in her discussion of the famous Innocenti hospital in Florence, which in the eighteenth century saw both an expansion in its facilities for orphans and an increase in the rate of abandonment. Given that wet-nurses were the most expensive part of the operation – despite their notoriously low pay – various experiments were introduced to save money. A cheaper alternative adopted in the 1740s was to feed infants with cows' milk. Indeed this was also recommended by the famous Florentine medical reformer, Antonio Cocchi, as part of a light diet. But the practice was abandoned because, as had been discovered elsewhere, it led to an increase in infant mortality.[73] This was also the effect of a second innovation, an attempt to reduce the number of wet-nurses employed. Their supply was always prone to shortage, particularly in the summer, when agricultural labour proved a more profitable alternative. However, as Levene concludes, the only solution to ensuring the long-term survival of infants was to place them promptly with external wet-nurses.

Mortality lies also at the heart of the final chapter in this book, in which Diego Ramiro Fariñas turns our perspective upside down. Instead of adopting the more normal approach of examining how far exogenous factors affected the mortality regime of the institution, he asks how far hospitals contributed to the mortality of the cities in which they were situated. Thus in late nineteenth-century Spain, 17 to 19 per cent of the mortality of urban areas took place in institutions, including hospitals, foundling homes, prisons and lunatic asylums. In some places mortality was even higher. In Toledo, for example, which in 1877–8 had a population of 20,000 inhabitants, a third of the population died in institutions. All this returns us to the wider question, considered above, of the relationship between town and country and in particular the provenance of the patient population. Ramiro contends that the high level of migration into Spanish cities was a partial cause of the high institutional mortality – a particular type of the much-discussed 'urban graveyard effect'. Towns attracted large numbers of people from the countryside in search of work. Rather like the 'Columbian exchange' they brought diseases that contributed to the ill health of impoverished locals, who lived in crowded unsanitary conditions alongside the new arrivals. The broad conclusion to Ramiro's chapter is that we must question the long-held assumption that cities had much higher mortality than rural areas: it was the deaths of migrants which swelled urban institutional mortality, especially those of foundlings.

An overarching theme, then, of many of the chapters of this book, as of some of the recent historiography on the subject, is the imperative of examining the hospital within a wider context to understand its impact on the environment, whether in terms of its effects on the local population, or of its major role in the local economy as a purchaser of goods or an investor in property or banks.[74] The importance of the hospital as a local employer has also begun to be examined. That extends the analysis of its charitable role to include employing the able-bodied poor, as exemplified by the 'corrodians' of many medieval hospitals, who entered into a life-time contract; board, lodging and care in sickness was provided in return for their labour and property. All this leads to a reconsideration of the relationship between formal (institutional) and informal (domestic) systems of support. And that in turn implicates wider questions about the changing relationship between in-patients and out-patients, seen in the context of demographic regimes and social and family structures.[75]

Superficially, it might be possible to conclude that these chapters suggest a certain uniformity of experience over the period examined, from late antiquity and the early Middle Ages to the present day. This stems partly from the very nature of the subject: we are examining a single institution (or a 'family resemblance group' of institutions). Yet, another way of interpreting the phenomenon is that the traditional Whiggish vision of hospital history has been abandoned. In other words, we are not seeing here a form of progressive development towards the triumph of modern biomedicine in hospitals. Rather, the very repetition of the same themes in different periods points to a long series of reactions to previous forms of 'indoor' solutions to the problems of poverty and sickness, though these reactions in their turn might lead to the imitation of past models, just as post-modern hospitals contain architectural elements of earlier designs. But even when earlier models or those imported from other countries were being adopted, the process led to transmutation, whether in terms of hospital regulations, therapies, or design. As the English Baroque may have been inspired by Italian architecture but was altered in its transplantation to England, so the Savoy Hospital and the London Foundling Hospital were different from their original models, the Florentine hospitals of Santa Maria Nuova and the Innocenti.

In the post-postmodern age in which we now live, globalisation is everything. For the old hospital history 'the hospital is our world', and that world is narrowly conceived. For the 'new' hospital history, which goes back to Granshaw and Porter and their fellow scholars, but which we try to extend and elaborate in what follows, 'the world' – Eliot's 'whole earth' – 'is our hospital'. In studying impacts of – and on – the hospital over the *très longue durée*, there are no frontiers to the contexts that we must invoke.

Notes

1   What follows is an essay in overview and interpretation. References are therefore minimal, offering only some background and guidance through controversies. For the section that follows see G.B. Risse, 'Before the Clinic was "Born": Methodological Perspectives in Hospital History', in N. Finzsch and R. Jütte (eds), *Institutions of Confinement: Hospitals, Asylums, and Prisons in Western Europe and North America, 1500–1950* (Cambridge, 1996), pp.75–96, at 87–91 (to which we are heavily indebted); Risse, *Mending Bodies, Saving Souls: A History of Hospitals* (New York, 1999), pp.257–88; A. Cunningham and R. French (eds), *The Medical Enlightenment of the Eighteenth Century* (Cambridge, 1990); P.P. Bernard, 'The Limits of Absolutism: Joseph II and the Allgemeines Krankenhaus', *Eighteenth-Century Studies*, 9 (1975–6), pp.193–215; D. Jetter, *Wien von den Anfängen bis um 1900*, Geschichte des Hospitals vol. 5 (Wiesbaden, 1982); B. Pohl-Resl, *Rechnen mit der Ewigkeit: das Wiener Bürgerspital im Mittelalter* (Vienna and Munich, 1996). We do not know of a monograph for Austria comparable to M. Lindemann, *Health and Healing in Eighteenth-Century Germany* (Baltimore, MD, 1997).

2   Though see T.H. Broman, *The Transformation of German Academic Medicine 1750–1820* (Cambridge, 1996), pp.59–63, for some qualifications of the conventional narrative.

3   The introduction of clinical hospital teaching is now normally attributed to Giambatista da Monte; see J.J. Bylebyl, 'The School of Padua: Humanistic Medicine in the Sixteenth Century', in C. Webster (ed.), *Health, Medicine and Mortality in the Sixteenth Century* (Cambridge, 1979), p.348.

4   See Risse, 'Before the Clinic', pp.92–3, for medical and surgical education in the Hôtel-Dieu at the time.

5   *System einer vollständigen medicinischen Polizey*, 4 vols (Mannheim, 1780–88), trans. E. Vilim from 3rd revised edn as *A System of Complete Medical Police* (Baltimore, 1976).

6   See n.3.

7   See A. Pastore, *Le regole dei corpi: medicina e disciplina nell'Italia moderna* (Bologna, 2006).

8   The best recent overview is L. Granshaw, 'The Hospital', in W.F. Bynum and R. Porter (eds), *Companion Encyclopedia of the History of Medicine* (London and New York, 1993), pp.1180–203. The various monographs of D. Jetter con-

tain much valuable detail. See e.g. his *Das europäische Hospital: von der Spätantike bis 1800* (Cologne, 1986); and *Grundzüge der Krankenhausgeschichte, 1800–1900* (Darmstadt, 1977).

9   For what follows see P. Horden, 'The Earliest Hospitals in Byzantium, Western Europe, and Islam', in M. Cohen (ed.), *Journal of Interdisciplinary History*, special issue, 'Poverty and Charity: Judaism, Christianity, Islam', 35 (2005), pp.361–89; T.S. Miller, *The Birth of the Hospital in the Byzantine Empire*, 2nd edn (Baltimore and London, 1977).

10   For western European overviews see J. Imbert, *Les hôpitaux en droit canonique* (Paris, 1947); M. Mollat, *The Poor in the Middle Ages* (New Haven and London, 1978); B. Bowers (ed.), *The Medieval Hospital and Medical Practice* (Aldershot, 2007).

11   P. Mitchell, *Medicine in the Crusades: Warfare, Wounds and the Medieval Surgeon* (Cambridge, 2004), ch. 2, and the new interpretation and survey of F.-O. Touati, 'La terre sainte: un laboratoire hospitalier au Moyen Age?', in N. Bulst and K.-H. Spiess (eds), *Sozialgeschichte Mittelalterlicher Hospitäler* (Ostfildern, 2007), pp.169–211.

12   J.W. Brodman, *Charity and Welfare: Hospitals and the Poor in Medieval Catalonia* (Philadelphia, 1998), pp.94–8.

13   J. Henderson, *The Renaissance Hospital: Healing the Body and Healing the Soul* (New Haven and London, 2006); J. Arrizabalaga, J. Henderson, and R. French, *The Great Pox: The French Disease in Renaissance Europe* (New Haven and London, 1997).

14   C. Rawcliffe, *Medicine for the Soul: The Life, Death and Resurrection of an English Medieval Hospital* (Stroud, 1999).

15   See T.J. McHugh, 'Establishing Medical Men at the Paris Hôtel-Dieu, 1500–1715', *Social History of Medicine*, 19 (2006), pp.209–24.

16   C. Jones, 'The Construction of the Hospital Patient in Early Modern France', in Finzsch and Jütte (eds), *Institutions of Confinement*, p.68; L. Brockliss and C. Jones, *The Medical World of Early Modern France* (Oxford, 1997), pp.689–700.

17   For brief synthesis and further references see S. De Renzi, 'Policies of Health: Disease, Poverty and Hospitals' in P. Elmer (ed.), *The Healing Arts: Health, Disease and Society in Europe 1500–1800* (Manchester, 2004), pp.150–60.

18   Granshaw, 'The Hospital', p.1195.

19   H. Marland, 'The Changing Role of the Hospital, 1800–1900', in D. Brunton (ed.), *Medicine Transformed: Health, Disease and Society in Europe 1800–1930* (Manchester, 2004), p.239.

20   For what follows, convenient syntheses are: U. Tröhler and C.-R. Prüll, 'The Rise of the Modern Hospital', in I. Loudon (ed.), *Western Medicine: An Illustrated History* (Oxford and New York, 1997), pp.160–75; L. Granshaw, 'The Rise of the Modern Hospital in Britain', in A. Wear (ed.), *Medicine in Society: Historical Essays* (Cambridge, 1992), pp.197–218. See also the very useful sec-

tions on hospitals in W.F. Bynum et al., *The Western Medical Tradition 1800 to 2000* (Cambridge, 2006), pp.53–64, 84–5, 150–62, 269–81, 349–52, 439–50.

21   Brockliss and Jones, *Medical World*, pp.269–72, 686; M. Rhodes, 'Women in Medicine: Doctors and Nurses, 1850–1920', in Brunton, *Medicine Transformed*, pp.164–76; C. Jones, *The Charitable Imperative: Hospitals and Nursing in Ancien Regime and Revolutionary France* (London and New York, 1989); S. Broomhall, *Women's Medical Work in Early Modern France* (Manchester, 2004).

22   See, for example, the discussion in Henderson, *The Renaissance Hospital*, ch. 6, and C. Rawcliffe, 'Hospital Nurses and their Work', in R. Britnell (ed.), *Daily Life in the Middle Ages* (Stroud, 1998), pp.43–64.

23   H.C.E. Midelfort, *A History of Madness in Sixteenth-Century Germany* (Stanford, 1999).

24   A. Scull, 'A Convenient Place to get rid of Inconvenient People: The Victorian Lunatic Asylum', in A.D. King (ed.), *Buildings and Society* (London, 1980), p.38, cited by J. Andrews, 'The Rise of the Asylum in Britain', in Brunton, *Medicine Transformed*, p.301.

25   Brockliss and Jones, *Medical World*, p.677.

26   R. Porter, *Blood and Guts: A Short History of Medicine* (London, 2002), p.152.

27   For what follows see further M.J. Vogel, 'The Transformation of the American Hospital,' in Finzsch and Jütte (eds), *Institutions of Confinement*, pp.39–54; M.J. Vogel, *The Invention of the Modern Hospital: Boston, 1870–1930* (Chicago, 1980); J.H. Warner and J.A. Tighe (eds), *Major Problems in the History of American Medicine and Public Health* (Boston, 2001); C.E. Rosenberg, *The Care of Strangers: The Rise of America's Hospital System* (New York, 1987); D. Rosner, *A Once Charitable Enterprise: Hospitals and Health Care in Brooklyn and New York, 1885–1915* (Cambridge, 1982); R. Stevens, *In Sickness and in Wealth: American Hospitals in the Twentieth Century* (Baltimore, 1999).

28   R.L. Numbers (ed.), *Medicine in the New World: New Spain, New France, and New England* (Knoxville, 1987); G. Risse, 'Shelter and Care for Natives and Colonists: Hospitals in Sixteenth-Century New Spain', in S. Varey, R. Chabrán, and D.B. Weiner (eds), *Searching the Secrets of Nature: The Life and Works of Dr. Francisco Hernández* (Stanford, 2000), pp.65–81 (a reference we owe to Andrew Wear).

29   See M. Harrison (ed.), *From Western Medicine to Global Medicine: The Hospital beyond the West* (forthcoming), the 'Introduction' to which was kindly shown to us by the editor in advance of publication.

30   J. Van Alphen and A. Aris (eds), *Oriental Medicine: An Illustrated Guide to the Asian Arts of Healing* (Boston, 1995), p.234.

31   Horden, 'Earliest Hospitals', with bibliography for this and what follows.

32   J. Legge, *A Record of Buddhistic Kingdoms, being an Account by the Chinese Monk Fâ-Hien of his Travels in India and Ceylon (AD 399–414) [...]* (Oxford,

1966, repr. New York, 1965), cited by D. Wujastyk, *The Roots of Ayurveda*, revised edn (London, 2003), p.xv.

33   *Ibid.*

34   H. Scogin, 'Poor Relief in Northern Sung China', *Oriens Extremus*, 25 (1978), pp.30–46, a reference we owe to Peter Brown.

35   M. Giteau, *The Civilization of Angkor* (New York, 1976), p.234, drawing on G. Cœdès, 'La stèle de Ta-Prohm', reprinted in his *Articles sur le pays Khmer*, vol. 2 (Paris, 1992), pp.11–49.

36   G. Attewell, 'Authority, Knowledge and Practice in Unani Tibb in India *c.* 1890–1930' (unpublished PhD thesis, University of London, 2004).

37   H. Sigerist, 'An Outline of the Development of the Hospital', *Bulletin of the History of Medicine*, 4 (1936), pp.573–81.

38   Risse, *Mending Bodies, Saving Souls*.

39   Granshaw, 'The Hospital'.

40   N. Jewson, 'The Disappearance of the Sick Man from Medical Cosmology 1770–1870', *Sociology*, 10 (1976), pp.225–44.

41   C. Jones, 'The Construction of the Hospital Patient in Early Modern France', in Finzsch and Jütte, *Institutions of Confinements*, p.66.

42   *Ibid.*, p.69.

43   L. Granshaw and R. Porter (eds), *The Hospital in History* (Routledge, 1989).

44   For the older historiography see the review article on a sample of it by J. Guy, 'Of the Writing of Hospital Histories there is no End', *Bulletin of the History of Medicine*, 59 (1985), pp.415–43.

45   Granshaw and Porter (eds), *Hospital in History*, pp.1–2, 24, 29, 51, 94, 110, 123, 150, 182, 221, 243.

46   *Ibid.*, pp.221–41.

47   M. Garbellotti, 'Ospedali e storia nell'Italia moderna: percorsi di ricerca', *Medicina e Storia*, 3 (2003), pp.116–17.

48   Cf. J. Frangos, *From Housing the Poor to Healing the Sick: The Changing Institution of Paris Hospitals under the Old Regime and Revolution* (Madison and London, 1997); O. Keel, *L'avènement de la médecine clinique moderne en Europe, 1750–1815: politiques, institutions et savoirs* (Montreal and Geneva, 2001).

49   See e.g. Finzsch and Jütte (eds), *Institutions of Confinement*; Y. Kawakita, S. Sakai, and Y. Otsuka (eds), *History of Hospitals: The Evolution of Health Care Facilities. Proceedings of the 11th International Symposium on the Comparative History of Medicine East and West* (Osaka, 1989), which does look back to the Middle Ages, but is essentially a (very welcome) comparison of modern Japanese and modern western hospitals; J. Barry and C. Jones (eds), *Medicine and Charity before the Welfare State* (London and New York , 1991), not wholly, of course, about hospitals.

50   Cf. S. Cherry, *Medical Services and the Hospitals in Britain 1860–1939* (Cambridge, 1996).

54   *John Henderson, Peregrine Horden and Alessandro Pastore*

51   Harrison, 'Introduction: From Western Medicine to Global Medicine'.

52   Andrews, 'The Rise of the Asylum', surveys the major literature. It is enough to mention the names of Andrew Scull, Roy Porter, and Andrews himself. See e.g. R. Porter and D. Wright (eds), *The Confinement of the Insane: International Perspectives, 1800–1965* (Cambridge, 2003).

53   See e.g. S.C. Lawrence, *Charitable Knowledge: Hospital Pupils and Practitioners in Eighteenth-Century London* (Cambridge, 1996); K. Waddington, *Medical Education at St Bartholomew's Hospital, 1123–1995* (Woodbridge, 2003).

54   On leprosy see now C. Rawcliffe, *Leprosy in Medieval England* (Woodbridge, 2006), with F.-O. Touati, *Maladie et société au moyen âge: la lèpre, les lépreux et les léproseries dans la province ecclésiastique de Sens jusqu'au milieu du XIVe siècle* (Brussels, 1998). For an outline of the evolution of *lazzaretti* for plague see C.M. Cipolla, *Public Health and the Medical Profession in the Renaissance* (Cambridge, 1976), ch. 1; on isolation hospitals for the Great Pox see Henderson in Arrizabalaga, Henderson, and French, *The Great Pox*, chs 2, 7 and 8; R. Jütte, 'Syphilis and Confinement: Hospitals in Early Modern Germany', in Finzsch and Jütte (eds), *Institutions of Confinement*, pp.97–115; K.P. Siena, *Venereal Disease, Hospitals and the Urban Poor: London's 'Foul Wards', 1600–1800* (Rochester, 2004).

55   On state funding and care in Britain see J. Mohan and M. Gorsky, *Don't Look Back? Voluntary and Charitable Finance of Hospitals in Britain, Past and Present* (London, 2001), and M. Gorsky, *Patterns of Philanthropy: Charity and Society in Nineteenth-Century Bristol* (Woodbridge, 1999).

56   M. Berengo, *L'Europa delle città: il volto della società urbana tra medioevo ed età moderna* (Turin, 1999), pp.609, 611.

57   J.-P. Gutton (ed.), *Les administrateurs d'hôpitaux dans la France d'ancien régime* (Lyon, 1999).

58   C. Jones and R. Porter, 'Introduction', in C. Jones and R. Porter (eds), *Reassessing Foucault: Power, Medicine and the Body* (London and New York, 1998), p.4; R. Jütte, *Poverty and Deviance in Early Modern Europe* (Cambridge, 1996).

59   B. Pullan, 'The Old Catholicism, the New Catholicism, and the Poor', in G. Politi, M. Rosa, and F. Della Peruta (eds), *Timore e carità: i poveri nell' Italia moderna* (Cremona, 1982), pp.17–18.

60   Risse, *Mending Bodies, Saving Souls*, pp.218–19, though for the counter-example of Venice, which during the course of the sixteenth century gradually developed an integrated charitable system in response to poverty in general and to sickness in particular, see R. Palmer, 'L'assistenza medica nella Venezia cinquecentesca', in B. Aikema and D. Meijers (eds), *Nel regno dei poveri: arte e storia dei grandi ospedali Veneziani in età moderna, 1474–1797* (Venice, 1989), pp.35–42.

61 I.W. Archer, *The Pursuit of Stability: Social Relations in Elizabethan London* (Cambridge, 1991), pp.154–5; A. Pastore, 'Introduction', in *Sanità e società: Friuli-Venezia Giulia, secoli XVI–XX* (Udine, 1986), pp.17–18.

62 N. Wachtel, *La foi du souvenir: labyrinthes marranes* (Paris, 2001).

63 Cited in A.-M. Piuz, 'Pauvres et pauvreté dans les sociétés pré-industrielles', *Revue suisse d'histoire*, 23 (1973), p.547.

64 Rawcliffe, *Medicine for the Soul*; P. Horden, 'Religion as Medicine: Music in Medieval Hospitals', in P. Biller and J. Ziegler (eds), *Religion and Medicine in the Middle Ages* (Woodbridge, 2001), pp.135–53; idem, 'A Non-Natural Environment: Medicine without Doctors and the Medieval European Hospital', in Bowers (ed.), *The Medieval Hospital*, pp.133–45; Henderson, *The Renaissance Hospital*.

65 See also A. Hayum, *The Isenheim Altarpiece: God's Medicine and the Painter's Vision* (Princeton, 1989).

66 See, for example, C. Stevenson, *Medicine and Magnificence: British Hospital and Asylum Architecture, 1660–1815* (New Haven and London, 2000); J. Taylor, *The Architect and the Pavilion Hospital: Dialogue and Design Creativity in England, 1850–1914* (Leicester, 1997); Aikema and Meijers (eds), *Nel regno dei poveri*.

67 J.D. Thompson and G. Goldin, *The Hospital: A Social and Architectural History* (New Haven and London, 1975). See also Jetter, *Das europäische Hospital*; H. Richardson (ed.), *English Hospitals 1660–1948* (London, 1998). For the medieval and early modern periods, see now F.-O. Touati (ed.), *Archéologie et architecture hospitalières de l'antiquité tardive à l'aube des temps modernes* (Paris, 2004).

68 Henderson, *The Renaissance Hospital*.

69 D. Hickey, *Local Hospitals in Ancien Régime France: Rationalization, Resistance, Renewal, 1530–1789* (Montreal and London, 1997), esp. pp.200–3. See also, on early modern Italian hospitals in small centres and rural areas, M. Garbellotti, *Le risorse dei poveri: carità e tutela della salute nel principato vescovile di Trento in età moderna* (Bologna, 2007).

70 P. Frascani, 'L'ospedale moderno in Europa e Stati Uniti: riflessioni sulla recente storiografia', *Società e storia*, 52 (1991), p.405.

71 Cf. R. Porter, 'The Patient's View: Doing History from Below', *Theory and Society*, 14 (1985), pp.175–98, and R. Porter (ed.), *Patients and Practitioners: Lay Perceptions of Medicine in Preindustrial Society* (Cambridge, 1985); more recently, G. Pomata, *Contracting a Cure: Patients, Healers and the Law in Early Modern Bologna* (Baltimore and London, 1998). For one of the few studies of the life of hospital patients see M. Louis-Courvoisier, *Soigner et consoler: la vie quotidiènne dans un hôpital à la fin de l'Ancien Regime, Genève, 1750–1820* (Geneva, 2000). More generally see J.S. Amelang, *The Flight of Icarus: Artisan Autobiography in Early Modern Europe* (Stanford, 1998), and

O. Niccoli, *Storie di ogni giorno in una città del Seicento* (Rome and Bari, 2000).

72　S. Cavallo, 'Family Obligations and Inequalities in Access to Care in Northern Italy, Seventeenth to Eighteenth Centuries', in P. Horden and R. Smith (eds), *The Locus of Care: Families, Communities, Institutions and the Provision of Welfare since Antiquity* (London and New York, 1988), pp.90–110; P. Horden, 'Family History and Hospital History in the Middle Ages', in E. Sonnino (ed.), *Living in the City (14th–20th Centuries)* (Rome, 2004), pp.255–82.

73　A. Cocchi, *Relazione dello Spedale di Santa Maria Nuova di Firenze*, ed. M. Mannelli Goggioli and R. Pasta (Florence, 2000).

74　O. Faure, *Genèse de l'hôpital moderne : les hospices civils de Lyon de 1802 à 1845* (Lyon, 1982), p.8; see also K. Waddington, *Charity and the London Hospitals, 1850–1898* (Woodbridge and Rochester, N.Y, 2000).

75　On this theme see Horden and Smith (eds), *The Locus of Care*; Horden, 'Family History and Hospital History'; M. Dupree, 'Family Care and Hospital Care: The Sick Poor in Nineteenth-Century Glasgow', *Social History of Medicine*, 6 (1993), pp.195–211. For a similar approach to the care of the mentally ill see P. Bartlett and D. Wright (ed.), *Outside the Walls of the Asylum: The History of Care in the Community 1750–2000* (London and New Brunswick, NJ, 1999).

Part One: The Impact of the Patron

PEREGRINE HORDEN

Chapter 1: Alms and the Man: Hospital Founders in Byzantium

'Pride and vanity have built more hospitals than all the Virtues together.'[1] So wrote the Dutch physician Bernard de Mandeville in *The Fable of the Bees* (1714). He added:

> Men are so tenacious of their Possessions, and Selfishness is so rivited in our nature, that whoever in any ways can conquer it shall have the Applause of the Publick.[2]

Mandeville was composing his satire on the eve of the 'voluntary hospital' movement in his adopted England. Georgian propertied classes found in the voluntary hospital a way of dignifying their pride and vanity and mitigating their possessiveness. Their subscriptions to hospitals purchased not only the esteem of their peers but the right to nominate suitable deserving patients. It was seen as prudent to help such people get back to work.[3] It was a social obligation, a Christian duty, a loan to God – Proverbs 19.17, but with extra resonance in the early Georgian economy – a loan that would be repaid at Judgement Day. Not least, it was a pleasure. As the *Gentleman's Magazine* put it in 1732, one year before Mandeville's death, charity was 'the most lasting, valuable and exquisite pleasure.'[4]

I

What would Mandeville have made of Byzantine hospitals and their founders? The *philanthropia* of the empire's inhabitants in general, and its particular expression in charitable institutions, has been lauded from early Byzantine times onwards. Most recently and influentially, some of those charitable institutions have been the subject of an 'upbeat', optimistic monograph by Tim Miller, *The Birth of the Hospital in the Byzantine Empire*. Yet, in all the literature, there has been surprisingly little discussion of founder's motives. It is as if it were enough to rehearse the Biblical and patristic proof texts on almsgiving, and then invoke economic circumstances – that is, clear need – as the demand that straightforwardly induced the charitable supply – compassion for the poor.[5] This confidence that the answer is obvious is one possible reason for lack of interest in the subject of motivation. Another, equally powerful, is paucity of evidence. The period of Byzantine history that concerns me runs from the fourth century to the twelfth, though with some excursion into the later, Palaiologan period (after the end of Latin rule in 1261).[6] Throughout that period, we mostly lack the kinds of personal detail that would give some glimpse of what really motivated founders. With a few exceptions, to which I shall return, we also lack even the more formulaic statements of founders' aspirations: what they wanted people to think were their motives. Yet it is, I think, still possible to recover something of the Byzantine founder's mindset.

The foundations to be considered here have been arbitrarily excerpted from the wider subject of charity in Byzantium. They were for the overnight accommodation of the poor, transients, the sick, lepers, the old, the orphaned, occasionally the blind, and others. I shall refer to all these for convenience as hospitals, generalising about them somewhat as Roman law did in its category of *piae causae* (literally pious causes) or *euageis oikoi* (holy houses) – a category that could, however, also include, as I shall not, churches and monasteries.[7] Such foundations were above all religious establishments. This was so not only in a basic legal sense: whatever their origin in the foundations of private individuals (clerical or lay), of churches, of monks, or of members of imperial families, hospitals tended to fall under ecclesiastical jurisdiction. More importantly, even in the most 'medicalised' hospital – the one with the most doctors – the Divine Liturgy was far more central to daily life than the ward round.[8] Yet it remains hard to pin down the particular way in which that religious aspect, and the theology underpinning it, affected, or reflected, Byzantine hospital founders' motivation.

Contrast for the moment the (as I see it) difficult topic of Byzantine foundations with the clearer picture that presents itself to a *later* medievalist studying, say, England.[9] In a typical later medieval hospital, as revealed elsewhere in this volume by Carole Rawcliffe – a hospital that housed a few paupers and pensioners – the chief beneficiary was not the inmates but the founder. The secular gratitude and recognition of the poor and all those (such as nurses, servants, and priests) who benefited from the hospital's existence could be expressed in prayer for the founder's soul. That gratitude was constantly renewed in the recitation of foundation statutes and rolls of benefactors, as well as in masses for the dead. The founder's name rang in the ears of the grateful poor, and his or her image assailed them on every side. Such was *memoria*, that (primarily liturgical) commemoration of the dead on which scholars, especially in Germany, have lavished such attention.[10] In these circumstances it was, perhaps, much harder to forget than to remember. And the purpose of remembering was theologically explicit; it was either to assure the founder's place in heaven or to abbreviate his or her passage through purgatory. The connection between one's own salvation and the almsgiving, prayers, fasting and (particularly) masses of other people was clear – even quantifiable. With its 'treasury of merits', its complex transactions between living and dead, this really was a 'spiritual economy' – aspects of which might have appealed to the Georgians if they could have overcome their Protestant aversion.[11]

Many facets of this western hospital scene are familiar to Byzantinists. How could they not be, given the common patristic roots of both eastern and western doctrinal traditions? But there is a temptation to see the less tightly coherent Byzantine scene as either a somehow incomplete version of Europe or as a completely alien religious culture. In this as in so many respects, however, Byzantium is both similar to and different from the West. The hard task is to disentangle those similarities and differences.

Pursuing them in what follows, I shall look first, for background, at the theology of almsgiving in late antiquity (section II). Then (section III), with reference to two of the most significant Byzantine hospitals, I shall explore the methodological problem of inferring founders' intentions from the various explanations that historians have been tempted to give of their foundations. Next (in section IV), I shall review some Byzantine evidence for the mixed motives of hospitals patrons – especially concern for reputation in this world as evidenced in the little-considered topic of the naming of hospitals. After that (section V), I shall give some examples of the most elaborate accounts of founders' aspirations that survive from Byzantium: those found in *typika* (foundation documents), with all their liturgical and commemorative specifications and their hopes of everlasting benefit to be derived from acts of philanthropy. Finally (in section VI), I shall ask what these benefits were thought to be in a religious culture which had no formal doctrine of purgatory. Why should hospital patients pray for a deceased founder?

II

First, the theology. The basic doctrine concerning almsgiving and its link with salvation, fortunately, is clear enough. The need for charity to the poor is emphasised again and again in the Judaeo-early Christian material from the Deuteronomic code onwards.[12] He who sows in almsgiving shall reap the fruit of life (Hosea 10.12). Almsgiving atones for sins (Sirach 3.30). This tradition Matthew especially among the gospel writers glosses with the familiar injunction to lay up treasures in heaven, not on earth. And he adds (at 25.31f.) the parable of the sheep and the goats, according to which, of course, the basis for the last judgement will be the treatment of Christ present in anyone who is hungry, thirsty, naked, and so on.

If anything, the emphasis on the salvific value of charity only increases in early Christian literature. 'Almsgiving is as good as repentance from sin, fasting is better than prayer; almsgiving is better than either.'[13]

When the rich man rests upon the poor [...] he believes that what he does for the poor can find a reward with God, for the poor man is rich in intercession.[14]

This is developed at great length in well-known homilies by, above all, John Chrysostom among the fourth-century Fathers. For him, alms erase post-baptismal sins, preserve from damnation, procure God's mercy; they are essential to salvation. These effects can be obtained for others: alms can be given vicariously – on behalf of the dead.[15] Commemoration of almsgivers came chiefly in prayers and in petitions in the liturgies of Chrysostom and Basil. 'Remember Lord those who are mindful of the poor. Give them your rich and heavenly gifts.'[16]

Such is the theological context for the emergence of Christian hospitals. Doubtless it is also a considerable part of the explanation for that emergence. In what follows I do not mean to cast aspersions on founders. Most, if not all, will have been deeply aware of the Bible's charitable imperative, will have felt some compassion for the poor, and will, especially, have been anxious about their prospects in the afterlife. A saint in the making will have been acutely – to us, perhaps disproportionately – aware of the tiniest spiritual blemish. For such a blemish might put the 'bosom of Abraham' beyond reach. A bishop or priest, answerable for his conduct towards the souls entrusted to his care, will have been hypersensitive to any pastoral failing on which divine judgement might focus. An 'ordinary' lay sinner, and still more an emperor with blood on his hands, will have wondered if hell could be avoided. Take for example the story recorded by John Moschus in the early seventh century, about how the Emperor Zeno was saved from the retribution of the Mother of God on behalf of a woman he had wronged. 'Believe me, woman,' says the Virgin appearing in a vision to the wronged woman's mother, 'I frequently tried to get satisfaction for you, but his [God's] right hand prevents me' – because, Moschus adds, the emperor was a very good almsgiver.[17] All – emperors, saints, others – in their different ways could seek spiritual merit, as well as earthly acclaim, through the founding of a hospital.

There must, however, be more to be said. Let us take two examples from opposite ends of my chosen period. First, some of the first hospitals we know about; second, the best documented, and most impressive, Byzantine hospital, from the early twelfth century.

III

To begin at the beginning, with the earliest Christian hospitals. It is not enough to see hospitals as an inevitable outgrowth of the early Christian charitable impulse, a natural development from doorstep distributions to overnight shelter, and therefore needing no particular explanation beyond the religious motives that I have just outlined. The early Christian hospital was an invention. It was, apparently, invented quite suddenly – not in Jewish communities of the first three centuries CE, not in *pre*-Constantinian Christian communities, not even in the reign of Constantine himself, for all his lavish patronage of the Church. It was an invention of (roughly) the 350s, in the reign of Constantius II, and in the heart of Anatolia, not just in Constantinople.[18]

Why? Many explanations have been offered. They have been couched in terms of the demography of the poor; of competition for support between Arian and Catholic; of the self-expression of an extremely ascetic form of urban monasticism; and, most recently, by Peter Brown, as an aspect of the fourth-century bishops' 'pitch' for urban leadership, and a visible 'quid pro quo' for imperial patronage.[19] 'Whom do we harm', wrote St Basil, founder of the first big philanthropic 'multiplex' at Caesarea around 370, 'if we build shelters for passers-by who need someone's attention because of ill health [...]?'[20] The answer is that quite a few will have been disturbed by his hospital's affront to traditional civic values, even to civic topography. And this despite the fact that hospitals can also be seen as traditional euergetism (civic beneficence) continued by non-traditional means. The bishop, according to Brown, was in a sense inventing the poor – and 'a fortiori' the hospital for the poor. He was seeing them as 'good to think with'. The hospital was not just a new type of building (it had precedents but few close analogues in the classical world). It was a conceptual tool in an urban revolution.

My purpose in reviewing these various explanations of what has rightly been called 'the birth of the hospital in the Byzantine empire'[21] is not to adjudicate among them. (We do not have to choose; several explanations will have applied; the hospital is always an 'overdetermined' phenomenon.) My purpose is, rather, to draw attention to a methodological problem. All these explanations offered by historians – essentially functional explanations – can, *mutatis mutandis*, be converted into guesses about founder's explicit or half-formed aspirations or motives. How we establish the criteria for a plausible guess is the methodological problem to which I have referred – and to which I am not sure that we yet have a solution.

A second illustration of the problem, as substitute for a solution. If Basil's is the first of the big foundations, the last, and in any ways the most impressive of them before the Latin conquest, is that of the Pantocrator founded, in effect jointly, by the Emperor John II Comnenos and his wife Irene in 1126. This monastery and its hospital is famed for its *typikon* or foundation charter (to which I return below) and for the number of doctors and support staff that the imperial couple planned for the hospital's patients – an almost 1:1 ratio.[22]

Some historians have seen this hospital as a fantasy that existed only on parchment; some as a short-lived experiment in intensive medical care; some as a symbol of the modernity of Byzantine community medicine and as a guide to the standard facilities of other, less well-documented establishments.[23] I align myself with those who see the hospital as highly unusual, at least in its medical aspect. I think that the medical presence planned for it can be analysed in terms of an imperial extension, to the medical profession, of what Paul Magdalino has called 'lordship over the professional classes'.[24] Indeed, through his patronage of hospital doctors, who were clearly not to be workaday quacks but 'consultants', the emperor can be seen as beginning to consolidate, even to create, the upper echelons of that profession.

I am encouraged in this interpretation by a comparison with a later hospital. The value of associating a major imperial foundation (and, as we shall see, family mausoleum) with a heavy medical presence in the monastery's hospital seems to have been as evident to the

Palaiologans as it was to the Comneni. Despite the eulogies of Michael VIII's *philanthropia* to have come down to us, the first clearly documented hospital foundation after 1261 was undertaken by Michael's widow, Theodora, towards the end of the century. She restored the tenth-century monastery established, it seems, by Constantine Lips, turning it into a large monastic multiplex with fifty nuns and a hospital for twelve female patients clearly modelled on the women's section of the Pantocrator hospital. Twelve patients were to be looked after by three male doctors and one assistant, one nurse, one head pharmacist and two others, six attendants, a phlebotomist, three servants, a cook and a laundress.[25]

It is one thing, though, for me to analyse all this in terms of imperial patronage of medicine; quite another to suggest that this was how the founders' thoughts ran as they drafted their *typika*. The methodological problem remains, ultimately, because of a lack of sufficiently intimate evidence about founders' ideas. In her splendid study of benefactors' motives in Turin, *Charity and Power in Early Modern Italy*, Sandra Cavallo takes religious motives as a standard lowest common denominator among benefactors.[26] She could thus leave religion virtually on one side, and look at how changing expressions of institutional charity reflected changing political structures and concomitantly changing aspirations among elite benefactors. None of this subtlety is possible for a Byzantinist concerned with the early and middle phases of the empire's history.

IV

Of course, Byzantine writers were as aware as any modern scholar that founders' motives were mixed. They also knew that those motives were not always commendable. In one of his sermons on loving the poor, Gregory of Nyssa, in the fourth century, for example, seemingly castigated those who saw hospitals as a means of getting beggars off the streets and out of sight.[27] The most emphatic identification of inappropriate motives for philanthropy comes in the well-known novel (new law) of the Emperor Nicephorus Phocas, perhaps drafted by Symeon Metaphrastes, and issued in 964 in a vain attempt to protect the empire's financial and military base from erosion by the tax dodges of 'the powerful'.[28]

> What is then the matter with the people who, moved by the wish to do something to please the Lord and to have their sins pardoned, neglect thus the easy commandment of Christ which enjoins them to be free of care and, selling their property, to distribute its proceeds among the poor? But instead of following this commandment they [...] subject themselves to more worries by seeking to establish [private] monasteries, hospitals and houses for the old. In times gone by when such institutions were not sufficient, the establishment of them was praiseworthy and very useful [...] But when their number has increased greatly and has become disproportionate to the need and people still turn to the founding of monasteries, how is it possible to think that this good is not mixed with evil [...]? And moreover, who will not say that piety has become a screen for vanity [Mandeville would have enjoyed this] when those who do good, do so in order that they may be seen by all the others? They are not satisfied that their virtuous deeds be witnessed by their contemporaries only, but wish also that future generations be not ignorant of them.

The emperor had his own reasons for exaggerating hospital founders' pursuit of worldly renown. When he asserted that the empire already had enough hospitals, he was not offering a considered estimate of the needs of the poor. Still, he raises for us the question of how easy it was in Byzantium to be remembered for having founded a hospital.

One way in which we can pursue this question is through the topic of hospital names. A late antique commentator on Aristotle's *Art of Rhetoric* puts hospitals first in a list – before churches – of things that perpetuate the memory of an individual after death.[29] Was the philosopher's advice heeded? St Basil's suburban philanthropic centre at Caesarea came to be called the *Basileias*, but not (one guesses) at his instigation. So far as we can tell from Procopius in his panegyric, *De Aedificiis*, the Emperor Justinian, one of the great founders and restorers of Byzantine hospitals, does not seem to have named any of them after himself: uncharacteristic modesty. The Pantocrator hospital, to which I have also already referred, was named for its monastery, not its imperial founder. As for other major establishments in Constantinople: the premier orphanage was St Paul's;[30] St Sampson did found the Sampson hospital, but exactly when is obscure and the name probably derived from popular association rather than the holy man's choosing.[31]

How many known hospitals in the early Byzantine Empire are in fact securely named after their founders as a way of preserving those founders' *memoria*? The apparent answer is: surprisingly few.[32] And this is not, as it would be in the West, because most hospitals are named for saints such as John the Baptist, although Theodore and George do have a few Byzantine adherents. Some 150 hospitals and similar establishments are known from the provinces of the empire from the fourth to the eighth centuries. Only about twenty of these are apparently named after their founders. Where a name is preserved at all, it usually identifies the hospital by its location or its mother religious house.

Now the figures that I have given are no more than rough estimates. There will have been many more hospitals founded than we know about. Of those that are known to us, only a few (about eight) are recorded in surviving inscriptions. But there must once have been many more of those inscriptions, each of which would presumably have announced the founder to all visitors and inmates. Even in the minority of cases in which the identity of a founder is recorded, that is not necessarily the same as the hospital's being named after him or her. The transmission of such information was not necessarily subject to the founder's control. Only in the Egyptian papyri do founders' names occur with any frequency, though still in a minority of the seventy-five references to hospitals now recovered.[33]

These crude statistics concern the provinces. In the capital, the picture is a little different. I think that twenty-three out of some fifty-eight establishments were known by the founder's name (or the founder's status, as with the 'Hospital of the King' (*tou Krale*), founded *c.* 1300 by the Serbian Stephan Milutin).[34] But in so many cases the evidence is ambiguous, and a fair number of these names are found in the strange writings of those not wholly reliable historians of urban folklore known as the patriographers.[35]

V

Ultimately, the renown that came from founding a hospital, whether it was transmitted orally, in the name of the establishment, or in an inscription over the door, was only a means to an end. Secular commemoration was principally valuable as an incitement to liturgical commemoration. I come back to the religious aspect of hospitals, shifting from the earlier to the later part of my period because that is where the evidence is. As John Thomas has commented,[36] after the papyri the most vivid evidence for Byzantine religious foundations comes from monastic *typika* or foundation documents. Here, in *typika* drawn up for houses with philanthropic establishments attached, we read founders' own characterisation of their religious motives. Naturally they write in acceptable and predictable formulae: these are not 'confessions'. But they are the nearest that we can come to the mentality of a hospital founder of the eleventh and twelfth centuries.

Thus in 1077 the senator and judge Michael Attaliates founds an almshouse and a monastery with two dependent poor houses.[37] He owes thanks to God for allowing him to rise from a humble and foreign background to the rank of senator, although he is a great sinner. He thinks daily about the account that he will have to render in the world to come, and wants to grant the Almighty some small pleasure. The poorhouses will, he hopes, propitiate his sins. (They would also effectively protect his family property.)[38]

A second example: in 1083 Gregory Pakourianos establishes a monastery in Bačkovo with three hospitals and with outdoor distributions.[39] He gives to God the ransom for his soul (Matthew 20.28), hoping to gain release from sins and from the threat of hell fire. On the anniversaries of his death and his relatives' deaths there are, for the salvation of their souls, to be offerings of the divine mysteries, memorial feasts, and distributions to the poor.

As we should expect from what can be learned about the Pantocrator hospital, the most elaborate provisions of this kind are to be found in that monastery's *typkon*.[40] In this mausoleum, monks, clerics, patients and doctors are all intercessors:

> Yet though I am not able to fathom the depths of thine incomprehensible wisdom which beneficially manages our lives, I [the emperor, somewhat suppressing the role of his wife Irene] give thanks for thy patience and at last according to my capabilities I unveil my enterprise, bringing thee a band of ascetics, a precious gathering of monks, whose duty it is to devote themselves to the monastery and propitiate thy goodness for our sins [...] Along with these I bring thee, the Lover of goodness, some fellow-servants, whom thou in thy compassion called brothers [Matthew 25.40], worn out by old age and toil, oppressed by poverty and suffering from diseases of many kinds [...] We bring thee these people as ambassadors to intercede for our sins; by them we attract thy favor and through them we plead for thy compassion.

The emperor's memory (*mnemosyne*), and that of his immediate family buried in the mausoleum, were to be lastingly preserved in several ways: (1) by regular mention in the daily services of the monastery and four times a week at services attended by hospital patients; (2) in two candles burning at the emperor's tomb; (3) by the offering of a daily communion loaf; (4) in weekly prayers for the dead at his tomb; (5) through annual commemorations associated with a visit to the monastery by a great icon of the Virgin.[41] And this was not all, because the *typikon* refers to other commemorations outlined in a separate confidential document, which does not survive.

It should not be thought that this kind of arrangement was at all new to the eleventh or twelfth century. The *typika* are bringing older practices into the light of our evidence. For instance, an edifying tale that is the sole survivor from the biography of a ninth-century recluse, Isaiah of Nicomedia, shows the extreme spiritual danger risked by a high-ranking official on the point of death. He had instructed his wife to distribute his fortune to the poor, but had oddly refused to pay fees to priests to celebrate the Divine Liturgy on the fortieth day after his demise.[42] A law of Leo VI (*c.* 900) expresses concern about private foundations that cannot support their complement of priests so that the divine mysteries are not celebrated. The 'memorial' consequences of that failing are clear: anniversaries of the dead pass unhallowed for lack of priests, to the detriment of both those who live here below and those 'who possess the life thereafter'.[43]

Founders rightly feared that their provisions would not meet the expenses of the commemorations that they planned. Some of John II's arrangements had apparently broken down within less than a decade after his death. As a monk wrote to the emperor's daughter-in-law, he

> desired very strongly [...] that his memory should not disappear into oblivion, and left no stone unturned in planning it and tried very hard in this connection, but failed.[44]

VI

If founders rightly feared such failures, they also feared that their foundations, however well intentioned and piously managed, would be insufficient to expiate their sins. What would happen to them? If they did not reach 'the bosom of Abraham', could they yet avoid the fires of hell? Orthodox thought, as I understand it, has always discouraged questioning what happens to the soul after death or formulating any precise or mechanistic connection between the fate of the dead and the prayers and memorial liturgies of the living. God is not to be bribed or bargained with in prayer.

Despite the endorsement of prayers for the dead by such figures as John the Almsgiver onwards,[45] and the clear evidence of liturgical commemoration, some monastic moralists and church authorities discouraged the idea that the prayers of others can have any affect on one's soul in the afterlife. Paul of Evergetis (d. 1054) in his *Synagoge* offers a stern warning: repent now, because there is nothing you or anyone else can do after death to change your fate in the other world. The second *hypostasis* of the first book of the *Synagoge*, which became the chief manual for the monastic and spiritual life, states categorically that, 'as long as we are in the present life, we must do good here, and not delay until the future. For after death, we cannot set things aright'.[46]

Within Orthodoxy there was thus room for a spectrum of opinion. The gaps that official pronouncements left were, for the ordinary believer, filled in by a variety of written 'questions and answers', hagiographical anecdotes, edifying tales, apocryphal revelations and visions that circulated throughout Byzantine history in the penumbra of orthodoxy.[47] Some of the material was cautious. A question addressed to Anastasius of Sinai in the seventh century produced an answer to the effect that suffrages for the dead are of some use for light sins, but it is better to rely on one's own actions.[48] Other tales showed in more detail why the dead were worth remembering.[49] I give two visionary examples. The first concerns Philentolos. He was renowned both for his charity (he built a hospital) and for his sexual conquests. After his death an archbishop was consulted about the fate of his soul but, with true orthodoxy, claimed not to know. Instead a hermit was granted a vision of Philentolos suspended between Paradise and Hell.

The second example is a vision attributed to a nun Anastasia, in an apocalypse of *c.* 1000. This shows how the charity and good behaviour of the living does actually determine the condition of the dead – the dead in a zone of interim punishment that is not hell, but is not some hitherto undetected Byzantine purgatory either.[50]

And again the angel turned back to where the sinners were being punished, and said to them, 'Behold! Here is a person from this life [Anastasia], and I am about to return her again to there, by the command of God.' And all [the sinners] raised a great voice to me, saying, 'We have left behind parents and children and wives. Passing over, send a message to them, so that they might be vigilant, lest they also come into these fearsome places of punishment – but truly, also, *so that they might make supplication to God on our behalf, and [do] almsgiving, namely that very money that we designated for the salvation of our souls. They have not given it, and we do not find any respite.* [Tell them]: you will come here too, where we are being punished. Look – do not be condemned by the righteous judge, because of our designations!'

Then I saw someone else, and they threw him into the pitch, which boiled over a thousand fathoms deep. And the angel said to him, 'She is from the vain world, and I am about to return her back there again, so send a message, if you wish.' And [the sinner] cried out with weeping and lamentation and gnashing, saying, 'I am from the west, Peter by name, from the *kastron* of Corinth, by rank *protospatharios*. And in my presence a person neither rejoiced nor obtained anything, but I wronged many in the vain life, and snatched away estates, wronged widows and orphans, arranged murders and did not judge justly because of money. *I never practised almsgiving, and the earth did not accept my body*, but God did not conceal my soul. I left behind wealth and much treasure. Report these things to my wife and to my children: be vigilant, lest you enter these fearsome places of punishment! *Be zealous through almsgiving, and supplicate God, and give these things on my behalf, that I might have rest from this bitter torment!'*

In his message from the place of punishment, the sinner did not mention hospitals as a form of almsgiving. But clearly if he had founded a hospital, or if his family at once proceeded to found one, his punishments would not be so severe. That was a message indeed worth remembering. It reveals to us a Byzantium that we do not find in the usual kinds of evidence. It is a Byzantium that is closer to the West in its theology of prudential hospital foundation than we might have expected – the West in the earlier Middle Ages, before the 'birth of Purgatory'.[51]

Notes

1   With the permission of the publishers, Akademie Verlag, this paper draws on material first presented in my 'Memoria, Salvation, and Other Motives of Byzantine Philanthropists', in M. Borgolte (ed.), *Stiftungen in Christentum, Judentum und Islam vor der Moderne* (Berlin, 2005), pp.137–46.

2   *The Fable of the Bees, or, Private Vices, Publick Benefits*, ed. F.B. Kaye (Oxford, 1924), 1, pp.261.

3   R. Porter, 'The Gift Relation: Philanthropy and Provincial Hospitals in Eighteenth-Century England', in L. Granshaw and R. Porter (eds), *The Hospital in History* (London and New York, 1989), pp.162–3.

4   Quoted by Porter, 'The Gift Relation', p.162.

5   T.S. Miller, *The Birth of the Hospital in the Byzantine Empire*, 2nd edn (Baltimore and London, 1997). See also D.J. Constantelos, *Byzantine Philanthropy and Social Welfare*, 2nd edn (New Rochelle, NY, 1991), esp. pp.15–21 on founders' motives, and E. Patlagean, *Pauvreté économique et pauvreté sociale à Byzance 4e–7e siècle* (Paris, 1977), pp.185–8, 231–5, for the initial demographic and political setting. For more recent work, see P. Horden, 'The Earliest Hospitals in Byzantium, Western Europe, and Islam', *Journal of Interdisciplinary History*, 35 (2005), pp.361–89.

6   On which see D. Stathakopoulos, 'Stiftungen von Spitälern in spätbyzantinischer Zeit (1261–1453)', in M. Borgolte (ed.), *Stiftungen in Christentum, Judentum und Islam vor der Moderne* (Berlin, 2005), pp.147–57.

7   A.P. Kazhdan et al. (eds), *The Oxford Dictionary of Byzantium*, 3 vols (New York and Oxford, 1991), s. v. 'euageis oikoi'.

8   P. Horden, 'Religion as Medicine: Music in Medieval Hospitals', in P. Biller and J. Ziegler (eds), *Religion and Medicine in the Middle Ages* (Woodbridge and Rochester, NY, 2001), pp.135–53.

9   C. Rawcliffe, *Medicine for the Soul: The Life, Death and Resurrection of an English Medieval Hospital* (Stroud, 1999), pp.103–32. See also S. Sweetinburgh, *The Role of the Hospital in Medieval England: Gift Giving and the Spiritual Economy* (Dublin, 2004).

10   K. Schmid and J. Wollasch (eds), *Memoria: der geschichtliche Zeugniswert des liturgischen Gedenkens im Mittelalter* (Munich, 1984); O.G. Oexle, 'Memoria und Memorialüberlieferung im früheren Mittelalter', *Frühmittelalterliche Studien*, 10 (1976), pp.70–95.

11   J. Chiffoleau, *La comptabilité de l'au delà: les hommes, la mort et la religion dans la région d'Avignon à la fin du moyen âge (vers 1320–vers 1480)* (Rome, 1980), remains classic.

12   R.M. Grant, *Early Christianity and Society* (London, 1978), pp.124–45. For what follows see now also R. Finn, *Almsgiving in the Later Roman Empire: Christian Promotion and Practice (313–450)* (Oxford, 2006), esp. pp.29–30, 177–82.

13   *II Clement* 16.4, ed. and trans. B.D. Ehrman, *The Apostolic Fathers*, 2 vols, Loeb Classical Library (Cambridge, MA, and London, 2003), 1, p.122. Trans. quoted is from Grant, *Early Christianity*, p.128.

14   Hermas, *The Shepherd* 51 (Parable 2), 5–7, ed. Ehrman, *Apostolic Fathers*, 2, pp.310–12; Grant, *Early Christianity*, p.130.

15   Finn, *Almsgiving*, pp.150–5; more generally O. Plassmann, *Das Almosen bei Johannes Chrysostomus* (Münster in Westfalen, 1961).

16   Constantelos, *Byzantine Philanthropy*, p.49.

17   John Moschus, *The Spiritual Meadow* (*Pratum spirituale*), p.175, in J.-P. Migne (ed.), *Patrologia cursus completus, series graeca* (hereafter *PG*), 161 vols (Paris, 1857–66), 87, col. 3044B, trans. J. Wortley, *The Spiritual Meadow of John Mochos* (Kalamazoo, 1992), p.144.

18   For what follows, see P. Horden, 'The Christian Hospital in Late Antiquity – Break or Bridge?' in F. Steger and K.P. Jankrift (eds), *Gesundheit-Krankheit: Kulturtransfer medizinischen Wissens von der Spätantike bis in die Frühe Neuzeit*, Beihefte zum Archiv für Kulturgeschichte, 55 (Cologne and Weimar, 2004), pp.77–99.

19   P. Brown, *Poverty and Leadership in the Later Roman Empire* (Hanover and London, 2002), pp.26–35.

20   Letter 94, *Saint Basile, Lettres*, ed. Y. Courtonne, 3 vols (Paris, 1957–66), 1, p.206.

21   Miller, *Birth*.

22   P. Horden, 'How Medicalised were Byzantine Hospitals?', *Medicina e Storia*, 5 (2005, published 2006), pp.45–74; Miller, *Birth*, pp.14–21, with further bibliography.

23   Contrast E. Kislinger, 'Der Pantokrator-Xenon, ein trügerisches Ideal?' *Jahrbuch der Österreichischen Byzantinistik*, 37 (1987), pp.173–9; Miller, *Birth*.

24   P. Magdalino, *The Empire of Manuel I Komnenus 1143–1180* (Cambridge, 1993), p.220.

25   J.P. Thomas and A. Constantinides Hero (eds), *Byzantine Monastic Foundation Documents: A Complete Translation of the Surviving Founders' Typika and Testaments* (hereafter *Typika*), 5 vols (Washington DC, 2000), also at <www.doaks.org/etexts.html>, no. 39, vol. 5, pp.1254–86, at 1281; Stathakopoulos, 'Stiftungen', pp.152–3.

26   S. Cavallo, *Charity and Power in Early Modern Italy: Benefactors and their Motives in Turin, 1541–1789* (Cambridge, 1995).

27   S.R. Holman, *The Hungry are Dying: Beggars and Bishops in Roman Cappadocia* (Oxford, 2001), pp.147, 203.

28   J. Zepos and P. Zepos, *Jus graecoromanum*, 8 vols (Athens: Phexe, 1931), 1, pp.251–2, trans. P. Charanis, 'Monastic Properties and the State in the Byzantine Empire', *Dumbarton Oaks Papers*, 4 (1948), pp.56–7. The text is also translated in E. McGeer, *The Land Legislation of the Macedonian Emperors* (Toronto, 2000), p.95.

29   H. Rabe (ed.), *Anonymi et Stephani in Artem Rhetoricam commentaria* (Berlin, 1896), p.52, cited by P. van Minnen, 'Medical Care in Late Antiquity', in P.J. van der Eijk, H.F.J. Horstmanshoff, and P.H. Schrijvers (eds), *Ancient Medicine in its Socio-Cultural Context*, 2 vols (Amsterdam and Atlanta, 1995), 1, pp.153–69, at 163 n. 39.

30   T.S. Miller, *The Orphans of Byzantium* (Washington, DC, 2003), pp.176–246.

31   T.S. Miller, 'The Sampson Hospital of Constantinople', *Byzantinische Forschungen*, 15 (1990), pp.101–35.

32   What followers derives from my reading of the often ambiguous evidence usefully collected by K. Mentzou-Meimare, 'Eparchiaka evage hidrymata mechri tou telous tes eikonomachias', *Byzantina*, 11 (1982), pp.243–308.

33   Van Minnen, 'Medical Care'.

34   R. Janin, *Les églises et les monastères*, La geographie ecclésiastique de l'empire byzantin, I.3, 2nd edn (Paris, 1969), pp.552–69; M. Živojinović, 'Bolnica Kralja Milutina u Carigradu', *Zbornik Radova Vizantoloshkog Instituta*, 16 (1975), pp.105–17; Stathakopoulos, 'Stiftungen', pp.156–7.

35   On whom see G. Dagron, *Constantinople imaginaire* (Paris, 1984).

36   J.P. Thomas, *Private Religious Foundations in the Byzantine Empire* (Washington, DC, 1987), p.171. For what follows see also R. Morris, *Monks and Laymen in Byzantium, 843–1118* (Cambridge, 1995), pp.122–30.

37   Thomas and Hero, *Typika*, no. 19, vol. 1, pp.326–76, at 333–4, 336–7, 349.

38   Thomas, *Private Religious Foundations*, pp.179–85.

39   Thomas and Hero, *Typika*, no. 23, vol. 2, pp.507–63, at 522, 544–56, 549–50. See also E. Patlagean, 'Les donateurs, les moines et les pauvres dans quelques documents byzantins des XIe et XIIe siècles', in H. Dubois, J.-C. Hocquet, and André Vauchez (eds), *Horizons marins, itinéraires spirituels (Ve–XVIIIe siècles)*, 2 vols (Paris, 1987), 1, pp.223–31.

40   Thomas and Hero, *Typika*, no. 28, vol. 2, pp.725–81. For the hospital, see pp.757–66.

41   See also A.W. Epstein, 'Formulas for Salvation: A Comparison of Two Byzantine Monasteries and their Founders', *Church History*, 50 (1981), pp.385–400; E.A. Congdon, 'Imperial Commemoration and Ritual in the *Typikon* of the Monastery of Christ Pantocrator', *Revue des Études Byzantines*, 54 (1996), pp.161–99.

42   D. Sternon, 'La vision d'Isaïe de Nicomédie', *Revue des Études Byzantines*, 35 (1977), pp.5–42 at 25.

43   P.-B. Noailles and A. Dain (eds), *Les novelles de Léon VI le sage* (Paris, 1944), p.25, no. 4.

44   M. Jeffreys and E. Jeffreys, 'Immortality in the Pantokrator?' *Byzantion*, 64 (1994), pp.195–6. For wider context, see J. Thomas, '*In perpetuum*: Social and Political Consequences of Byzantine Patrons' Aspirations for Permanence for their Foundations', in Borgolte (ed.), *Stiftungen*, pp.129–32.

45   *Life of John the Almsgiver* 24, in A.-J. Festugière (ed), *Léontios de Néapolis, Vie de Syméon le Fou et Vie de Jean de Chypre* (Paris, 1974), pp.375–6. See also the 'Oration on those who have fallen asleep in the faith' and on the value of alms for the salvation of their souls, once (wrongly) attributed to John of Damascus, *PG*, 95, cols. 247–78.

46   V. Matthaios (ed), *Evergetinos etoi Synagoge [...] tomos protos* (Athens, 1957), p.42; Bishop Chrysostomos et al. (ed. and trans.), *The Evergetinos: A Complete Text. Volume I of the First Book* (Etna, CA, 1988), p.57.

47   J. Wortley, 'Death, Judgement, Heaven, and Hell in Byzantine "Beneficial Tales"', *Dumbarton Oaks Papers*, 55 (2001), pp.53–69, at 55, and N. Constas, '"To Sleep, Perchance to Dream": The Middle State of Souls in Patristic and Byzantine Literature', *ibid.*, pp.91–124.

48   (Pseudo-)Anastasius of Sinai, *Questions and Answers* 22, in *PG*, 89, col. 536C.

49   F. Halkin, 'La vision de Kaioumos et le sort éternel de Philentolos Olympiou', *Analecta Bollandiana*, 63 (1945), pp.56–64.

50   R. Homburg (ed.), *Apocalypsis Anastasiae* (Leipzig, 1903), pp.27–30, trans. J. Baun, *Tales from Another Byzantium: Celestial Journey and Local Community in the Medieval Greek Apocrypha* (Cambridge, 2007), p.41, adapted, and with italics added.

51   J. Le Goff, *The Birth of Purgatory* (Aldershot, 1984); M. McLaughlin, *Consorting with Saints: Prayer for the Dead in Early Medieval France* (Ithaca and London, 1994).

Kevin C. Robbins

Chapter 2: Patrimony, Trust, and Trusteeship: The Practice and Control of Burgundian Philanthropy at Beaune's Hôtel-Dieu, *c.* 1630

The analysis of patronage as a socio-political phenomenon has become an integral part of historical writing about France in the old regime.[1] However, it is the function of patronage as a modulator and structuring force of high political power that has commanded most attention. To be sure, historians of French painting and literature have also explored the cultural and aesthetic aspects of elite art patronage. Yet this scholarship, so often devoted to questions of formal influence, protégés flattering protectors, and the decoding of intricate master-works revealing a 'French school', tends to rarify patronage, removing it from the quotidian material and political existence of ordinary French people.[2] Moreover, the generally esoteric description of patronage, whether in high art or high politics, makes it difficult to assess how this variable and contested socio-economic practice connected with more common trends in the development of the early modern French polity. This is especially true when we seek to know how historic forms of patronage interacted with the formation of an early modern 'public sphere' increasingly shaped by the mores of law-abiding, literate, trustworthy, and bourgeois households.[3] This essay reassesses one interesting and contentious history of Burgundian hospital patronage, examining in detail the capacity of former protégés (here a sorority of lay nurses and allied commoners) to challenge legally and successfully the designs of their titular noble patron. Contention between these apparently mismatched adversaries over the proper use and administration of the hospital reveals the lay sisters' increasingly sophisticated and judicially advantageous assertion of empowering stewardship over a public trust. Their effective claim to real trusteeship of the hospital legitimates legal combat with their nominal aristocratic patron, demonstrating how seventeenth-century struggles to define 'public interest' (especially by women) prefigure the later consolidation of a broader 'public sphere'.

Investigation of this conflict over internal control of Burgundy's greatest hospital can also broaden and deepen a growing history of nurses and nursing in early modern France.[4] The bulk of existing scholarship on this subject focuses on various orders of Catholic nuns devoted to nursing as a pious and self-abnegating vocation. The charitable work of professed Augustinian sisters, who staffed a majority of France's hôtels-dieu, figures most prominently in recent studies. This literature emphasises the increasing subordination of nuns as nurses to the male governors of French churches and cities, especially after 1650. The 'docility' of avowed nursing sisters and the low cost of their mainly spiritual services allegedly made them irresistible to authoritarian city fathers and senior prelates intent on enlisting them in the cheapest possible defence of traditional secular and sacred governing bodies.[5]

By contrast, evidence from Beaune in the 1630s shows the vitality and expansion of an entirely lay sorority of nurses. These women were far less vulnerable to clerical influence than their cloistered sisters. More importantly, nurses in Beaune grew bolder in asserting a vital connection between their own practical skills as caregivers, making the sick poor well, and public support, even veneration, for the hospital where they worked. Beaune's lay nurses capitalised on this linkage to defend in writing and at law an exceptional degree of power-sharing with men in the governance and operation of the hospital. Far from being the submissive handmaidens of traditional male authorities, sacred or secular, medical or political, Beaune's nurses actively redefined the meaning and social utility of a hospital, emphasizing the efficiency, success, and public awareness of the ward and pharmaceutical treatments they dispensed.

These historic events reveal a wide diversity of actresses among early modern French nurses. Lay caregivers at Beaune made no pretence of submission to local churchmen, to the aristocratic male heirs of their hospital's first great patron, nor to city fathers. These working women, strengthened in a sorority of charitable public service, challenged many traditional authorities. They made nursing, as an endeavour at physical as well as spiritual welfare, a means of personal empowerment and institutional transformation.[6]

Among the accoutrements of French nobility, the noble prerogative of generosity bulked large in the lives of ordinary people. While charity was the duty of every Christian, *largesse* on a grand scale became a signifier of exalted rank. As Georges Matoré has noted, 'la *liberalité* est une qualité inhérente au statut social'.[7] More recently, Jean Starobinski, has tracked the visual history of philanthropy (especially in early modern France). He emphasises how traditional and humiliating asymmetries of power and status between propertied donors and humbler recipients provoked enlightened social theorists, like Rousseau, to posit more egalitarian systems of gift exchange as a better basis of modern democratic politics.[8] Since classical times, magnificence in giving defined the noble soul and worked, ultimately, to define the nobility itself.[9]

In the realm of ducal Burgundy, late medieval feats of noble charity were especially prized as manifestations of cultural superiority (*vis-à-vis* the French) and as bulwarks of a socio-political order conceived and celebrated in chivalric terms. Such gestures of socio-political distinction captivated Nicolas Rolin, the chancellor and aspiring courtier of Philip the Good. In 1443, Rolin created the Hôtel-Dieu, or private charity hospital, in the Burgundian city of Beaune. Ennobled by Philip, an intimate of the glittering Burgundian court, and endowed with numerous seigneurial properties, Rolin moved impressively in the highest echelons of the duchy's political elite. By investing his heirs in perpetuity with patronage and administrative control of the Hôtel-Dieu, Rolin, through his various testaments and detailed operating memoranda for the hospital, clearly intended perpetual family governance of the institution to become an indelible sign of the clan's generous nobility.

Sustained by an endowment comprised of premier Burgundian vineyard properties and perpetual rents on the Burgundian salt monopoly, the Hôtel-Dieu in Beaune prospered throughout the early modern period. However, the administrative history of this wealthiest private charity in Burgundy is marked by prolonged seventeenth-century legal controversies over the proper use and government of the institution. These disputes pitted two generations of the de Pernes

family (counts d'Epinac), aristocratic heirs by marriage to the founding patron Rolin, against the hospital's staff, comprised of operating
officers from Beaune's *haute bourgeoisie* and the well organised lay
nursing sisters doing all of the institution's actual charitable medical
care. These protracted judicial struggles ultimately involved the
Parlement of Burgundy and elicited extensive legal commentary from
a host of local and Parisian secular and ecclesiastical authorities.
These battles evoke conflicting early modern ideas about the nature of
charitable institutions, their operation, their socio-political significance, and their proper capacity to empower over time those who
created, supervised, and served in them.

Here, I would like to explore briefly the existing archival record
of friction at Beaune's hospital between the two opposing legal
parties. The aristocratic d'Epinacs and their lawyers espoused traditional notions of pious bequests centered on the material and spiritual
benefits supposedly accruing to the family and soul of the noble benefactor. Their opponents, male and female commoners running the
Beaune hospital, advocated more modern understandings of philanthropy and trusteeship as inherently social and public acts empowering
living servants or practitioners of these benefactions with decisive
control over charitable institutions established by deceased donors.
Depositions from the episodically contending parties in the Beaune
hospital case reveal nascent early modern French conceptions of trust,
trusteeship, and the capacity of differing social orders to execute
faithfully the posthumous philanthropic intentions of distinguished but
dead benefactors. Building upon the notable contributions of Jean-
Pierre Gutton and Daniel Hickey to the social and political histories of
early modern French charity hospitals, I would like to address here the
broader cultural history of Burgundian philanthropy and its conflicts
with older conceptions of noble patronage.[10]

Beginning in the 1430s, Chancellor Nicolas Rolin worked tirelessly to make the Hôtel-Dieu in Beaune his hospital. Rolin devoted
years to the patient acquisition of free title to all land in Beaune on
which the structure sat and then, at great cost, gained for the hospital
ten potent papal bulls exempting the institution in perpetuity from any
church surveillance, investigation or control whatsoever. Other papal
dispensations obtained by Rolin accorded a plenary indulgence to any-

one dying in the hospital and extensive remissions of sin for those who either visited the building's chapel or who made their own contributions to the charity. To stimulate such attention, Rolin, at exorbitant cost, also equipped the Hôtel-Dieu with an impressive suite of reputedly powerful relics purchased in Rome and expedited to him by papal secretaries.[11] Finally, Rolin also obtained multiple, comprehensive fiscal exemptions for the hospital from the dukes of Burgundy he so capably and so discretely served.

Rolin worked hard to endow his charitable medical institution with a durable administrative structure. He established a master to superintend the hospital, a rector to oversee its finances, a headmistress to organise the work of nursing sisters, a chief surgeon to coordinate medical care, and a father confessor to supervise the spiritual needs of staff and patients. The master, mistress, rector, surgeon, and confessor formed the governing board of the hospital and Rolin instructed them to report annually to and to take non-binding advice from Beaune's mayor and town councilmen. Rolin personally revised the operating statutes of the Hôtel-Dieu at least twice in his lifetime, seeking always to insulate the institution from the avaricious designs of grasping civic magistrates, jealous local churchmen, regional episcopal authorities, parlement officers, and royal agents.

The headmistress was charged by Rolin to direct the work of lay nursing sisters who, in turn, were ordered by the first patron to swear forever their devotion to the hospital, its founder, his heirs, and their headmistress while explicitly rejecting all outside church affiliations. The sisters did not take holy orders, were not cloistered, and retained all legal rights to the use and administration of personal or familial assets maintained outside of the Hôtel-Dieu.[12] Sisters could freely renounce their profession and leave the institution at will. Daughters from notable but not noble Beaunois patrician families figured prominently in this prestigious sorority. Nicolas Rolin eventually accorded the sisters the free right to elect their own confessor from among Beaune's higher clergy, reserving the right as patron to confirm the election and to stipulate precisely the clerical tasks and emoluments to which the confessor might lay claim. Rolin's son, Jean, a cardinal and bishop of Autun, succeeding as patron of the Hôtel-Dieu in 1461, extended the sisters' privileges. He gave them the right to elect their headmistress by secret ballot, subject to his or his heirs' ultimate confirmation of the candidate chosen in open elections.

By 1500, Beaune's lay nurses enjoyed an exceptional degree of autonomy in the day-to-day operations of the hospital. Moreover, through their elected headmistress, who served *ex-officio* on the hospital's governing board, they already exercised a deliberative voice in the general administration of the institution. Compared to the professed nuns serving obediently in other French hôtels-dieu, Beaune's lay nurses possessed more personal freedoms, greater powers of self-government, and stronger influence over defining the hospital's mission. These rights were not an anomaly in French hospital administration. As the lay sisters' renown for effective medical care grew, they began to receive invitations from civic authorities elsewhere to found new hospitals on the Beaune model. Ultimately, nurses from Beaune organised and operated more than thirty similar hospitals in other French and Swiss cities.[13]

Given an impressive, custom-designed, and richly decorated ensemble of buildings and administrative statutes by the Rolin family, the Hôtel-Dieu in Beaune thrived. Hospital administrators amassed a large endowment comprised of extensive vineyards, rural and urban rental properties, decorative art objects, furniture, and cash donated by a wide cross-section of Burgundian society. From its opening, the Hôtel-Dieu, in its structure and operations, seems to have awed observers (no doubt as intended by the founding patron). In 1494, the Abbot of Citeaux, a fine builder himself and a connoisseur of architectural beauty, called the Hôtel-Dieu, 'a splendid and famous hospital established on a plan so vast and so perfect as to compel the admiration of the most powerful seigneurs and foreign nobles'.[14] In 1619, another observer called the Hôtel-Dieu

> one of the rarest and most superb structures in France which more resembles the residence of a prince than a hospital for the poor, renowned throughout the world, firstly for the great charity and hospitality extended there to all types of sick people, but above all for the buildings, singular structures and so well ordered with a hall, for ill commoners, so marvellously grand, so richly furnished and maintained and so clean where the poor sick are served with the utmost civility.[15]

The legal problems recounted here began when one seventeenth-century seigneur, apparently much impressed by the hospital's actual resemblance to a princely residence, tried indeed to move in and install his entire household there. In 1639, Louis de Pernes was a *chevallier du Roy*, royal *conseiller*, governor of the city and chateau of Saintes, seigneur of nine noble estates, husband to the granddaughter of Nicolas Rolin, and, by this match, titular patron of the Hôtel-Dieu. That year de Pernes asserted his right both to live at the hospital and to lodge there with his full retinue of family and servants whenever visiting his many Burgundian properties.

The master, confessor, headmistress, nursing sisters, and town council of Beaune formed an immediate opposition to this plan. Antoine Vorvelle, confessor (or *père spirituel*) at the hospital, addressed a long letter of protest to de Pernes, bluntly contending that the patron's residence at the Hôtel-Dieu would ruin the institution's vital fund raising campaigns without which the current scale of medical services to the poor could not be maintained.[16]

'Your entrance here', Vorvelle wrote to de Pernes,

> would close the door on all the legacies and donations one might otherwise expect [...] you could not prevent a common belief that donations for the poor would now go to your own expenditures and that gifts to the hospital would become gifts to the seigneur of the hospital. You will watch this fountain of mercy and charity dry up.[17]

De Pernes' household might also include 'disreputable and untrustworthy servants'. Their presence, Vorvelle warned, would discourage recruitment of new nursing sisters.

> What father would allow a daughter or kinswoman to enter into this confusion of valets, sommeliers, cooks, stableboys, lackeys, and others who ordinarily are so insolent and often so licentious?[18]

The staff of the Hôtel-Dieu actively solicited the opinions of senior Burgundian jurists and Parisian clerics on the legitimacy of de Pernes' claim to residence at the hospital. They feared that the Hôtel-Dieu, which was not legally a religious house in any way obliged to cloister its nursing sisters, might indeed be subject to invasion by the patron's domestic suite. Examining Nicolas Rolin's original charter of the institution, lawyers to the Burgundian Parlement concluded that de Pernes' 'pretention' was not only groundless, but also scandalous, capable of causing a 'prejudice perpetuel et successif' to the Hôtel-Dieu despite de Pernes' direct familial connection to the founder.[19] They urged de Pernes not to sully the 'bien et honneur' of the Hôtel-Dieu, an edifice they regarded as a 'maison de Dieu'.[20] The presence of his retinue would dispossess the poor of 'their house' given to them and donated to God as an unencumbered gift in perpetuity by Nicolas Rolin, original patron of Burgundy's 'most charitable institution'. As the Dijonnais lawyers concluded, the intangible 'bien spirituel' of the organization would be ruined by de Pernes lodging there.

The nursing sisters of the Hôtel-Dieu also filed multiple, vigorous written protests of de Pernes' residential bid, taking the lead in local opposition to their nominal patron's invasion [21] Labelling themselves as 'servants of the poor', these key staff members hardly behaved in a servile manner. Arguing in more secular terms than their eloquent lawyers, the nurses sought to protect the 'bien et honneur' of their house from the presence of the patron and his suite. But the conception of 'honnor' they advanced was not traditional nor static. It did not rely on conventional notions of aristocratic or clerical comportment. Lodging a supposedly noble house in the Hôtel-Dieu would offend, the nurses claimed, not only the rules of the hospice's operation as set down in the foundation charter itself, but would also intolerably violate the 'honnêteté publique' of the charity hospital.[22] Although dutiful servants themselves, they feared the presence, familiarity, and misbehaviour of unscrupulous servants in de Pernes' employ. According to the sisters, their honour, as distinguished yet humble philanthropic actors, and the good repute of the institution they served for public benefit were under double threat.

Common in these counter-attacks against de Pernes' move can be found his female opponents' emphasis on the public honour or public integrity of the Hôtel-Dieu. The nurses boldly defended the institution's 'honnêteté publique', an acquired title of distinction for the corporate entity of the hospital superior in value and worthy of precedence over any familial rights of patronage claimed by de Pernes. Installation of the titular patron's household would unconscionably besmirch the institution's own public honour and freeze out any future alms or pious bequests by destroying the public's trust in the hospital's actual philanthropic status.

De Pernes' opponents, especially among the nurses, stress their own trustworthiness and the trustworthiness of the institution they serve while casting grave doubt upon the virtue and integrity of the count's noble retinue. The governing board and sisters of the Hôtel-Dieu present themselves as the defenders of a public trust, as trustees in essence of the Hôtel-Dieu (by office or by work experience). They derive from trustee status a legitimation of their combat against a noble lord, their nominal patron, and a member of France's aristocratic governing elite. The capacity of early modern French urban charities publicly to empower even the humblest and female members of their personnel in this fashion should be counted among the most significant aspects of their political and cultural histories.

As Matoré notes, the personal expression 'honneste homme' appears first in French usage circa 1538. Novel connotations of 'honneste' are developed by Montaigne, especially in the *Essais* (1580). The term acquires more elaborate adjectival meanings – with reference to human subjects – in Nicot's *Thresor de la Langue françoyse* of 1606.[23] However, the more impersonal, corporate, and public usages of 'honneste' and 'honnêteté' encountered fluently in the legal briefs Beaune's nurses filed against de Pernes are not elucidated in these earlier lexicons. This strongly suggests that – at least in Beaune – the actual practice and legal defence of caring service to the indigent by lay charitable actors expanded the civil meaning of these terms. The net result is a modified vocabulary of civic action through which former protégés, even women, can express and legitimate their opposition to the dictates of powerful noble patrons. Female nurses in Beaune did this by collectively and loudly avowing their dignified maintenance of a public trust through voluntary charitable service. This adroit publicizing of 'honnêteté' by the hospital's lay sisters in the 1630's (with serious local political repercussions) antedates by nearly a hundred years the efforts of contentious southern French males to use royal and municipal tribunals to enforce an enlightened code of 'honnêteté.[24]

Nor was the sisters' opposition to de Pernes limited to the housing issue. When the count sought to dismiss Antoine Vorvelle, their
father confessor, for insubordination in August 1639, all the sisters,
including four novices, fired off an angry, signed, and notarised letter
of protest. Here, they advised de Pernes of their intent to retain legal
counsel in the matter and denounced his renewed attack on 'the liberty
and repose of our consciences'.[25] Confronted by de Pernes' repeated
'violences and constraints' against them, the sisters swore once again
to protect the integrity of the Hôtel-Dieu, 'their house' as they explicitly and more frequently called it. In this lexicon, supplanting
references to patrons and protégés and eschewing meek religious
terminology, the sisters sought to identify the hospital as essentially
their place of work. Through their combined petitions, trustees of the
Hôtel-Dieu convinced the Prince de Condé, governor general of the
province of Burgundy, to intercede with de Pernes on their behalf.
Under Condé's pressure, the count promptly abandoned his plans to
move in and his efforts to fire Vorvelle.[26]

This resolution of the matter temporarily diminished but did not
eradicate the animosities the de Pernes family directed against the
female personnel of the Hôtel-Dieu. In 1652, this rancour again boiled
over. This time, it was the son of Louis de Pernes, also named Louis,
who sought revenge on the nursing sisters instrumental in thwarting
the commands of his own noble father twelve years before. The new
count d'Epinac sought to annul the recent election of Nicole Bourgeois as headmistress of the Hôtel-Dieu. Bourgeois had been a leading
opponent of lodging the de Pernes household at the hospital in 1639.
Moreover, the new count also sought to abolish entirely the traditional
election of headmistresses and claimed the right, as titular patron, to
appoint all successors to this office.[27] De Pernes now sought confirmation of this prerogative from the Parlement of Burgundy. This ploy,
although instigated by a lay nobleman, clearly parallels contemporary
efforts by senior French churchmen to expand and tighten their control
over the nursing orders of women religious.

De Pernes backed his claim to pre-eminence in the selection of
headmistresses with the argument that the patron's chief duty was the
maintenance of order within his institution. All office appointments,
crucial to this order, thus could only be legitimately decided by the

patron himself, acting in his traditional role as an aristocratic leader. De Pernes drew this line of reasoning from an even more fundamental axiom. 'Order', he asserted, 'is the soul of charity'.[28] De Pernes complained that his fidelity to this principle, so complementary one might add to post-Tridentine equations of charity and police, earned him only the insolent disrespect of the nurses and commoners running the Hôtel-Dieu in Beaune.

De Pernes' new bid to control the appointments of headmistresses met strong opposition from the staff members of the hospital led by Hughes Guyard, the headmaster who also held office as an *avocat* accredited to the Burgundian Parlement. Guyard counter-sued de Pernes before the Parlement, arguing that the count's attempt to deny the sisters their traditional voting rights in the election of headmistresses violated the charters of the Hôtel-Dieu as amended by Jean Rolin in 1461.[29] Moreover, Guyard contended that the vengeful new count, a 'patron laic' removed from the daily operations of the hospital, could not presume to know who, among the more experienced sisters, would be most capable of shouldering the heavy responsibilities of the headmistress. Guyard argued that only the sisters themselves could rightly make that judgment. This was not just because they had been previously invested with this right. It was mostly because the nurses were eminently trustworthy women with practical expertise in the sick wards and a superior knowledge of their patients' and their community's real needs in medical care.

Even worse, Guyard alleged, should de Pernes get to name new headmistresses, a patron less pious, less scrupulous, might name any woman he pleased to the post. This admirable position concentrating public regard might become 'the recompense of a *femme de chambre* or a mistress *d'intelligence avec son bienfaiteur*'.[30] And then, sadly, 'the resources of this house of God, given for the subsistence of the poor, could easily be turned to luxury and profane use'.[31] By such clever insinuations of aristocratic malfeasance, Guyard sought to undercut his opponent's public persona of trustworthiness or integrity while amplifying the honesty, devotion, and reliability of the lay nursing sisters in their medical conduct and electoral activity. Here Guyard joins with earlier defenders of the Hôtel-Dieu against the de Pernes clan by advocating the superior capacity of the hospital's diligent female staff to behave as respectful and respectable trustees of the founding patron's true charitable wishes.

Senior Parisian jurists, retained by Guyard to render an opinion in the case, found for the plaintiffs, arguing that the count's particular or private interest to control appointments could not supercede the public interest served by the nurses' internal election of the woman most capable for the job of headmistress.[32] The judges decided that this public interest in the Hôtel-Dieu also deserved the strongest possible defence because, over decades, generous public donations to the hospital had come to constitute its largest source of funding. The heirs of Nicolas Rolin, including the counts d'Epinac, now provided a dwindling proportion of the hospital's total gift capital. Shifts in institutional funding further undercut the pretensions of the hospital's nominal noble patron. Therefore, as the Hôtel-Dieu's best legal advisors concluded, 'There is good reason to argue that the public is the founder in part, and in the largest part, of the resources given to the said hospital'.[33] Thus the prime source of this endowment required that the public interest, defined and defended in the existing electoral procedures of the sisterhood, should prevail over the private interest of the Louis de Pernes, Count d'Epinac. Here the sisters finally achieved popular and judicial acknowledgments as superior trustees of that public interest whose diligence rendered them immune to the challenges of the count. His assertion of increasingly antique patronage rights proved unavailing in this novel public contest of integrity and honourable philanthropic service to the community and its needy.

Even in summary, as presented here, the conduct and discourse of these legal confrontations clearly evoke the capacity of French philanthropic institutions of the old regime to concentrate and amplify the political powers of their lay, non-noble directors and servants. Through empowering affiliation with and devotion to these charities, a diversity of provincial philanthropists, not limited to local governing elites and including large numbers of bourgeois lay women, could derive notable reputations as guardians of the public interest. Their stature as trustees rather than as patrons of good works enabled them successfully to oppose the strictures local nobles (and encroaching monarchs) sought to impose on the governance of charity and the articulation of conscience in early modern France. Conversant with the 'honnêteté publique' of the institution they maintained, these lay trustees construed a hospital as a vital constitutive element of a nascent public sphere detached from aristocratic pretensions to know and to patronise public welfare better than anyone else.

The legal contests at Beaune thus contrast with some of the conclusions Daniel Hickey drew from his meticulous comparative analysis of French provincial hospitals. Such institutions could regularly anchor opposition by influential townsmen against outsiders' attempts to meddle in local fiscal affairs and to systematise care and control of the needy.[34] Hinkey finds that local hospitals were often bastions in 'the maintenance of the social patterns and value structures upon which small town communities were based'.[35] However, close analysis of the language and ethos of the nurses' defence of their place in the Hôtel-Dieu at Beaune indicates that battles over hospital control did not always result in the mere reinforcement of traditional social hierarchies and established parochial values. To the contrary, at Beaune, such contests catalyzed progressive mutations in traditional notions of honour, confirmed vocational expertise as most conducive to social welfare, and enabled a sorority of experienced lay nurses to assert themselves as superior guardians of the public's trust in communal institutions.

In the case of the nursing sisters of the Hôtel-Dieu in Beaune, the public service they performed and the empowerment they derived from conservation of a public trust should not be construed as singular, anomalous, or transient. This is because the sisters tirelessly exported their model of hospital organisation, administration, and trusteeship to over thirty satellite care centres in towns and bourgs throughout eastern and southeastern France and western Switzerland. Often specifically invited by parish officials and conscientious civic magistrates in other towns to create new urban hospitals replicating Beaune's Hôtel-Dieu, the nursing sisters, by 1700, had implanted similar organisations in neighbouring communities such as Beaujeu, Besançon, Chalon-sur-Saône, Châtillon, Dôle, Pont-de-Vaux, Vesoul, and Villefranche-sur-Saône.[36] Comprehensive assessments of the socio-cultural and socio-political repercussions of this expansion have never before been attempted. However, newer scholarship documents the central role of women religious in the modernisation of European states after 1750, especially in the domains of schooling, health care, and social services. These discoveries suggests that lay sororities – like the nurses of the Hôtel-Dieu – deserve far closer scrutiny themselves as potent agents of modernity responsible, in part, for creating both the institutions and the rhetoric of the European, urban public sphere well before the Enlightenment.[37]

Notes

1   See, for one fine and representative example, S. Kettering, *Patrons, Brokers, and Clients in Seventeenth-Century France* (Oxford, 1986).
2   See, for example, A. Chastel, *French Art: The Renaissance 1430–1620* (Paris, 1995).
3   The absence of patronage (*Begünstigung* or *Gönnerschaft*) and its socio-political shifts and significance over time as subjects of sustained discussion in J. Habermas, *The Structural Transformation of the Public Sphere* (Cambridge, 1989), seems representative to me of this occlusion.
4   See, for examples, S. Broomhall, *Women's Medical Work in Early Modern France* (Manchester, 2004), esp. ch. 4, 'Hospital Nursing by Women Religious: The Hôtel-Dieu in Paris'; M. Dinet-Lecomte, 'Les religieuses hospitalières à Blois aux XVIIe et XVIII siècles', *Annales de Bretagne et des pays de l'Ouest*, 96 (1989), pp.15–40; idem, 'Les soeurs hospitalières au service des pauvres malades au XVIIe et XVIIIe siècles', *Annales de démographie historique* (1994), pp.277–92; idem, 'Les religieuses hospitalières dans la France moderne', *Revue d'histoire de l'Eglise de France*, 80 (1994), pp.195–216; idem, 'Les hôpitaux sous l'Ancien Régime: des enterprises difficiles à gerer?', *Annales. Histoire, économie et société*, 18.3 (1999), pp.527–45; C. Jones, *The Charitable Imperative: Hospitals and Nursing in Ancien Régime and Revolutionary France* (London, 1989).
5   See, in particular, Dinet-Lecomte, 'Les religieuses hospitalières à Blois', p.18.
6   The capacity of early modern French hospital administrators and staff members to create new bodies of law and to effect the modernization of society outside the bounds of medical care is emphasized by P.-J. Hesse, 'Les recteurs d'hôpitaux, créateurs de droit dans l'Europe moderne', in J.P. Gutton (ed.), *Les administrateurs d'hôpitaux dans l'Europe moderne* (Lyon, 2002), pp.101–29. The histories of French nurses, lay and religious, should be scrutinized for similar signs of their ability to change institutions and communities while serving within them.

7   G. Matoré, *Le vocabularie et la société du XVIe siècle* (Paris, 1988), p.151, emphasis in the original.

8   J. Starobinski, *Largesse* (Chicago, 1997). See in particular ch. 3, 'Charity', and pp.66–8.

9   See, for examples, the great classical treatises on giving such as Aristotle, *Nicomachean Ethics*, Book 4, and Seneca, *On Benefits*. For a history of public benefactions conducing to the perfection of patrician souls in Hellenistic cities, see P. Veyne, *Bread and Circuses* (London, 1990), ch. 1.

10   See J. –P. Gutton, *La société et les pauvres: L'exemple de la généralité de Lyon 1534–1789* (Paris, 1971); idem, 'La mise en place du personnel soignant dans les hôpitaux français (XVIe–XVIIIe siècles)', *Bulletin de la Société Française d'Histoire des Hôpitaux*, 54 (1987), pp.11–19; and D. Hickey, *Local Hospitals in Ancien Régime France: Rationalization, Resistance, Renewal, 1530–1789* (Montreal, 1997).

11   A. Boudrot, *L'Hôtel-Dieu de Beaune* (Beaune, 1881), p.13.

12   The nursing sisterhood at Beaune did not become professed nuns until 1939. Before this date, nurses at Beaune exercised all the rights lay French females possessed under local customary law and subsequent French national legislation. The lay nursing sisters in the Hospices Civils of Lyon enjoyed similarly broad rights of personal autonomy and employment. This congruity with their counterparts in Beaune suggests that lay nurses in Lyon may also have worked the kinds of transformations in local power-political relationships and in the articulation and guardianship of public trusts that I attribute to the nurses of Beaune's Hôtel-Dieu. For Lyon, see A. Croze, *Les soeurs hospitalières des Hospices Civils de Lyon* (Lyon, 1933). Note that Croze's claims about the unique freedoms of the nursing sisters in Lyon are mistaken.

13   See A. Leflaive, *L'Hôtel-Dieu de Beaune et les hospitalières* (Paris, 1959), pp.181–94.

14   Boudrot, *Hôtel-Dieu de Beaune*, p.108.

15   *Ibid.*, p.155.

16   Archives de l'Hôtel-Dieu (henceforward AHD), Beaune, 2264A, unpaginated.

17   *Ibid.*

18   *Ibid.*

19   AHD, 2264C, unpaginated.

20   *Ibid.*

21   AHD, 2264D, unpaginated.

22   *Ibid.*

23   Matoré, *Vocabulaire et société*, p.147 and n. 1. Even far more recent scholarly lexicons of the French language continue to discuss *honnêteté* in primarily personal terms, as an attribute of 'cultivated' or 'polite' individuals especially prized since the later eighteenth century. See, for example, G. Cabourdin and G. Viard, *Lexique historique de la France d'ancien régime* (Paris, 1990), s.v. 'Honnêteté'.

24   See the now classic text by Y. Castan, *Honnêteté et relations sociales en Languedoc, 1715–1780* (Paris, 1974), especially 'Le concept d'honnêteté', pp.22–8. Note also that the eighteenth-century political neutralization of *honnêteté* (through its increasing conflation in the public mind with *politesse*,) did not operate in the earlier era when the feisty sisters of the Hôtel-Dieu used novel conceptions of the term to build up the concept of a public trust and to limit and eventually to rebuff the pretensions of their noble lord.

25   AHD, 2264C, unpaginated.

26   AHD, 2265D, Excerpts of Deliberations of the Chambre de Ville of Beaune, 9–12 August 1639.

27   AHD, 2266B. The new count's case is also set forth extensively in a dossier of papers related to this case. See the Archives Départementales de la Saône et Loire, G 638, 1–20.

28   AHD, 2266B, unpaginated.

29   AHD, 2266C, unpaginated.

30   *Ibid.*

31   *Ibid.*

32   AHD, 2266D, unpaginated. Written legal opinion of Brodeau and Montholon in Paris dated 10 September 1652

33   *Ibid.*

34   Hickey, *Local Hospitals*, pp.198–208.

35   *Ibid.*, p.202.

36   Leflaive, *L'Hôtel-Dieu de Beaune et les Hospitalières*, pp.181–94.

37   For the place of nuns in creating the infrastructure of modernizing European states see the review article of P. Harrigan, 'Women Teachers and the Schooling of Girls in France: Recent Historiographical Trends', *French Historical Studies*, 21.4, (1998), pp.593–610; M. Magray, *The Transforming Power of the Nuns: Women, Religion, and Cultural Change in Ireland 1750–1900* (Oxford, 1998); and R. Rogers, 'Reconsidering the Role of Religious Orders in Modern French Women's Education', *Vitae Scholasticae*, 10.1–2 (1991), pp.43–55.

MATTHEW THOMAS SNEIDER

Chapter 3: The Treasury of the Poor: Hospital Finance in Sixteenth- and Seventeenth-Century Bologna

In 1601 the governors of the hospital of Santa Maria della Vita were gratified by the completion of a new and comprehensive register of their institution's property. This book, one of a series of such documents produced over the course of the sixteenth and seventeenth centuries, exhaustively describes the location and condition of each of the hospital's possessions. The reader is led through the dark and narrow streets east of the Piazza Maggiore – past the hospital and its ancient church and into a warren of fish-stalls, apartments, houses and shops. Radiating outward from this urban core are the gates of the city, and the reader is lead through each of them in turn to inspect Santa Maria della Vita's impressive rural holdings – vast estates as well as small farms. This proud patrimony has heavenly origins: 'the lord has favoured this hospital with temporal goods [...] for its sustenance, and that of the poor infirm'. Divine aid and good government have continually improved the hospital's condition – '[things have] always gone from good to better' – so that the poor no longer need to rely on the charity of Bologna's citizenry but can support themselves from their own resources. Although this optimistic document contains an allusion to past *stretezz[e]* caused by famine, contemporary records suggest that economic difficulties continued to plague the hospital.[1]

Just how well did the city's institutions of charity function economically? What were the sources of their income? Was this income always sufficient to cover their needs? What expedients did they adopt during periods of crisis? My paper reports the results of an ongoing research project into these questions and focuses on a period stretching from the late sixteenth to the mid-seventeenth centuries.[2]

The Origins of Institutional Wealth

Bologna's hospitals succoured the full panoply of early modern poverty.[3] Santa Maria della Vita and Santa Maria della Morte treated the injured and the sick,[4] San Biagio and San Francesco aided wandering pilgrims,[5] Santa Maria del Baraccano housed orphaned girls, San Giobbe aided sufferers from syphilis, and the Opera dei Poveri Mendicanti housed the Bolognese indigent.[6]

These charitable activities were rooted in large patrimonies brought together over the course of a centuries-long effort to expand resources. The institutions' wealth originated in the gifts they received from pious donors; this wealth was then invested in patrimonial expansion. Donation was the first channel by which property flowed to the institutions. The citizens of Bologna were extraordinarily generous patrons. It seems likely that institutions began receiving gifts immediately after their foundations, with the number of gifts swelling as they grew in size and reputation. Gifts were very diverse and reflected the world in which their donors lived: farms, bushels of wheat, noble urban *palazzi*, animals, *scudi*, orchards, bedclothes and government securities. Although the immediate value of these gifts to the institutions was probably limited, taken collectively they provided the capital which fuelled the purchase of property.[7]

Fig. 3.1 reveals the early fourteenth century to have been a period of relative languor in purchasing; institutional operations were most likely funded by income from a constant stream of donations.[8] The number of purchases begins to rise in the mid-fourteenth century and peaks in the mid-fifteenth, the mid-sixteenth, and the mid-seventeenth centuries. How do we explain patrimonial expansion? Historians have long recognized that the fifteenth and sixteenth centuries were a period of transformation in social welfare. Smaller hospitals were folded into larger hospitals and the treatment of particular social ills became fixed in particular institutions; institutional activities became more intensive and expensive; new institutions were created.[9] These changes have been traced for the charitable institutions of Bologna: we have noted how the hospital of Santa Maria della Vita focused on

the care of the sick; we have noted how Santa Maria della Vita and
Santa Maria della Morte provided themselves with effective spaces
and staffs; we have noted the transformation or creation of charitable
institutions in the sixteenth century. Such changes required large and
reliable revenues; expansion was likely aimed at providing institutions
with patrimonies capable of supporting their responsibilities.[10]

Figure 3.1
Purchases by six hospitals, 1270–1700

Year	SMV	SMM	OSF	OSB	Barr	ODM	Total
1250–	4	–	–	–	–	–	4
1300–	5	0	0	0	–	–	5
1350–	17	7	0	0	–	–	24
1400–	22	19	0	7	0	–	48
1450–	37	29	3	13	10	–	92
1500–	31	16	6	5	1	–	59
1550–	56	4	7	5	8	12	92
1600–	12	1	12	3	20	12	60
1650–	18	25	10	0	21	10	84

SMV=Ospedale di Santa Maria della Vita, SMM=Ospedale di Santa Maria della
Morte, OSF=Ospedale di San Francesco, OSB=Ospedale di San Biagio,
Barr=Ospedale di Santa Maria del Baraccano, ODM=Opera Pia dei Poveri Mendicanti

The acquisition of property, however, was only the *material* part
of the long effort to construct effective patrimonies. Equally important
was the 'fixing' of its ownership and control. Property belonged to the
collectivity of a hospital's poor inmates. Whether it was explicitly
donated to them or purchased in their name, the purpose of property
was to fund the assistance of the poor – a hospital's governors were
merely prudent factors for their afflicted masters.[11]

The records of several Bolognese hospitals suggest that this conception grew only gradually, in reaction to what seems to have been
considerable ambiguity about the proper use of institutional property.
If one may judge from calumnies and calls for reform property may
sometimes have been used for personal ends. On the 8 July 1408 the

brothers of Santa Maria della Vita learned of a 'scandalous rumour': '[...] the poor of the said hospital and their goods and rights are not being managed in an honest or proper manner'. We lack details about the mismanagement, but a measure passed on the same day, condemning 'those who unjustly hold or control [...] [the] [...] goods of the company', suggests that the problem was the usurpation of institutional property.[12] An undated provision appended to a 1408 copy of the hospital's statutes describes illicit exploitation of its real estate. It laments that transactions with members of the confraternity are causing scandal in Bologna. It is said that sales are being contracted for less than the just value of the property and that leases are being contracted for overly low rates and overly long terms.[13] The issue raised by both of these scandals was the nature of institutional property: did it belong to the poor and to the benefactors or to the members of the confraternity?

The hospitals answered this question by enacting a series of regulations aimed at preserving

> the languishing poor in that which our ancestors left them and to save the souls of those who from time to time seek, with great subtlety, to occupy the goods of [...] the poor, to the detriment and prejudice of the [...] poor and the worship of God.[14]

The regulations placed strict controls on the permanent or long-term alienation of property belonging to the hospital, they distinguished between proper and improper financial involvement by members of the confraternity, they limited the amount of money that governors could spend without the approval of the broader membership of the confraternity, they instituted procedures for overseeing the accounts of outgoing financial officers, they fulminated against members of the confraternity and hospital employees who wasted institutional resources. Such reforms were the final steps by which the institutions created patrimonies out of their numerous and disparate properties.[15]

Figure 3.2
Sources of income for the hospital of Santa Maria della Morte,
1564–90, in lire

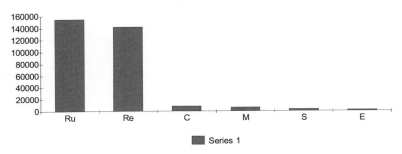

Ru=Rural holdings, Re=Rented properties, C=Credits on Monti di Pubblica Prestanza,
M=Miscellaneous, S=Sales, E=Alms or testamentary payments

Figure 3.3
Sources of income for the hospital of Santa Maria della Vita,
1690, in lire

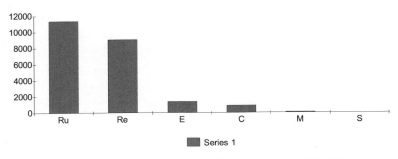

Ru=Rural holdings, Re=Rented properties, C=Credits on Monti di Pubblica Prestanza,
M=Miscellaneous, S=Sales, E=Alms or testamentary payments

The Use of Institutional Wealth

Income

The period stretching from the mid-fourteenth through the mid-seventeenth centuries was one of patrimonial expansion and consolidation for the hospitals of Bologna. The generosity of the city's inhabitants and the shrewd purchases of the administrators made them ever wealthier.[16]

The copious documentation available from the mid-sixteenth century onward makes it possible to describe this patrimonial wealth. Figs 3.2 and 3.3 represent the revenue available to the hospital of Santa Maria della Morte from 1564 through 1590 and to Santa Maria della Vita in 1690.

Charitable institutions throughout Italy tended to rely on real estate for a large part of their income.[17] This was certainly the case for the two medical hospitals of Bologna. The hospitals were surrounded by a close network of properties, ranging in size from mere stalls and shops to imposing houses. All were leased for short terms to a wide variety of tradesmen and tenants and generated respectable profits in liquid money and in goods. Of greater importance for the two institutions, however, was property in the countryside – in the hills to the south of the city or in the broad plain, which stretched toward the Po River. Many rural properties were leased for money rents, but some were managed directly by the hospitals themselves.[18] Such estates, worked by sharecroppers who were constantly supervised by the institutions' officers, were capable of producing impressively large harvests of grain, wine, wood and hemp. Much of this produce was, of course, directed to the fulfilment of the hospitals' alimentary and charitable needs but surpluses were frequently sold on the urban market.[19]

Early modern Italian taxation and public finance – *dazi, gabelle,* and *monti di pubblica prestanza* – provided contemporary hospitals with another important source of income.[20] Santa Maria della Vita and Santa Maria della Morte earned a growing share of their income from credit on the city's *monti di pubblica prestanza*.[21] By the late sixteenth century the governors of Bologna's hospitals were shifting their attention to this form of investment, which they evidently saw as more economically sagacious than physical property. The returns on these investments were more regular and predictable than those on real estate: they did not depend on the vagaries of the local economy or the weather and they did not require close management.

Real estate and *monte* credit were supplemented by several less regular sources of income. Alms from the pious citizens of Bologna, although not central to the balances of Santa Maria della Vita and Santa Maria della Morte, were still important. Figs 3.4 and 3.5 reveal the degree to which two other Bolognese hospitals – San Francesco and San Biagio – relied on alms for income. These institutions did not wait idly for their collection boxes to be filled. They engaged in an intense and constant effort to provoke the consciences and open the purses of their city: their needs were publicised from the pulpits of the city's most important churches, collection boxes were affixed to the walls of their chapels, influential politicians were exhorted to favour the cause of the *poveri*, and collectors were hired to tour the city and countryside gathering money, food and clothing.

The generosity of Bologna's inhabitants was joined by the generosity of Bologna's government. Nicholas Terpstra's work on the history of charity in early modern Bologna has underscored how the city's government and governing classes cultivated the development of its hospitals. The financial dimensions of this patronage were manifested in many ways. The city's hospitals received regular exemptions from the payment of certain taxes and duties.[22] Provision was made by the city's spiritual authorities to ensure that the zeal of Bologna's donors did not slacken – from the earliest days special indulgences were given to those pious citizens who gave to the hospitals.[23] More substantive aid was sometimes given to hospitals which were temporarily or permanently incapable of funding their operations. This was the case when, in the sixteenth century, the Bolognese Senate offered a regular annual payment of 100 *lire* to the hospital of San Giobbe.[24]

The revenues of charitable institutions were not limited to those produced by their large patrimonies or raised by appeals for alms. In

Matthew Thomas Sneider

Figure 3.4
Sources of income for the hospital of San Biagio, 1596–1600,
in lire

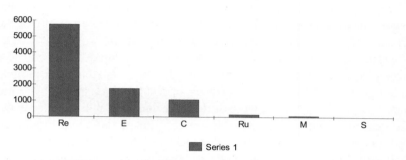

Ru=Rural holdings, Re=Rented properties, C=Credits on Monti di Pubblica Prestanza,
M=Miscellaneous, S=Sales, E=Alms or testamentary payments

Figure 3.5
Sources of income for the hospital of San Francesco, 1586–94,
in lire

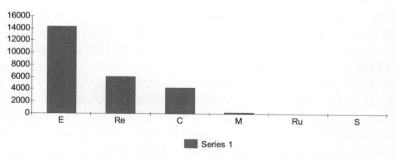

Ru=Rural holdings, Re=Rented properties, C=Credits on Monti di Pubblica Prestanza,
M=Miscellaneous, S=Sales, E=Alms or testamentary payments

good times they always held a certain quantity of capital – capital which was not crystallized in bricks or cultivated soil – which they repeatedly loaned to a series of borrowers. Such loans were almost always hidden behind fictitious sales and leases of property. Thus a hospital would 'purchase' a borrower's property for the amount of the loan, and then lease it back to that same borrower for a rent which corresponded to the interest payments. The term of the loan was the term of the 'lease'. Another common technique was the purchase of a *censo*, or the right to partake in the profits of an enterprise or a piece of remunerative property. The institution would 'purchase' this right from a borrower, who would then make regular payments for a certain period of time.[25]

Expenditure

The same documents which permit us to determine the sources of income available to these hospitals permit us also to discover the basic uses of this income. Fig. 3.6 divides regular expenses for Santa Maria della Morte and Santa Maria della Vita into three categories – liturgy, patrimony and charity.

The most dramatic of the liturgical expenses were public rituals: the processions and celebrations which marked the feast of a patron saint. Institutions spent money on the decoration of their churches, on wax torches, on food for ritual exchanges, on musicians. The quantity of money spent in these celebrations sometimes occasioned scandal and reproof by administrators or by authorities. A substantial share of the liturgical budget was taken up by 'internal' expenses. This included the spiritual life of the institution itself: the masses which were said for the spiritual health of the poor and the staff. It also included the observances which constituted the chief link between a confraternity and its dead members and patrons – masses of remembrance.[26]

Figure 3.6
Expenditure by Santa Maria della Morte (1564–90), Santa Maria della Vita (1690), San Biagio (1596–1600) and San Francesco (1586–94), in lire

Category	SMM	SMV	OSB	OSF
Liturgy	40938	3417	2314	1066
Patrimony	54087	2195	400	2139
Charity	179688	14549	3864	7533
Other	41445	4403	2058	2328

Also burdensome were costs related to a hospital's patrimony. Institutions like Santa Maria della Vita and Santa Maria della Morte were reliant on their patrimonies for much of their income. Regular outlays were therefore made to continue the cycle of production in the countryside and to maintain and improve properties. From the mid-sixteenth century through 1624, for example, the hospital of Santa Maria della Vita spent a total of 11,680 *lire* on the improvement of its rural property.[27] Less common, but certainly more dramatic, were the expenses incurred by institutions when they chose to build property from scratch. The 1620 decision to build a new women's infirmary, for example, involved the hospital of Santa Maria della Vita in costs which exceeded 6260 *lire*.[28]

Unsurprisingly the hospitals spent the most in their provision of charity. A chief component of this expense was the food given to the poor. Although meals were certainly not lavish – their diet consisted mainly of bread, wine, and *minestre* – their sheer number made them a heavy burden on the balances. Hospitals such as Santa Maria della Vita and Santa Maria della Morte were provided with much food from their own rural possessions. Less wealthy hospitals, however, were likely forced to purchase their foodstuffs or rely on the charity of the Bolognese citizenry. Added to this expense was money spent in the provision of the hospitals' particular form of charity. Hence Santa Maria della Vita and Santa Maria della Morte each paid the salaries of doctors – surgeons and physicians – and their assistants. They also purchased whatever medicines were deemed necessary for the treatment of the patients. Finally, charity in all hospitals depended on a small army of employees – servants, nurses, chaplains, cellarers, guardians – who were paid salaries and maintained at the hospital's board.[29]

Crises

We have reviewed the revenues and the expenses of Bolognese hospitals. What was the balance between these two things: how effective were patrimonies in meeting the demands of hospital activities?

Figure 3.7
Income and spending for Santa Maria della Morte 1564–90,
1614–43, 1654–60 and 1662–7, in lire

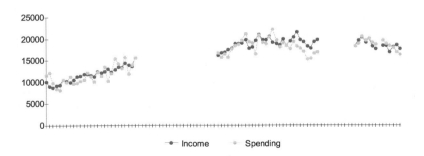

Fig. 3.7 traces income and expenditure for the hospital of Santa Maria della Morte from the mid-sixteenth through the mid-seventeenth centuries.[30] The graph suggests that the revenues of the great medical hospital largely sufficed to cover its expenses – this was the case in forty-two out of the seventy years for which information is available. The truly striking feature of the graph, however, is the volatility of expenses – the sharp rises and falls in institutional

spending. One would like to know whether this kind of volatility ever caused hospitals like Santa Maria della Morte to 'go into the red'. A perusal of the administrative records of Bologna's charitable institutions provides evidence suggesting that this *was* a danger.[31]

In the event of a temporary shortfall one might imagine that an institution's governors would have recourse to saved money. Indeed, many of Bologna's hospitals had money deposited in their name – with private individuals and on the city's Monte di Pietà.[32] The documentation contains several examples of institutions withdrawing such money to cover unexpected expenses. In 1569, for example, the governors of Santa Maria della Vita withdrew 900 *scudi* from the Monte di Pietà to fund a purchase of wheat for the city of Bologna during a year of penury[33] and on another occasion the same hospital was forced to withdraw 1600 *lire* from the *banco* of Cornelio Malvasia to use 'for the needs of the house'.[34]

Hospitals sometimes resorted to the more dramatic expediency of borrowing. Hospitals borrowed money using the same techniques with which they leant money: they sold and rented their property with *pacti francandi*; they created and sold *censi*. Institutions also had recourse to a form of borrowing which occupied a shadowy space between charity and credit – a 'pious donor' gave a quantity of money to the borrowing institution in return for regular annual payments during his lifetime.

Institutions might be forced to borrow money by the financial demands of patrimonial expansion – this was the case for the hospital of Santa Maria della Vita. The purchase of large pieces of rural property would probably have been impossible had the hospital been forced to rely on its patrimonial income and it contracted a series of private loans to afford the property it desired.[35]

More revealing than this practice of borrowing investment capital are the occasions when institutions were compelled to contract loans during periods of crisis. Such crises arose on the 'supply side' when patrimonies proved incapable of providing for institutional needs. Sometimes this was the result of damage to normally remunerative property. A particularly dramatic example was the crisis which afflicted the orphanage of Santa Maria del Baraccano in 1606 when a hailstorm fell upon its rural possessions at Cadriano and Viadagola.

The administrators decided to accept a donation of 2000 *lire* from
Tommaso Muratori, a fishmonger who demanded an annuity of 200
lire for as long as he and his wife lived.[36] Bad harvests were another
cause of crisis. In 1648 the governors of Santa Maria della Vita faced
a bad harvest and a lack of ready money. The crisis, so acute that the
hospital lacked 200 *corbe* of grain, forced the administrators to
consider the contraction of a loan.[37] A year later the hospital of Santa
Maria della Morte considered the creation and sale of a *censo* in order
to 'get money [...] to buy grain, which has been lacking and which is
lacking in the present year, for the poor of both sexes in the said
hospital'.[38]

Still other crises flowed from the 'demand side'. Santa Maria
della Morte and Santa Maria della Vita weathered a crisis of this sort
in the early 1590s, a time of particular difficulty for Bologna. Santa
Maria della Morte was forced to sell a part of its possession at Budrio
to Niccolò Gabrielli for 1618 *lire* to meet the expenses of the 'great
number of poor who flocked to the said hospital' in 1590. The
proceeds from this loan – one of several that year – were used to purchase beds.[39] A year later Santa Maria della Vita's governors were
burdened by a doubling in the number of the hospital's inmates, by
requests for aid on behalf of the city, and by debts. On 24 May they
voted to seek out 2000 *scudi* by selling and leasing hospital property
or by accepting a donation in return for the payment of an annuity.[40] In
1592 Santa Maria della Morte sold a 1200 *lire* credit on the Monte
Residuo della Carne to acquire money 'to use in aiding the poor infirm
who in very great number flock [to the hospital] [...] in these calami-
tous times'.[41]

An increased number of poor combined with warfare and bad
weather to produce a crisis for Santa Maria della Vita in 1644. In that
year the hospital was forced to accept a donation of 6000 *lire* with an
attached annuity. The problem arose from the 'great expenditure on
the unusual number of sick people over the last two years, and [from
the] many injuries done to the possessions over the same two years by
war, snow, and frost'. In consequence the hospital was 'oppressed by
a notable quantity of debts'. The chief administrator of the hospital
sustained that it was necessary to find money 'not so much to satisfy

[the hospital's] obligations, but to maintain the credit which is most necessary for the affairs and the good governance of the hospital'.[42]

The last citation hints one effect of debt: the need to borrow from Peter to pay Paul. Sometimes debt resulted from borrowing undertaken in the maintenance of the patrimony, as when the hospice of San Biagio sold a valuable shop with a *pacto francandi* in order to have money needed to pay debts contracted during work on its properties.[43] Debt occasionally had its origin in the charitable mission of the institution. In 1622, for example, Santa Maria della Vita voted to name deputies to find money 'in any manner possible' to satisfy a 'great' debt it owed to its own *camerlengo* and to spend for the daily needs of the hospital.[44] Whatever its origin, the satisfaction of debt was a common motivation for borrowing.[45]

This fact speaks volumes about the sometimes shaky economic condition of hospitals in the sixteenth and seventeenth centuries. One finds allusion in the documentation. In 1548, for example, Santa Maria del Baraccano decided not to admit to its care any girls below the age of ten or any foreign girls. It also required each girl to pass a vote before she could be admitted. The hospital did this because, as the deliberation declares, it lacked the revenue to succour the floods of girls who come to the hospital during difficult times.[46] The same hospital, in 1567, declared itself incapable of repairing a house in Bologna 'given its poverty and great burdens'.[47] In 1588 the hospital of San Francesco decided not to spend its own money to ransom captives of the Turks 'because our hospital and company are poor and have do not have enough revenue to offer hospitality, nor [are we able] to give it to others'.[48]

Santa Maria della Vita seems to have suffered greatly at mid-century. A deliberation of 1654 refers to a situation in which 'in addition to the small and declining revenues [the hospital finds itself] burdened with many debts'. Here the great burden of past debt combined with the excessive demands of charity – in a broader context of Bolognese, and indeed European, crisis – to seriously harm the Vita's interests. The governors of the hospital – conscious of the great difficulty in which their institution found itself – reacted decisively. They named four deputies charged with reducing the expenses of the house, with leasing the institution's property more effectively, with reforming the oversight of property, and with augmenting revenue.[49]

Conclusion

The measures proposed by the governors in 1654 were worthy of the compilers of the 1601 property register. This document records a patrimony which is the product of collective generosity, a patrimony which is rigorously organized and carefully overseen by hospital administrators. Ordinarily it seems that such treasuries of civic charity were capable of providing for the poor. Although the records of the city's hospitals belie the optimism of Santa Maria della Vita's 1601 register, revealing that they were often dangerously close to crisis, one is struck by their determination to do whatever was necessary to continue serving their charges.

Notes

1   Archivio di Stato di Bologna (henceforth ASB), Archivio degli Ospedali, Arciconfraternita e Ospedale di Santa Maria della Vita, *Campioni libri amministrativi e miscellanee*, n.14, cc. 9r–12v, 1601.

2   The first section of this paper treats a process of patrimonial expansion and consolidation which I have traced in two earlier published articles – once for all urban institutions and once for the hospital of Santa Maria della Morte. The section on hospital income also includes information from these articles: M. Sneider, 'Charity and Property: The Wealth of *Opere Pie* in Early Modern Bologna', in V. Zamagni (ed.), *Povertà e innovazioni istituzionali in Italia dal Medioevo ad oggi* (Bologna, 2000), and idem, 'Il patrimonio dell'ospedale di Santa Maria della Morte in Bologna', in A. Pastore and M. Garbellotti (eds), *L'uso del denaro: patrimoni e amministrazione nei luoghi pii in Italia, secoli 15–18* (Bologna, 2001). The patrimonial history of Santa Maria della Vita has received the greatest share of historical attention. Anita Maremmi used the hos-

pital's earliest registers to trace its administrative and economic history, particularly the development of a 'patrimonial' as opposed to 'devotional' mentality in
the fourteenth century (A. Maremmi, *La confraternita di Santa Maria della Vita
nella prima metà del XIV secolo*, Tesi di Laurea, 1970–1, Università degli Studi
di Bologna). Roberto Fregna used property registers to trace the formation and
management of the hospital's urban patrimony: Fregna, 'Città e investimenti',
in *Cultura popolare dell'Emilia Romagna* (Bologna, 1979). Nicholas Terpstra
provides an overview of economic history of Bolognese institutions of charity
with a special emphasis on Santa Maria della Vita: N. Terpstra, *Lay
Confraternities and Civic Religion in Renaissance Bologna* (Cambridge, 1995),
pp.162–70.

3   I will refer to all these institutions as 'hospitals', adopting the early modern
sense of the term *ospedale*. For broad overviews of the 'system of charity'
operating in Bologna see M. Fanti, *Gli archivi delle istituzioni di carità e
assistenza attive in Bologna nel Medioevo e nell'Età moderna*, Istituto per la
storia di Bologna, 1 (Bologna, 1984), and F. Giusberti, 'Elementi del sistema
assistenziale bolognese in età moderna', in *Storia Illustrata di Bologna*
(Bologna, 1989).

4   The confraternities of Santa Maria della Vita and Santa Maria della Morte had
their origins in the tumultuous Bologna of the thirteenth and fourteenth centuries. They were founded in the wake of penitential processions – in 1260 and
in 1335 – aimed at bringing peace to a divided city. The charitable activities of
the two confraternities emerged early in their histories. The *congregatio dev-
otorum*, the society later known as Santa Maria della Vita, was given charge of
a hospital at Casalecchio in 1270 and founded its own hospital in the centre of
the city in 1289. By 1348 Santa Maria della Morte was offering care in its own
hospital. The capacity of the two hospitals grew over the course of the fifteenth
and sixteenth centuries. Santa Maria della Morte expanded its hospital in 1427,
1477, and 1561 and Santa Maria della Vita did the same in 1421, 1518, and
1569. The history of Santa Maria della Vita suggests that this physical growth
was accompanied by an increasing focus on medical care. The care of the poor
infirm was probably always the hospital's most important function, but other
classes of poor were also admitted. Additions to the hospital's statutes in the
fifteenth and sixteenth centuries precisely define the hospital's function as the
treatment of the sick; the same additions set limits on the use of the hospital by
pilgrims or the aged. The centrality of medical care was reflected in the size of
the staff: the 1553 statutes provide for a physician and a surgeon served by
three male nurses, two female nurses, and an apothecary. By the early seventeenth century Santa Maria della Vita and Santa Maria della Morte were the
largest medical hospitals in the city, central to the education of new generations
of doctors and to the care of the poor infirm. For the above see: the contributions of V. Sabena, M. Maragi, and V. Busacchi in *Sette secoli di vita ospitali-
era in Bologna* (Bologna, 1960); M. Fanti, 'Istituzioni di carità e assistenza a

Bologna alla fine del medioevo', in *Forme e soggetti dell'intervento assistenzi-ale in una città dell'Antico Regime* (Bologna, 1984), esp. pp.45–55; idem, 'La confraternita di Santa Maria della Morte', *Quaderni del centro di ricerca di studio sul movimento dei disciplinati*, 20 (1978), esp. pp.10–42, and Terpstra, *Lay Confraternities.*

5 The confraternities of Santa Maria dei Servi (San Biagio) and Santa Maria delle Laudi (San Francesco) were two of the many lay confraternities founded over the course of the fourteenth century. Their hospices offered lodging, food, and religious ritual to pilgrims of both sexes making their way through Bologna. For San Biagio and San Francesco see Terpstra, *Lay Confraternities*, p.10 and Fanti, *Gli archivi*, pp.34, 40.

6 These three hospitals represent changes in Bologna's sixteenth-century 'system of charity'. They were the fruit of an era in which prosperity was accompanied by new levels and forms of poverty. The city's ruling patricians met this challenge in innovative ways. As members of governing boards or as members of the city's government, they intervened to transform old and create new institutions. Santa Maria del Baraccano had been created in 1402 to guard a holy image along the south-eastern wall of the city and to manage its increaseingly important cult. Until the end of the second decade of the sixteenth century the company's characteristic form of charity was the lodging of pilgrims. In 1527, in the midst of a severe famine, the company shifted its attention to what would become its permanent charitable activity: the care of young female orphans. The orphanage provided lodging, food, and dowries for its charges. Santa Maria dei Guarini (San Giobbe) underwent a similar transformation in the late fifteenth century. It shifted from the lodging of pilgrims to the treatment of men and women suffering from *Mal Francese*. The creation of the Opera Pia dei Poveri Mendicanti reflected a profound shift in the way the poor were perceived across Europe in the late fifteenth and early sixteenth centuries. The breach between 'honest' and 'dishonest' forms of poverty, between 'biblical' and 'social' forms of poverty, between 'respectable' and 'shameful' forms of poverty seems to have widened. A series of reforms, instituted in many urban contexts throughout Europe, aimed at distinguishing those worthy of charity from those unworthy of charity, expelling foreign or disruptive vagabonds, rationalising the funding and distribution of charity and, most dramatically, 'enclosing' the truly poor within institutions. Bologna's political elite was not immune to this shift in mentalities. From the mid-sixteenth century an ever more elaborate series of anti-poverty measures were proposed and adopted by the government of Bologna – censuses of the poor, organized distributions of food, and expulsions of foreign beggars. In 1563 these efforts culminated in the enclosure of all able-bodied Bolognese beggars in a single hospital whose operations would be funded by contributions from other charitable and religious institutions. For Santa Maria del Baraccano see Terpstra, *Lay Confraternities*, pp.16–18, 190–6, and L. Ciammitti, 'Fanciulle, monache, madri. Povertà fem-

minile e previdenza in Bologna nei secoli XVI–XVIII', in *Arte e pietà. I patrimoni culturali delle opere pie* (Bologna, 1980). For San Giobbe see Terpstra, *Lay Confraternities*, pp.181–9. For the Opera Pia dei Poveri Mendicanti, see *ibid.*, pp.203–5 and idem, 'Apprenticeship in Social Welfare: From Confraternal Charity to Municipal Poor Relief in Early Modern Italy', *Sixteenth Century Studies*, 25 (1994), pp.101–20.

7   For the importance of testamentary charity for Florentine and Sienese charitable institutions, see J. Henderson, *Piety and Charity in Late Medieval Florence* (Oxford, 1994), and S. Cohn, *Death and Property in Siena, 1205 through 1800: Strategies for the Afterlife* (Baltimore, 1988). For donations to Santa Maria della Vita in the fourteenth century, see Maremmi, *La confraternita di Santa Maria della Vita*, pp.148–156. For donations in general, see Terpstra, *Lay Confraternities*, pp.160–2.

8   Fanti, 'Istituzioni di carità', pp.46–7.

9   For a general overview see B. Pullan, 'Povertà, carità e nuove forme di assistenza nell'Europa moderna', in D. Zardin (ed.), *La città e i poveri. Milano e le terre lombarde dal Rinascimento all'età spagnola* (Milan, 1995), pp.21–44. For the transformation of hospitals see A. Pastore, 'Strutture assistenziali fra chiesa e stato nell'Italia della Controriforma', in *Storia d'Italia, Annali 9* (Turin, 1986). For Bologna see Terpstra, *Lay Confraternities*, pp.179–205

10   This is Fregna's explanation for the expansion of Santa Maria della Vita's urban patrimony: Fregna, 'Città e investimenti', pp.282–4, 287–8. In the late fourteenth and early fifteenth centuries this hospital frequently sold land to meet pressing expenses. The situation seems to have reached a head towards the end of the first decade of the new century. The record of a sale made in 1407 eloquently describes the fiscal predicament in which the institution found itself – its possessions and rents were not producing foodstuffs in sufficient quantity for the inhabitants of the hospital. On the other hand, the same document continues, the hospital owned many *possessiones* from which it drew little profit – some were unimproved and others demanded much repair. The governors consequently resolved to alienate valueless properties in order to raise the capital necessary for the purchase of a possession from which they might have the grain necessary for the hospital. BCB, Fondo Ospedale, Ospedale di Santa Maria della Vita, n.4, c.19, 27.12. 1407. A possession – 88 *tornature* of improved land with a house in the commune of Prunaro – was in fact purchased on 30 April of the following year for a total of 1057 *lire* and 10 *soldi*. ASB, Archivio degli Ospedali, Arciconfraternita e Ospedale di Santa Maria della Vita, *Campioni libri amministrativi e miscellanee*, n. 4, cc. 27v–28v: 30.6.1408. The calculated sale of less valuable properties in order to purchase a single possession capable of providing for the alimentary needs of the hospital's poor seems to have been one aspect of a more general economic strategy in the early fifteenth century aimed at maximising patrimonial profits. Roberto Fregna notes that these same years saw the construction of a number of small bottegas along

the present-day Via Pescheria Vecchia and the beginning of a long and determined struggle on the part of the hospital's administrators to make them profitable. The construction of bottegas is described in the documentation as having been undertaken to provide for 'the necessities of the [...] poor' and it – like the purchase of property at Prunaro – seems to have been at least partially funded by the sale of property. For the construction of the *botteghe* and the subsequent struggle with the Fishmongers' Guild, see Fregna, 'Città e investimenti', pp.290–1.

11   M. Fanti, 'Istituzioni di carità e assistenza a Bologna alla fine del medioevo', p.52.

12   Fanti, 'Istituzioni di carità e assistenza a Bologna alla fine del medioevo', pp.52–3 in n. 60. ASB, Archivio degli Ospedali, Arciconfraternita e Ospedale di Santa Maria della Vita, *Campioni libri amministrativi e miscellanee*, n.4, cc. 31r-v, 8.7.1408.

13   BCB, Fondo Ospedale, Santa Maria della Vita, n.6, cap. 45, 1408.

14   *Ibid.*, cap. 63, 1408.

15   Anita Maremmi traces the first glimmerings of this 'managerial' or 'patrimonial' mentality in the mid-fourteenth century. Maremmi, *La confraternita di Santa Maria della Vita nella prima metà del XIV secolo*, p.129. R. Fregna discusses sixteenth-century regulation of sales and leases: Fregna, 'Città e investimenti', p.288.

16   The expansion and consolidation of institutional patrimonies was one part of a larger movement in Bologna and throughout the peninsula. B. Farolfi, for example, discusses the consolidation of patrician economic power in the countryside of Bologna by the early sixteenth century. In 1502 a narrow group of 82 families had come to control 65.65% of Bologna's countryside: B. Farolfi, *Strutture agrarie e crisi cittadina nel primo Cinquecento Bolognese* (Bologna, 1977). E. Stumpo discusses the expansion and consolidation of patrimonies for the great religious institutions of the peninsula in the seventeenth century: idem, 'Il consolidamento della grande proprietà ecclesiastica nell'età della Controriforma', in G. Chittolini and G. Miccoli (eds), *La Chiesa e il potere politico* (Turin, 1986).

17   M. Lecce and S. Epstein trace the tremendous importance of real estate for charitable institutions in Verona and Siena. M. Lecce, 'I beni terrieri di un antico istituto ospitaliero veronese (secc. XII–XVIII)', in *Studi in onore di Amintore Fanfani* 3 (Milan, 1962), pp.51–181, and S. Epstein, *Alle origini della fattoria Toscana: l'Ospedale della Scala di Siena e le sue terre (metà '200 – metà '400)* (Florence, 1986). Both works emphasize the meticulous planning and the long effort required to construct rural patrimonies; both works point out the importance of charitable institutions to the development of the countryside. The efforts of Santa Maria della Vita to knit together through purchase and exchange, to capitalize and develop, and to oversee large rural possessions are analogous. M. Dubini and M. Garbellotti describe the importance of real estate

112   *Matthew Thomas Sneider*

for charitable institutions in Como and in Trent. M. Dubini, 'L'ospedale gabelliere: le risorse economiche dell'Ospedale Maggiore di Como e degli istituti assistenziali dei baliaggi svizzeri', esp. p.181, and M. Garbellotti, 'Il patrimonio dei poveri: aspetti economici degli istituti assistenziali a Trento nei secoli XVII–XVIII', in Pastore and Garbellotti (eds), *L'uso del denaro* (Bologna, 2001), pp.196–206.

18   The question of whether to directly manage a rural property or lease it frequently occasioned debate in the councils of the hospital. An often employed argument in favour of renting, rather than directly working, properties, was the possibility of impelling the renter – by means of pacts carefully written into the lease – to improve the condition of a particular property at his own trouble. ASB, Archivio degli Ospedali, Arciconfraternita e Ospedale di Santa Maria della Vita, *Campioni libri amministrativi e miscellanee*, n.30, d.334, 14.5.1773. An even more interesting *relazione* argues the hospital can expect better cultivation from renters because by making improvements and working with greater attention they serve their own interest in getting greater revenue. *Ibid.*, d.327, undated.

19   See, for example, the 1558 sale by the hospital of Santa Maria della Morte of 60–70 *corbe* of *marzadelli* to take advantage of a price which is 'assai conveniente'. ASB, Archivio degli Ospedali, Ospedale di S. Maria della Morte, *Libri delle congregazioni*, n.1, 5.1.1558. See also ASB, Archivio degli Ospedali, Arciconfraternita e Ospedale di Santa Maria della Vita, *Libri delle congregazioni*, n.2, 6.12.1568.

20   M. Dubini notes the reliance of the Ospedale Sant'Anna of Como on *dazi*. Dubini, 'L'ospedale gabelliere', pp.182–91.

21   M. Carboni notes the increasing reliance of the charitable institutions of Bologna on investment in the public debt. M. Carboni, *Il debito della città: Mercato del credito fisco e società a Bologna fra Cinque e Seicento* (Bologna, 1995), pp.120–7.

22   See, for example, the exemption granted by the Cardinal Sforza Visconti to the hospital of Santa Maria della Vita from paying the *dazio* on milling 'up to three hundred pounds' of grain and from transporting 'up to fourteen pounds' of grain into the city. ASB, Archivio degli Ospedali, Arciconfraternita e Ospedale di Santa Maria della Vita, *Campioni libri amministrativi e miscellanee*, n.17, d.8, 21.11.1487. See also the 1497 exemption of granted by the government of Bologna, mindful of the 'tenuous and weak faculties and revenues' of the institution. *Ibid.*, bundle labelled '*Numero 6 Brevi e Decreti*', d.3, 27.10.1497. See also ASB, Archivio degli Ospedali, Santa Maria della Morte, *Istrumenti*, b.18, d.13, 1496. See also ASB, Fondo Demaniale, Ospedale di San Giobbe, 1, 6472, d.6, 9.11.1520.

23   See the series of indulgences rewarding those who donate to the hospital of Santa Maria della Vita and contained in ASB, Archivio degli Ospedali, Arciconfraternita e Ospedale di Santa Maria della Vita, *Campioni libri amminis-*

trativi e miscellanee, n.19, bundle marked *Indulgenze Diverse*. See especially d.15, d.16, d.17, d.24, d.25 and d.26.

24 Terpstra, *Lay Confraternities*, pp.188–9, and ASB, Senato, *Partiti*, b.2, c. 182r, 24.3.1526. For a renewal in the later sixteenth century see ASB, Archivio degli Ospedali, Ospedale di Santa Maria dei Guarini o di San Giobbe, *Miscellanea*, n.1, d.2, 20.11.1555 in which the Senate renews this payment until the year 1560.

25 Luisa Ciammitti notes that the real importance of Santa Maria del Baraccano's lending of dowry capital lay in the socio-political connections created by these loans. L. Ciammitti, 'La dote come rendita: Note sull'assistenza a Bologna nei secoli XVI–XVIII', in *Forme e soggetti dell'intervento assistenziale in una città di antico regime*, pp.124–7. Marina Garbellotti notes the same function of loans in Trent: Garbellotti, 'Il patrimonio dei poveri', pp.206–18.

26 When testators made donations they often burdened the receiving institution with the performance of posthumous religious ceremonies in perpetuity. One of the many such testaments was that of archpriest Andrea Capelli, who obliged the hospital of Santa Maria del Baraccano to celebrate a mass every week and one on every religious holiday in both its church and in an oratory to be built on one of the testator's possessions. ASB, Archivio degli Ospedali, Ospedale di Santa Maria del Baraccano, *Istrumenti*, b.57, d.29, 25.2.1633. Over the decades such testaments grew into exceptionally heavy burdens which provoked numerous petitions for relief. For these obligations see Terpstra, *Lay Confraternities*, pp.161–2.

27 The hospital spent this money on the construction of three houses, four *teggie*, two stone portals and on repairs to its subordinate hospitals at Barbarolo, Casalecchio and Salicetto. ASB, Archivio degli Ospedali, Arciconfraternita e Ospedale di Santa Maria della Vita, *Campioni libri amministrativi e miscellanee*, n.15, cc. 74v–81r.

28 *Ibid.*

29 Less important from a financial standpoint, but very important from a religious standpoint, was the charity which *opere pie* distributed to needy individuals – often members of the confraternity that governed the hospital – and institutions. Such charity was often given in response to direct solicitation by the recipient. Examples from the records of the hospital of Santa Maria della Vita include the 3 *corbe* of wheat which the hospital donated to a religious house, the 3 *scudi* which it donated to the rector of San Matteo for constructing a *baldachinum*. ASB, Archivio degli Ospedali, Arciconfraternita e Ospedale di Santa Maria della Vita, *Libri delle congregazioni*, n.2, 9.3. 1568 and 30.3.1568.

30 This figure must be used only while keeping firmly in mind the warnings about the 'common price' applied to agricultural products intended for internal consumption. This accounting practice could underestimate revenues from the land and expenditure on food. We must therefore admit the possibility that both lines should be higher. F. Landi, 'Per una storia dei falsi in bilancio: le contabilità

pubbliche dei conventi e dei luoghi pii', in Pastore and Garbellotti (eds), *L'uso del denaro*, pp.41–62.

31   For the economic difficulties of the traditional charitable institutions of Bologna in a later period see A. Giacomelli, 'Conservazione e innovazione nell'assistenza bolognese del Settecento', in *Forme e soggetti dell'intervento assistenziale in una città di antico regime*, 2 (Bologna, 1986).

32   For the Monte di Pietà see M. Fornasari, *Il Tesauro della città: Il Monte di Pietà di Bologna* (Bologna, 1993).

33   ASB, Archivio degli Ospedali, Arciconfraternita e Ospedale di Santa Maria della Vita, *Libri delle congregazioni*, n.2, 21.8.1569.

34   *Ibid.*, 31.5.1570.

35   For the purchase of an expensive property at Bagnarola see ASB, Archivio degli Ospedali, Arciconfraternita e Ospedale di Santa Maria della Vita, *Campioni libri amministrativi e miscellanee*, n.5, cc. 88v–90v, 13.6.1564. The hospital paid 1000 *scudi* towards the overall price of 5833 *lire* and 2 *soldi*. It promised to pay the remainder when it received money from a certain Giovanni Modesti. Three days later the hospital accepted a donation of 3000 *lire* from Modesti. The interest rate owed 'during his natural life' was 12 per cent. Modesti was a very frequent lender to the institution over the course of the late sixteenth century. ASB, Archivio degli Ospedali, Arciconfraternita e Ospedale di Santa Maria della Vita, *Istrumenti*, b.15, d.2, 16.6.1564. The burden of debt created by such loans was troubling to the administrators of the hospital and in 1568 they tried to control the practice. ASB, Archivio degli Ospedali, Arciconfraternita e Ospedale di Santa Maria della Vita, *Libri delle congregazioni*, n.2, 11.8.1568. See also *ibid.*, 16.10.1569.

36   ASB, Archivio degli Ospedali, Ospedale di Santa Maria del Baraccano, *Istrumenti*, b.53, d.2, 1.7.1606.

37   ASB, Archivio degli Ospedali, Arciconfraternita e Ospedale di Santa Maria della Vita, *Libri delle congregazioni*, n.5, 28.8.1648.

38   ASB, Archivio degli Ospedali, Arciconfraternita e Ospedale di S. Maria della Morte, *Libri delle congregazioni*, n.4, 23.3.1649.

39   ASB, Archivio degli Ospedali, Ospedale di S. Maria della Morte, *Miscellanea*, n.5, 1606.

40   ASB, Archivio degli Ospedali, Arciconfraternita e Ospedale di Santa Maria della Vita, *Campioni libri amministrativi e miscellanee*, n.24, d.2, 24.5.1591.

41   ASB, Archivio degli Ospedali, Ospedale di S. Maria della Morte, *Istrumenti*, n.36, d.12, 1592.

42   ASB, Archivio degli Ospedali, Ospedale di Santa Maria della Vita, *Libri delle congregazioni*, n.5, 5.12.1644.

43   ASB, Archivio degli Ospedali, Ospedale di Santa Maria dei Servi o di San Biagio, *Istrumenti*, n.10, d.43, 24.3.1575 and *ibid.*, n.11, d.7, 8.4.1580.

44   ASB, Archivio degli Ospedali, Arciconfraternita e Ospedale di Santa Maria della Vita, *Libri delle congregazioni*, n.4, 22.11.1622.

45   ASB, Archivio degli Ospedali, Ospedale di Santa Maria della Vita, *Libri delle congregazioni*, n.4, 5.1.1612; *ibid.*, n.4, 25.5.1612 (this vote was not successful); *ibid.*, n.4, 5.3.1614; *ibid.*, n.4, 16.8.1621; *ibid.*, n.5, 20.6.1652; ASB, Archivio degli Ospedali, Arciconfraternita e Ospedale di Santa Maria della Vita, *Istrumenti*, n.15, d.15, 17.6.1567. See also the 1585 decision by the governors of the hospital of San Biagio to borrow 600 *lire* to pay debts amassed in construction. ASB, Archivio degli Ospedali, Ospedale di Santa Maria dei Servi o di San Biagio, *Istrumenti*, n.11, d.11, 23.12.1585. See also the 1604 decision by the governors of San Francesco to accept a loan of 300 *lire* in order to pay a testamentary bequest for which they lacked the money. ASB, Archivio degli Ospedali, Ospedale di San Francesco, *Istrumenti*, n.13, d.53, 20.10.1604.

46   ASB, Archivio degli Ospedali, Ospedale di Santa Maria del Baraccano, n.44, d.46: 8.11.1548.

47   *Ibid.*, n.113, cc. 101r–108v, 13.7.1567.

48   ASB, Archivio degli Ospedali, Ospedale di San Francesco, *Libri delle congregazioni*, n.1, 27.11.1588.

49   ASB, Archivio degli Ospedali, Arciconfraternita e Ospedale di Santa Maria della Vita, *Libri delle congregazioni*, n.5, 4.3.1654. That the economic situation of the city around this time harmed the ability of the hospital to win revenue from its patrimony is suggested by deliberations in which hospital governors refer to difficulties in making money from urban property. In 1655 the governors of the Vita lament '[the difficulty of collecting] rent' on shops in the Contrada delle Pescarie. This difficulty may reflect an economic context which made it more difficult for tenants to pay their rents. ASB, Archivio degli Ospedali, Arciconfraternita e Ospedale di Santa Maria della Vita, *Libri delle congregazioni*, n.5, 18.1.1655.

MARINA GARBELLOTTI

Chapter 4: Assets of the Poor, Assets of the City: The Management of Hospital Resources in Verona between the Sixteenth and Eighteenth Centuries

Introduction

In 1526, J.L. Vives published what is probably his most famous work – *De subventione pauperum.*[1] This short essay is composed of forty-eight pages in octavo and outlined the measures that the city authorities should adopt to improve welfare and reduce the number of the poor. The suggestions of this Spanish humanist were addressed to the burgomasters of Bruges, the Flemish city where he was staying at the time, and they were the result of experiences in other towns, such as Ypres, Nuremberg and Strasbourg. They also stemmed from discussions with friends, including Thomas More, as well as from the influence of thinkers who had pondered over the problem of begging. Rather than suggesting innovative regulations, Vives interpreted the new policies of charity which had been implemented in many cities between the fifteenth and sixteenth centuries. These can be summarised in the basic principle according to which the authorities had to take care of people who were really in need. Therefore, the cities had to monitor the work of hospitals, check the management of charitable resources and implement repressive measures to turn away idle beggars. In particular, the many misuses found in the administration of alms, the misappropriation of funds in hospitals, the unplanned and sometimes thoughtless donation of subsidies led to reconsideration of the management and allocation of charity. Vives's solution was that all gifts, alms and legacies for the poor should be brought into one trust under the city administration and that appointed officers should then allocate them to the real poor. This trust or 'common chest' – called 'Gemeinde Kasten' in the German territories, 'cassa comune' in Italy and Aumône générale in France – was introduced especially in the reformed cities, although some examples can be found in the Catholic cities which accepted the plan to centralise and municipalise the resources for charity.[2] Some administrations, like the ones in the Protestant cities of Leisling and Wittenberg, applied this measure strictly and ordered that the common chests should also absorb the endowments of hospital institutions, thus depriving them of any administrative authority.[3] In other places, although a common chest was used to subsidise welfare, the hospitals continued to maintain and manage their patrimony.

In the Italian peninsula from the fifteenth and sixteenth centuries princes and city councils started to deal directly with welfare issues and took charitable institutions under their jurisdiction. Welfare plans were drawn up to regulate, limit and, hopefully, try to eliminate begging. However, in Italy the aim of bringing all funds for the poor into one common chest was not achieved, although some weak attempts were made to centralise and rationalise charitable resources. In fact, in some cities specific offices were set by the territorial authorities, such as the Provveditorati alla Sanità (Health Board) in Venice and the Ufficio dell'elemosina dei poveri (Office for Alms to the Poor) in Genoa, which were in charge of collecting and re-allocating the alms to the poor like the 'common chest'.[4]

But, it was impossible to unify hospital patrimonies under one single administration. The charitable institutions were independent bodies, managed by councils who ran them freely and administrated their assets. Basically, the city authorities intervened or conditioned the appointment of hospital councillors and influenced their boards, but they did not take part in the hospital council meetings nor did they discuss welfare policies or give any indications about administration. The city authorities, however, acknowledged the major social role of charitable institutions which were rewarded with measures safeguarding their economic situation. For instance, in 1528, the Venetian authorities, fearing that the outbreak of the epidemic would increase the numbers of the poor, helped to establish alms-houses and levied a tax to support them.[5] To face up to the economic disaster caused by the 1575 plague, the city of Verona decided to levy a tax in favour of the poor.[6] To support hospitals at the beginning of their activity or in the event of extraordinary calamities, the Italian cities adopted other measures, too, such as the transfer to charitable institutions of the right to collect duties;[7] and quite often they approved the transfer of part of the money penalties in favour of charitable institutions or the granting of short or long term tax relief.[8] However, these were only temporary measures, dictated by the precarious circumstances and not by a thought-out welfare programme guaranteeing a charity 'chest'.

All available research concerning the Italian states in the fifteenth and sixteenth centuries underline the active role played by the municipality in the management of hospital foundations[9] – to what extent and in what way is not always clear. The scarcity of information on this subject may depend on the fact that Italian studies of the history of welfare have been focused on the development, the internal and external activities of hospitals, and the relationships between hospital governors and management, ignoring the role of political institutions in the welfare sector. For example, an active and significant participation of the Verona Municipality can be seen in its administration of the patrimony of charitable foundations.

Welfare organisation

From 1500, the Veronese welfare system went through a considerable period of reform, shared by other Italian cities to a greater or lesser extent. In this period, welfare policy in favour of the poor and hospital networks changed. In the 1530s, the city council set up the 'Società di carità' (Society of Charity) aimed at helping the really poor.[10] To subsidise its activity, special boxes were placed in the city parishes and monasteries to collect alms and 'bulletins', i.e. papers on which the poor indicated their needs. The representatives of the Society had to check the reliability of the bulletins, make a survey of the poor and allocate alms. In those same years, the city council enforced measures of control and repression of beggars.[11] Four municipal officers had to accompany the poor people found begging to the most suitable alms-house. If a beggar refused to enter the house, was found begging again or was not eligible to be considered really poor, then he/she was sent to prison or exiled. The legislation was very straightforward and strict, but loopholes in enforcement rules left ample space for infringement.

As to the hospital network in Verona, as in other Italian cities in the fifteenth and sixteenth centuries, some small hospitals were closed, some were refurbished and new ones were built. A rational and co-ordinated welfare structure was established.[12] From 1500 the hospital of Sts Giacomo and Lazzaro[13] ended its original medieval function as a leper house and started to treat patients with scabies. In 1426, the Casa della Pietà was founded with two separate wards, one for generic patients and one for foundlings under the age of five. The hospital of Santa Casa della Misericordia, built in 1515, had a double role – assisting and bringing up Veronese orphans (in the age group of seven to twelve), and treating syphilis, TBC and incurable patients in a special ward. The Opera dei Derelitti e dei Mendicanti, set up in the second half of the 1500s, housed children and poor people who had not found a place to stay in other charitable institutions.

The reorganisation of the charitable network came especially from private initiative. In fact, citizens and confraternities, with the collaboration of the city council and the bishop's approval, founded hospitals with the aim of checking and coordinating health care and charitable activities. During this stage of reorganisation, the city council established its jurisdiction over hospitals relatively early on. First, it intervened in the appointment of governors. From 1500 the management of the hospital of Sts Giacomo and Lazzaro was en-trusted to a steering committee composed of seven counsellors appointed by the city council and chosen among the representatives of the most notable families in the city.[14] As for the Casa di Pietà, its statute ordered that the seven governors had to be elected from among the members of the city council and those of the Board of Notaries.[15]

Moreover, the city council became involved in the financial resources of hospitals. In the early modern period, the so-called patri-mony of the poor, i.e. the real estate and capital accumulated by charitable institutions thanks to gifts and legacies, was the primary financial source, if not the exclusive one, of the welfare sector. Unsurprisingly, the management of hospital patrimonies had always been the subject of special attention both from lay and Church authorities – the Council of Trent obliged the bishops to collect the 'redde rationem' from ecclesiastical institutions. This, together with the duty of visiting, was an essential aspect of ecclesiastical hospital legislation.[16]

Management of the Patrimony of the Poor

The Venetian Republic, to which Verona had been subject since 1405, granted considerable autonomy to its subject cities in the administration of the various sectors of public life, including welfare.[17] Although the Venetian government did not play a major role in the social policy of its subject cities, it drew up some directives concerning the administration of the assets of charitable institutions which strengthened the guidelines of the Veronese municipality's social policy rather than opposed them.

The directives published in 1667, which established the rules for the 'good government' of confraternities, lay schools and charitable institutions in the Veronese territory, is an excellent example of the above.[18] This booklet contains a series of norms to safeguard the patrimony of charitable institutions. The governors of pious places are urged to administer them correctly and to provide accurate accounts. Ecclesiastical representatives – parish priests, chaplains and others – were again banned from interfering in the administration of lay schools, thus confirming the markedly lay policy of the Venetian government. Of special interest, is the obligation for the administrators of charitable foundations to deposit surpluses exceeding 4 ducats in the city's pawnshop; this took place at the end of the year when the administrators calculated their income and expenses. The legislation does not specify the purpose of the deposit opened at the pawnshop, but these surpluses are likely to have been diverted into a health and 'public' care trust, following a practice since the sixteenth century. Thus although it might be an exaggeration to speak of a 'common chest', an integrated system of welfare resource management did certainly exist.[19]

In Verona, the hospital of Sts Giacomo and Lazzaro, more than any other, deposited significant sums in the pawnshop on a regular basis. According to the city chronicles, the hospital was always 'at the disposal of the city' and the two large shields with the communal coat-of-arms placed on the building in 1420s to 1430s represented the symbolical patronage of the municipality of the hospital.[20] Official support was also reflected in a policy of protectionism. On many occasions, the city municipality saved the hospital from the clergy's attempts to include it among ecclesiastical fiscal assets, but, at the same time, it used the hospital's capital freely to help finance policies measures taken during the city's emergencies and to subsidise other pious institutions.

From the beginning of the fifteenth century, the municipality took income from the hospital of Sts Giacomo and Lazzaro to give to the *Domus Pietatis*, which the hospital also provided with stocks of cereals and medicines. Other sums were provided for plague victims, to the Santa Casa di Misericordia and to poor religious institutes.[21] The hospital of Sts Giacomo and Lazzaro was a kind of charitable and communal public chest and this role was consolidated and better defined in the seventeenth century, and became subject to specific regulations by the municipality.

In the first few years of the seventeenth century, by order of the city council, the hospital's prior or manager, who was personally in charge of the administration and handling of revenues and expenses, every year had to deposit in the pawnshop part of the money coming from the management of the hospital's property.[22] The city council's regulation on the matter was very clear: all the money 'exceeding the hospital's needs' shall be deposited every year in the pawnshop'.[23] In other words, before 1662, the prior had to deposit the rents of some properties in the pawnshop but, after that date, he had to transfer the annual budget surplus to the pawnshop account.[24] The capital deposited could not be removed or utilised without the city council's approval. In an attempt to prevent corruption and embezzlement, accounts of which were recorded frequently in the chronicles of the time, the city council ruled that any operation relating to this capital had to be approved by a majority of five of its six counsellors. In the first decades of the seventeenth century, the capital accumulated in the pawnshop was divided into three separate deposits and employed by the city council to fund three specific sectors – public health, charitable institutions and the municipality. Public health was managed by the Ufficio di Sanità (health board) annexed to the hospital of Sts Giacomo and Lazzaro from the fifteenth century. The health office depended on the city, but it was funded by the hospital. In the case of an emergency created by an epidemic, like that of 1576, the establishment of sanitary cordons, the control of people, animals and goods entering the city, the doctors' pay, the distribution of medicines, food and whatever else was necessary, were financed with the capital from the hospital of Sts Giacomo and Lazzaro deposited in the pawnshop. Again, when a new lazzaretto had to be built at the beginning of the seventeenth century, the city council collected huge sums of money from this same deposit.[25]

As far as the integration of hospitals was concerned, some of the profits from Sts Giacomo and Lazzaro were employed yearly to subsidise city hospitals in financial difficulty. At the beginning of the seventeenth century, for instance, the pawnshop account of Sts Giacomo and Lazzaro amounted to 10,000 ducats which yielded an annual interest 500 ducats. Each year, the city council decided to allocate this sum to other hospitals. In 1617, some officers appointed by the city council visited the Casa di Pietà and confirmed its serious financial difficulties. Their report made the city council allocate a subsidy of 500 ducats to the Casa di Pietà,[26] which, however, was not enough to cover the Pietà's deficit. The following year, in order to pay the Pietà's debts, the city council voted, with forty-eight votes in favour and five against, to withdraw 2,000 ducats from the pawnshop account of Sts Giacomo and Lazzaro. This diminished the 10,000 ducat deposit, which the council decided to compensate by passing two measures. First, the prior of Sts Giacomo and Lazzaro had to deposit in the pawnshop the subsidies, amounting to 400 ducats, which were traditionally distributed to the poor at Easter and Christmas; otherwise he would lose his salary. Secondly, the interest from the capital of Sts Giacomo and Lazzaro deposited in the pawnshop had to be employed to make good the deficit, so that the hospital could start distributing Christmas and Easter alms again as soon as possible.[27]

The decision to grant the 500 ducats to one institution rather than to another caused discontent. When the city council decided to benefit the Casa della Pietà, another hospital, the Misericordia, which had enjoyed that contribution in the previous years, wrote a complaint to denounce the serious consequences caused by the lack of the annual subsidy. The governors of the Misericordia had been forced to stop the distribution of medicines to syphilitic patients and pleaded for help.[28] The city council was not insensitive to their requests and, considering the terrible effects which a lack of medicines would have had, granted a subsidy to the Misericordia. The money was withdrawn from one of Sts Giacomo and Lazzaro's deposits. When the Casa della Pietà, thanks to a series of measures passed by the city council, put its accounts in order, the subsidy was granted to other institutions. From 1624 to 1628, the Mendicanti was a beneficiary.[29]

The 'city' was the third sector financed by the deposits of the Sts Giacomo and Lazzaro hospital in the pawnshop, especially in exceptional circumstances. In 1693, for example, the Venetian Republic asked the city of Verona for 12,000 ducats to deal with urgent financial problems – probably due to the war waged against the Turks a few years before (1686–7). The city council withdrew the sum from the pawnshop deposit and decided to deposit four annual instalments of 3,000 ducats to build it up again.[30] This enabled the city of Verona to recover a significant sum in a short time and, above all, without paying any interest. In other Venetian cities, like Vicenza and Padua, the authorities helped themselves to the capital in the local pawnshop to solve their financial emergencies. It does not appear, however, that the owners of these deposits were hospitals.[31]

The money deposited in the pawnshop by the Sts Giacomo and Lazzaro yielded in different ways. The 10,000 ducats, whose interest was given to hospitals in need, were interest-bearing and yielded an annual interest of 5 per cent. On the other hand, the deposit for the city was, as the sources remind us, 'unprofitable', that is non-interest-bearing. It was a sort of reserve that the pawnshop took care of. These large sums were useful for the pawnshop, too, because it could grant more loans and, since it applied a 6 per cent interest rate, could increase its revenue derived from interest.[32] As for the deposit used to finance the Health Office, it is not certain whether it was interest or non-interest bearing.

Some initial comments can be made concerning the above data. The city council knew about the economic situation of hospitals and intervened whenever the situation was precarious or in an emergency. The choice of contributing to the economic resources of one hospital rather than another reflected the welfare policy followed by city authorities. In 1618, the city council decided to allocate to the Casa di Pietà the sum of 500 ducats and this testifies to its concern about the decline of the only institution for abandoned children, which was an increasingly acute social problem. Moreover, the Sts Giacomo and Lazzaro hospital enjoyed an unrivalled financial stability vis-à-vis other charitable institutions. Sometimes, the other hospitals were asked to contribute to welfare expenses. In 1539, for instance, in consideration of the significant increase in poor people, the city council met and deliberated to withdraw from the hospitals 8,000 ducats to be converted into alms.[33] However, no other institution managed to contribute so constantly and significantly to the 'common chest' as the Sts Giacomo and Lazzaro hospital. The reasons for its sound economic situation did not depend only on the considerable landed property accumulated throughout the centuries,[34] but can also be attributed to its limited charity work. The Sts Giacomo and Lazzaro hospital accepted patients with scabies and had about forty beds. It was open only seven to eight months a year. During the other months, it only distributed medicines and alms.[35] The welfare expenses were therefore more limited compared to those borne by hospitals with the same number of beds, such as the Casa della Misericordia and the Casa di Pietà. These two foundling hospitals were open all year round and as the flow of abandoned children could not be regulated, they often had to take in a number that exceeded their financial resources. For example, in the 1620s, the Pietà's welfare account was considerable as it had to look after almost 160 foundlings. At the Sts Giacomo and Lazzaro, the allocation of the extraordinary funds and alms (such as those for the Easter and Christmas festivities) could be interrupted or devoted to another sector, depending on the necessities or priorities identified by the city council.

Safeguarding the Property of the Poor

It was essential that the land and real estate of charitable institutions did not decrease and was administered profitably, if resource integration was to be effective and hospitals were to function. So, for those who, for different reasons, had the poor at heart, the safeguarding of hospital assets was a constant and primary goal.

Hospital statutes dedicated some chapters to administration, especially to that of the bursar, who was personally in charge of hospital accounts. They also stated that the council should, collectively and periodically, control the budgets drawn up by the bursar to avoid misappropriation and waste. Other parts concerned land maintenance. The governors of Sts Giacomo and Lazzaro, for instance, periodically appointed two members of the board of directors to visit the premises, the infirmaries and the hospital church, but also its properties to ascertain that they were cultivated and exploited in the best possible way.[36] However, these measures were not enough to avoid misappropriation, and the city council's attention was drawn to the risk of economic conditions getting irreparably worse. During the 1662 meeting, the city council remarked that the city aimed

> con occhi vigilantissimi non solo alla diligente curatione degl'infermi [...] ma alla conservatione insieme di quei capitali e proventi che in occorrenza di contaggio a sovegno dei miseri languenti sono destinati[37]

('with attentive eyes not only at the diligent treatment of the sick [...] but also at the preservation of capital and profits which, in the case of epidemics, are destined to the miserable and diseased'). At that time, the counsellors were concerned about the Sts Giacomo and Lazzaro hospital and the charitable sectors which depended to a various extent on this institution. So, to avoid theft and waste, any decision concerning the Sts Giacomo and Lazzaro property, including the sale of land, the signing of rent and loan agreements or any movement of money, had to be approved jointly by the city council, who also decided on the buyer's means of payment and on any type of capital investment.[38]

From the beginning of sixteenth century, similar rules were approved for the Casa di Pietà and it is also significant that the city council's decisions were added to the hospital statute, published in 1699, to underline their official status.[39] In the 1540s, following a check of the Pietà's management, city council representatives found the usual disorder: the sale of property even when cash was not really needed; the deteriorating state of the land; exchange of pieces of land to the disadvantage of the institution and in favour of the other parties, some of whom were relatives or friends of the hospital's governors;[40] loans were granted too easily, often without the approval of the institution's council; and negligence in collecting rents.[41] In 1543, to remedy this, the majority of the city council forbade the Pietà to exchange or alienate any property without its consent.[42] In 1572, referring to legislation on the renting of ecclesiastical assets,[43] it stipulated that the lease contracts signed by the Pietà could not be valid for more than three or five years depending on the area. The lease contract was generally used for infertile land and envisaged that the owner entrusted the cultivation and maintenance of the soil to a leaseholder in exchange for an annual rent, which was usually of modest value. The agreement had an average validity of twenty years and was often renewed and passed on to the heirs who came to consider themselves the owners of the land.[44] The reduction of the lease contract time aimed at preventing the leaseholder from claiming ownership of the property for himself.

Conservative ideas about how to exploit property dominated in statutory chapters and in the city council's directives. No methods to increase productivity and to obtain better financial investments were suggested, but controls and restrictions were imposed to avoid hospital assets being eaten away or dispersed until all welfare policy resources were drained. The city council's interventions can also be explained by its duty to safeguard the community, to which the poor belonged, however marginally. In fact, the property of the poor belonged to the poor only nominally. Although they were real persons, they were at the same time anonymous, with no juridical identity. The community of the poor could not directly administer the properties acquired in its name and the task of managing them was entrusted to charitable institutions, which merely administrated assets belonging to third parties. In a certain sense, the city council ensured that this task was carried out correctly.

The interest of the Venetian Republic and the ecclesiastical authorities for the assets belonging to hospitals was based on the same principle. The 'Dominante' safeguarded assets financing welfare and, in mainland cities, published edicts against anybody jeopardising their value. The detailed list of prohibitions contained in these edicts is quite surprising. It was forbidden to ruin buildings and properties, cut down trees, steal wood and products, graze animals, use water or even cross the land on foot and with carriages. The proclamation was signed by the Venetian governors in 1778, but had already been published in 1645.[45] In addition to being condemned to the traditional punishment for similar crimes and having to pay an immediate reimbursement, whoever damaged the land of the Sts Giacomo and Lazzaro hospital or took possession of it illegally, was condemned, if a man, to three lashes and sent to the galleys for three years, and if a woman or child, was whipped and exiled for ten years. Punishment was very severe. In fact, exile meant temporary exclusion from the community. Whoever acted against the property of the poor, thus damaging the whole community, was expelled from their social group.

The lack of an effective control network lessened judicial persecution and offenders were rarely denounced, arrested, tried and condemned. However, it is important to note how the lay authorities paid special attention to the property of the poor as they considered it 'a public asset'. In 1600, Verona's city council deliberated that anyone in default towards the Casa della Pietà could be compared to city debtors and, as such, undergo the same sanctions. The Pietà debtors, like those of the city and community, were to be excluded from public appointments and deprived of any honour and public benefit until they had settled their debts.[46] The same punishment was reserved to the Casa della Pietà administrators who had not submitted the hospital accounts when due. In 1717, according to the same principle, the city council established that every three months, the revenue collectors of the Sts Giacomo and Lazzaro hospital should publish the names of debtors.[47] Before their possessions were seized, the first punishment was to make public the names of those who acted against the assets of the poor. They lost their reputation and were subject to immediate 'public condemnation'.

Conclusion

Considering the many interventions of the city council to safeguard and to prevent dispersal of hospital funds and resources, welfare measures were very few. If periods of calamity are excluded, the city council rarely issued any directives on the matter, such as checking the professionalism of house physicians, ensuring there were enough of them to satisfy the patients' needs, and obliging the hospital governors to privilege the treatment of a specific category of patients. In the early modern period, although hospitals had medical staff and were 'specialised' in treating specific diseases, in the mind of city authorities they were considered part of the framework of public order, acting as 'receptacles' for the poor and diseased, who would otherwise have crowded the streets, threatened law and order and spread diseases. For this reason, during their rare inspections of hospitals, municipal officers pointed out administrative irregularities and also the ineffective measures which compromised the functioning of charitable institutions. In 1617, during the visit to the Casa della Pietà, the representatives of the city council complained that the hospital housed poor elderly patients and boarders, women who were not ill and who paid a regular fee to contribute to their stay. These two categories were not included in the statutory rules, since the old people should have gone to the 'Mendicanti' and the women to the 'Franceschine' institute. Their stay in hospital took away resources from foundlings and generic patients for whom the hospital had been founded. The surveillance of the city council focused primarily on the property of the hospitals under its protection and management. These measures limited the autonomy of institutions with their own board of directors, but, at the same time, this system of monitoring and earmarking hospital financial resources in excess made it possible to centralise resources for welfare, create a kind of 'common chest', optimise resources and reduce the risks of misuse and dispersion. The city council played a monitoring and coordinating role. In fact, it controlled the hospitals' financial situation and allocated the sums for charity according to contingent priorities.

Notes

1   J.L.Vives, *De subventione pauperum*, ed. A. Saitta (Florence, 1973); see the Introduction for a discussion of the political and cultural context.

2   For a thorough analysis of the subject matter see: J.E. Olson, *Calvin and Social Welfare: Deacons and the 'Bourse française'* (London and Toronto, 1989); C.H. Parker, *The Reformation of Community: Social Welfare and Calvinist Charity in Holland 1572–1620* (Cambridge, 1998); T.G. Fehler, *Poor Relief and Protestantism: The Evolution of Social Welfare in Sixteenth-Century Emden* (Aldershot, 1999).

3   B. Geremek, *La pietà e la forca: Storia della miseria e della carità in Europa* (Rome and Bari, 1995), pp. 190–1.

4   B. Pullan, 'Povertà, carità e nuove forme di assistenza nell'Europa moderna (XV–XVII centuries)', in D. Zardin (ed.), *La città e i poveri: Milano e le terre lombarde dal Rinascimento all'età spagnola* (Milan, 1995), pp.26–7. The author describes the welfare reforms which took place at the beginning of the early modern period and compares and discusses two historiographic traditions which he defines as northern European and southern European (especially Italy), p.24.

5   Geremek, *La pietà*, pp.138–9.

6   L. Vecchiato, 'La vita politica economica e amministrativa a Verona durante la dominazione veneziana (1405–1797)', in *Verona e il suo territorio*, Istituto per gli studi storici veronesi (Verona, 1995), 5, p.179. Other taxes for the poor were levied in 1586, 1587, 1591, 1594, 1597 and 1601.

7   In 1460, the Florentine government promoted the recent foundation of the Innocenti hospital and gave it the right to collect a duty: L. Sandri, 'La gestione dell' assistenza a Firenze nel XV secolo', in *La Toscana al tempo di Lorenzo il Magnifico: Politica, economia, cultura, arte* (Pisa, 1996), p.1378. Generally, these grants were time-limited, but sometimes hospitals – and this is the case of the St Anna hospital in Como – became the owners of the duties which they had originally obtained as temporary privileges; see M. Dubini, 'L'ospedale gabelliere: Le risorse economiche dell'Ospedale Maggiore di Como e degli istituti assistenziali dei baliaggi svizzeri (secoli XVI–XVIII)', in A. Pastore and M. Garbellotti (eds), *L'uso del denaro: Patrimoni e amministrazione nei luoghi pii e negli enti ecclesiastici in Italia (secoli XV–XVIII)* (Bologna, 2001), pp.179–94.

8   On tax exemptions and the conflicts that these privileges might cause with other taxable persons, see the case of Padua studied by I. Pastori Bassetto, 'Fiscalità e opere pie a Padova nei secoli XVI–XVIII', in Pastore and Garbellotti (eds), *L'uso del denaro*, pp. 63–88. The Venetian Senate intervened in many ways to favour the social function of the Pietà foundling home and, among the privileges granted in 1530, it assigned the institute the right to receive a commission from the penalties: C. Grandi, 'L'assistenza all'infanzia abbandonata veneziana: i "fantolini della pietade" (1346–1548)', in A. Grieco and L. Sandri (eds), *Ospedali e città: L'Italia del centro-nord, XIII-XVI secolo* (Florence, 1997), p.104.

9   For a historical and historiographical description of the Italian welfare history, see A. Pastore, 'Strutture assistenziali nell'Italia della Controriforma', in G. Chittolini and G. Miccoli (eds), *La Chiesa e il potere politico*, Storia d'Italia: Annali, 9 (Turin, 1986), pp. 435–62; G. Albini, *Città e ospedali nella Lombardia medievale* (Bologna, 1993); B. Pullan, *La politica sociale della Repubblica di Venezia 1500–1620*, 2 vols (Rome, 1982); G. Politi and M. Rosa, F. Della Peruta (eds), *Timore e carità: i poveri nell'Italia moderna* (Cremona, 1982); Grieco and Sandri (eds), *Ospedali e città*; V. Zamagni (ed.), *Povertà e innovazioni in Italia: dal Medioevo ad oggi* (Bologna, 2000).

10   P. Lanaro Sartori, 'Radiografia della soglia di povertà in una città della terraferma veneta: Verona alla metà del XVI secolo', *Studi veneziani*, n.s., 6 (1982), pp. 46–7, n.5.

11   Archivio di Stato di Verona (hereinafter ASVr), *Ospedale Santi Giacomo e Lazzaro*, n.11, fol.19v.

12   See A. Pastore et al. (eds), *L'Ospedale e la città: Cinquecento anni di arte a Verona* (Verona, 1996). For the 'political' relationship between hospitals and municipalities on the Venetian mainland and the evolution of the hospital system in these cities, see G.M. Varanini, 'Per la storia delle istituzioni ospedaliere nelle città della Teraferma veneta nel Quattrocento', in Grieco and Sandri (eds), *Ospedali e città*, pp. 107–55.

13   The hospital had two main buildings with two functions. Its administrative centre was located inside the city walls and housed the archives and the Health Office which was linked to the city council and funded with the revenue of the Institute of Sts Giacomo and Lazzaro. The welfare centre was outside the city walls, in the Tomba district, and from the sixteenth century it treated leper and scabies victims: M. Repetto Contaldo, 'La chiesa e le chiese dell'ospedale dei Santi Giacomo e Lazzaro "pro honore divino et dignitate civitatis": arredi interni e decorazioni pittoriche dal Cinque al Settecento', in Pastore et al. (eds), *L'Ospedale e la città*, p.149.

14   S. Faccini, 'L'ospedale dei Santi Giacomo e Lazzaro alla Tomba in età moderna', in Pastore et al. (eds), *L'Ospedale e la città*, p.64.

15   ASVr, *Istituto Esposti* (hereinafter *IE*), *Capitula, et ordines Domus Sanctae Pietatis Veronae* (hereinafter *Capitula*), n.60, fols 3–4 (1699).

16   The Council of Trent gave the bishop the right to visit hospitals (sess. XXII, c. 8 *de ref.*) and the administrative *potestas* (sess. XXII, c. 9 *de ref.*), i.e. the obligation for the governors of charitable institutions to report annually on their administration: A. Turchini, 'I "loca pia" degli antichi stati italiani fra società civile e poteri ecclesiastici', and M. Garbellotti, 'Visite pastorali e pia loca tra legislazione e prassi: il caso di Trento', both in C. Nubola and A. Turchini (eds), *Fonti ecclesiastiche per la storia sociale e religiosa d'Europa: XV-XVIII secolo* (Bologna, 1999), pp.369–409 and 411–40.

17   The direct representative of the Venetian domination *in loco* was the captain of the city who, together with the Podestà represented the executive branch of the Venetian authority. For the role of the Venetian governors, see G. Benzoni, 'Tra centro e periferia: il caso veneziano', in *Studi veneti offerti a Gaetano Cozzi* (Vicenza, 1992), pp. 97–108.

18   ASVr, *Antico Archivio del Comune, Registri*, n.803, *Ordini et provisioni dell'illustrissimo et eccellentissimo signor Francesco Contarini capitanio di Verona, per il buon governo, administrationi et essattioni delle confraternità, scuole laicali et altri luoghi pii del territorio di Verona. Confermati dall'eccellentissimo senato con ducali 11 maggio 1667* (Verona: Giovanni Battista Merlo Stampatore Camerale, undated).

19   G.M. Varanini, 'La carità del municipio: gli ospedali veronesi nel Quattrocento e primo Cinquecento', in Pastore et al. (eds), *L'Ospedale e la città*, p.26.

20   ASVr, *Ospedale Santi Giacomo e Lazzaro*, n.1, *Breve discorso di Antonio Vidali I. C. del dominio et governo che ha la città di Verona sopra l'hospitale de Santi Giacomo [...]* (hereinafter *Breve discorso*), fol. 4: 'questo hospitale è sempre stato da principi dominanti di tempo in tempo confermato nel dominio de suoi beni, privilegiato d'essenzioni, liberato totalmente dalla giurisdittion ecclesiastica et lasciato in libera disposition della magnifica città' ('this hospital has always been confirmed, from time to time, in the owners of its assets by the ruling princes, privileged with exemptions, completely free of the ecclesiastical jurisdiction and at the disposal of the magnificent city').

21   Varanini, 'La carità del municipio', pp. 26–7.

22   ASVr, *Ospedale Santi Giacomo e Lazzaro*, n.11, f.ol. 20.

23   From the report drawn up in 1629 by the Podestà Lorenzo Suriano, it appears that the pawnshop's revenue constantly subsidized the welfare sector. At the end of the year, the pawnshop's administrators had to deduct from the revenue the costs for renting the office and for employees' salaries. The remaining sum was to be distributed to the other pious places of the city, *Relazioni dei rettori veneti in Terraferma*, vol. 9: *Podestaria e capitanato di Verona* (Milan, 1977), p.301 (report of the Podestà Lorenzo Suriano, 7 December 1629). I have not found any traces of these accounts in the documents I consulted.

24   ASVr, *Ospedale Santi Giacomo e Lazzaro*, n.11, fols 20v, 22r.

25   Faccini, 'L'ospedale dei Santi Giacomo e Lazzaro', p.63.

26   ASVr, *Antico Archivio del Comune, Registri*, n.676, fol. 66r. The city council's initial solution envisaged the levy of a temporary tax to be collected on the assessment, but this proposal was rejected with a large majority (23 votes for and 39 against). The city council did not intend this to be a burden on the city's taxpayers and preferred getting the money from the funds which had already been allocated for welfare.

27   ASVr, *Antico Archivio del Comune, Registri*, n.676, fols 68–9.

28   ASVr, *Santa Casa della Misericordia*, n.35, n.n.

29   ASVr, *Ospedale Santi Giacomo e Lazzaro*, n.1, *Breve discorso*, fol. 7r.

30   ASVr, *Ospedale Santi Giacomo e Lazzaro*, n.11, fol. 24. The city council had to obtain the 3,000 ducats by levying a tax on tax-free and taxable people as well as from privileged and unprivileged people.

31   For this and other aspects relating to the activity of the Venetian pawnshops, see P. Lanaro Sartori, 'L'attività di prestito dei monti di pietà in terraferma veneta: legalità e illeciti tra Quattrocento e primo Seicento', *Studi storici Luigi Simeoni*, 33 (1983), pp.172–3.

32   *Relazioni dei rettori veneti in Terraferma*, 9, p.295 (report of the Podestà Leonardo Donato, 6 July 1628). The Veronese pawnshop was founded in 1490 and was then divided into two institutes called 'monte piccolo' (small pawnshop) and 'monte grande' (big pawnshop). The 'small' pawnshop had its own capital, made up of gifts and legacies; it also granted free loans for pledges of small value (less than 4 'mocenighi'). The capital of the 'big' pawnshop was made up of deposits.

33   ASVr, *Antico Archivio del Comune*, Processi, b. 11/2513, c. 1.

34   For the creation and evolution of the land holdings of the Institute of SS. Giacomo and Lazzaro see: M. Lecce, *I beni terrieri di un antico istituto ospitaliero veronese (secoli XII–XVIII)* (Milan, 1962).

35   Faccini, 'L'ospedale dei Santi Giacomo e Lazzaro', p.66.

36   ASVr, *Ospedale Santi Giacomo e Lazzaro*, n.32, fols 112r, 117r.

37   ASVr, *Ospedale Santi Giacomo e Lazzaro*, n.11, fol. 21r

38   In 1717, the city council approved the sale of one of the hospital's properties to
      Francesco Campagna at the price of 5,000 ducats. It also established that
      Campagna should deposit 4,000 ducats in the pawnshop, interest-free and with-
      in 4 months – in the case of delay, a 4 per cent interest rate should be applied,
      and he could deposit the remaining 1,000 ducats when to wanted to, but with a
      4 per cent interest rate, ASVr, *Ospedale Santi Giacomo e Lazzaro*, n.40,
      Terminazioni (1707–18), fol. 180.

39   A copy of the Casa di Pietà statutes, published in 1699, includes both the 1444
      statutory version with 1546 vernacular additions and the city council
      resolutions.

40   P. Lanaro Sartori, 'Carità e assistenza, paura e segregazione: Le istituzioni
      ospedaliere veronesi nel Cinque e Seicento verso la specializzazione', in
      Pastore et al. (eds), *L'Ospedale e la città*, p.50.

41   ASVr, *IE*, *Capitula*, n.60, fols 22–3.

42   The Casa di Pietà counsellors had to vote it jointly to alienate or lease a
      property, submit a request to the city council, wait for the approval of the city
      council and of the prior of the board of notaries with two thirds of votes. As
      from the city council's decision in 1589, this complicated procedure was
      applied only to properties whose extension exceeded three fields, ASVr, *IE*,
      Capitula, n.60, fols 24–5.

43   ASVr, *IE*, *Capitula*, n.60, fol. 24

44   Lecce, *I beni terrieri*, p.77.

45   ASVr, *Ospedale Santi Giacomo e Lazzaro*, n.16, fol. 8r.

46   ASVr, *Antico Archivio del Comune, Registri*, n.676, fols 50–1.

47   ASVr, *Ospedale Santi Giacomo e Lazzaro*, n.40, *Terminazioni* (1707–18), fol.
      181. The practice of making public the names of those who had damaged the
      property of the poor can be found in other places, too. In Venice during the
      1528 epidemic, the parish priest read out the names of those who had delayed
      the payment of a tax for the poor, Geremek, *La pietà e la forca*, p.139.

ANDREA TANNER

Chapter 5: Too Many Mothers? Female Roles in a Metropolitan Victorian Children's Hospital

Introduction

Victorian voluntary children's hospitals were, by and large, male creations.[1] The first children's hospital in Britain, The Hospital for Sick Children, Great Ormond Street (HSC) has been portrayed as the fulfilment of the dream and vision of one man, Dr Charles West, inspired by his experiences of sick children's hospitals in Europe. By contrast, the Evelina Hospital in Southwark was the monument of Baron Rothschild to his dead wife.[2] Children's hospitals in Manchester, Edinburgh, Southampton and Bristol can also be attributed to the efforts of a single guiding male medical ambition.[3] Once established, the management of these specialised institutions was largely in masculine hands, as was the clinical care of the patients, and the all-important fundraising.[4] Given the overarching emphasis of the time on the centrality of women in childcare, it seems a little curious, to say the least, that women did not play a more obvious part in the setting up and management of these relatively small establishments. This paper explores the opportunities for women's involvement in the running of children's hospitals before 1900, and argues that the part female hospital supporters were allowed to take was firmly rooted in the central maternal role considered best suited to their sex by the patriarchal tenets of the time. This is also true for the hospital nurses, whose most valued personal trait was neither proficiency nor intelligence, but kindness to their patients. Ironically, the women who were denied a maternal role in the care of the child in hospital were the mothers of the patients themselves. It is the tension between these three groups of women, as played out at HSC, that will be explored here.

The Hospital opened its doors on St. Valentine's Day, 1852 at 49 Great Ormond Street, a mansion that had once belonged to Dr Richard Mead, physician to Queen Anne. At that time it had only ten beds, and its medical establishment consisted of two part-time physicians, Charles West, and the well-connected Dr William Jenner, and one surgeon, G.D. Pollock. A female matron was in charge of the complement of three nurses and the domestic staff. One of the avowed aims of the new institution was to educate working-class mothers in childcare by raising the standards of expectation of care in the child patient. If the hospital recreated a comfortable middle-class home in the hospital ward, then the patients would take home with them the values – material, moral and spiritual – of the middle-class. This philosophy of behavioural education was found in other children's hospitals; Miss Alice Cross, lady superintendent at the Evelina Hospital in Southwark from 1879 to 1901 reinforced the cultural imperialism implicit in the regime of her institution:[5]

> [T]he thing that struck me most was the apparent neglect of the wretched children, sometimes the women with frousy shawls huddling something to their tattered bosoms. Occasionally, but very rarely, I heard a merry cry or an honest burst of laughter, but for the most part the children of these Southwark streets, swarming in every direction, dirty, tangled, ragged, bandy and rickety, were left to themselves to get under the horses' heels or to play in the gutter, to catch and spread their infant diseases as fate ordered it and to look upon a warm and comfortable nursery as a destiny as improbable as the arrival of some beneficent creature scattering largesse of sugar plums in the kennel of Southwark Bridge Road. It was like coming from darkness to light, to change from all this wretchedness, to the airy, well lighted and comfortable nurseries of the Evelina Hospital.

At the HSC, the children and their mothers were to be educated by the examples of the nursing staff, who, in their turn, had learnt the catechism of cleanliness and godliness from the female volunteers who interested themselves in the new institution. The arena for social change was the hospital ward, a neutral space compared to the homes of the poor familiar to the women volunteers of domestic visiting societies. The interface between the 'do-gooders' and the poor mothers was facilitated by the medical function of the building, and by the presence and actions of an intermediate tier of women – the lady superintendent and the nurses – that might make the educative process more palatable to all.[6]

The Lady Visitors

The HSC, from the very beginning, encouraged middle and upper-class women to support the hospital.[7] There were no British women medical doctors at that time, and women were not allowed to sit on the board of management, but the following plea, written by the HSC's Honorary Secretary, H.A. Bathurst, in February 1859, reveals what was expected from the female supporters:[8]

> The kindly feelings of every Lady must be with the children of the poor in infancy and sickness, whilst the interests of the rich must ever be associated with the advancement of Medical knowledge, in respect of children's diseases, and with the growth of a class of highly qualified nurses […] If children, in poverty and sickness, find not friends in the Ladies of England, whence can help be expected for those who most require it.

The ladies of England were indeed kindly disposed towards the fledgling institution, but they wanted more of a say in the management of this most homely of hospitals. All suggestions that women supporters join the management committee were rebuffed by the laymen who dominated the board of management, and the male medical staff. The ladies' committee that was eventually set up in 1860, to co-ordinate female voluntary effort and liaise with the nursing staff, lasted only three years. This was in stark contrast to other children's hospitals, which relied on women's committees to manage nursing matters and almoner functions.[9] The subordinate role of educated women at HSC, as opposed to other children's hospitals, was noted by at least one female journalist,[10]

> Surely if woman's quick and ready sympathy, woman's tenderness of heart and
> hand and voice, woman's ingenuity in soothing pain and devising a thousand
> ways and means of adding inexpensively to comfort, order and regularity, be
> anything more than a poet's dream or a lover's fancy, here. Of all places in the
> world, is her ministering presence needed, here, in virtue of the maternal quali-
> ties of her nature, should she surely be found. And we cannot help thinking that
> the benevolent men who form the management committee would find their
> hands strengthened, their hearts comforted, and the funds of the hospital en-
> larged, by admitting women side by side with them as fellow-labourers in the
> same field of love and charity, which has for its harvest here the succour of
> those of whom Christ says, 'Of such are the kingdom of Heaven'.

The principal role of women supporters of HSC was in day-to-day
fund-raising. They were barred from attending the grand annual dinner
as full guests (it was strictly a men-only affair), but were allowed in to
sit in the gallery to listen to the speeches.[11] While this jamboree was
the principal fund-raising event for most of the nineteenth century, it
was women who organised the year-round bazaars, collections and tea
parties in support of specific cots, or for the general running of the
hospital.[12] They sent in the cast-off clothes, toys and books of their
own children, and made Garibaldi jackets, nightshirts and bed-jackets
for the patients. In addition to raising subscriptions towards the hospital, they were encouraged to make visiting the wards part of the
social round of London ladies' society. The advantages were clear.
Apart from offering a new place to visit on long out-of-season
afternoons, going along to the HSC gave middle-class women of little
status the opportunity to rub shoulders with women of much greater
social standing.[13] The patron of the hospital, Queen Victoria, and her
daughters were regular visitors, and often sent in consignments of fruit
and items of clothing sewn by the female members of the royal household.[14] On one occasion, the Queen sent hundreds of toys, ordered
from a toy factory that she had visited while on holiday in Germany.[15]
Victoria's gifts were not only a publicity dream, but her example
encouraged her lesser subjects to give to the institution.

The royal visits tended to occur in isolation, but the socially-
conscious lady visitor might hope to encounter women of high status
on open afternoons. These occurred every day, except Sunday afternoon, between two and five.[16] Titled ladies feature prominently, com-

pared to men and women professionally linked to hospital management or to medicine. In addition to the Great and the Good, the visitors' books record attendances at the hospital by the wives of prominent politicians, by journalists (male and female), foreign diplomats (including a delegation from Siam), industrialists and the families of such 'Men of Letters' as Charles Dickens, William Thackeray and Thomas Carlyle.

Visitors were encouraged to write their impressions of the HSC in the visitors' book. The comments are generally restricted to 'much pleased, very much pleased, and highly gratified', but, occasionally, a longer entry reveals the attitude of the visitors to the patients and the staff. Those ladies at the higher end of the social scale tended to comment on the apparent happiness and contentment of the children, but their more humble sisters were a little more exacting in their requirements. They looked in the linen cupboards, ran their hands along surfaces looking for dust, and scrutinised the dress and attitude of the nurses. Miss Arnott of Chatham was typical in the great interest she took in the running of the hospital:[17]

> Went over the Establishment, and finding the rooms clean and the children as comfortable as they could well be, I think the arrangements of the House and the control of the nurses do a great credit to the matron and the superintendent of the nurses.

The nurses were not seen as the social equals of the visitors, and their cleanliness, attitude and competence were viewed critically by the ladies who came into the wards. One reason for this scrutiny was that the ladies were looking at the nurses as potential employees, as the training at HSC was viewed as an excellent grounding for privately-employed children's nurses.[18] In order to make money, the hospital hired out their nursing staff to care for the children of wealthier families. These children were ineligible for treatment at Great Ormond Street, but, for a weekly fee, the HSC nursing staff could be hired to look after the sick offspring of the middle-class hospital supporters.[19] A close inspection of a nurse's skills, personal hygiene and demeanour would hold a mother in readiness for the application to the HSC for paid help.

The disruption caused to ward routines by visitors was often resented by the nurses. A book of cartoons by Ada Bois, a late nineteenth-century nurse, illustrates this.[20] In one double cartoon, the HSC secretary, Adrian Hope, is drawn showing society ladies round the hospital, with nurses acting as maids carrying the tea and cakes round.[21] The legend reads, 'We greatly enjoy waiting on the distinguished visitors and Adrian Hope, and found the novelty of directing them delightful'. There is some suggestion in the book that the ladies were ultra careful in not letting their skirts touch the hospital floors. The author gives her feelings about this full rein:

> 'Mind the germs, mind the germs!
> They stick for quite a week!'
> If it's the germs on our floors they mean?
> We think it's beastly cheek.

The attention lavished on the visitors by the management of the hospital was another cause for resentment. The managers' smiles were rationed to the visitors, and management thought nothing of bringing them unannounced into the nurses' quarters, but the hospital management clearly felt that it was worthwhile upsetting the nurses for the sake of the benefits that the ladies brought. Lady visitors tended to become subscribers (or, as they were termed, governors) of the HSC, or to persuade their husbands to become such. To be a governor of the Hospital was not to sit on any board of committee, but to have certain privileges of recommending patients to the institution. They brought other ladies to visit, who, in turn, became subscribers. They and their children made clothes for the patients, they passed on used bed-linen, clothing and toys to the HSC, and, if sufficiently moved by the plight of the patients, they visited on specific days and read to them, played with them, fed them, and taught them their lessons. This *ad hoc* education was resolutely Christian in character and content. Much of the reading and teaching matter was supplied by the Religious Tract Society and similar organisations, and many of the afternoon visitors quizzed the children on their knowledge of the scriptures.[22]

One such visitor was Mrs Margaret Gatty, a vicar's wife from Sheffield, children's author, and editor of a children's newspaper called *Aunt Judy's Magazine*. Mrs Gatty wrote about the patients in her publication, and launched an appeal among her readership to sponsor a cot in perpetuity. The venture was so successful that two cots were sponsored, and the stories of the occupants of these cots provided much editorial copy in the years to come. The Gatty family were regular visitors to the HSC, always checking on the current occupants of 'their' cots.[23]

One visitor who became a subscriber, and is fairly typical of the lady supporters, was Mrs Lee of Grove Hall in Yorkshire, who endowed a cot, named 'the Alice Cot' in memory of her dead daughter. She asked permission to recommend patients to occupy the cot from time to time, and to be sent the details of the children who were placed in it. The grieving mother also asked that she might send these specific patients clothes, toys and books.[24] The loss of her daughter was the catalyst for this mother to support sick poor children, and the personal connection enabled her to have news about each of the occupants of her cot, and to maintain a long-distance relationship with these patients.

The financial benefits of the lady visitors were not underestimated by the matrons of the main hospital and the convalescent home. The lady superintendent at Cromwell House (the convalescent home in Highgate opened in 1868) complained about the consequences to the HSC's reputation by lack of consideration shown by the doctors:[25]

> It is most perplexing to arrange our hours when some of the Medical Officers come in the morning and some in the afternoon [...] For the Visitors and the Ladies who come to read to and amuse the children the inconvenience is obvious to all who know how much benefit is done to the Hospital by Visitors being able to see the children pleasantly, and talk to them, thus exciting very frequently great sympathy in our work – & you yourself know the results of this sympathy. The visitors are told that they may come in the afternoon after 2 o'clock, but I am sorry to say that owing to the presence of the MOs, we are frequently obliged to hurry the visitors through the wards, or perhaps not let them in except for a moment, or pain them with the cries of children who have just been examined.

The Lady Volunteers and Lady Nurses

From the ranks of the lady visitors grew a committed band of women who regularly gave of their time and service. In addition to the mother-substitutes and fairy-godmothers who read and played with the children, a group of ladies supervised the nurses, acting, in effect, as ward sisters. In the 1850s and 1860s they had no formal nurse training, but their experience in running their own households was deemed qualification enough. They were not answerable to the male medical establishment, but were under the direct control of the lady superintendent, who was herself, for most of the nineteenth century, a volunteer of the same social standing as the members of the management committee.[26] At the annual fundraising dinner, the hospital consultant surgeon, Thomas Smith, paid homage to these ladies:[27]

> [T]here are those ladies who give up their time so unselfishly to the management of the wards. The public scarcely know what those ladies do. They administer prescriptions and carry out the behests of the medical officers, and by their care, which is not medical, but rather maternal, and by the gentle and tender love which they exhibit to their patients, I believe they can deprive the physician's prescriptions of more than half their nauseousness, and I am quite sure than half deprive the surgeon of his terrors. We, as medical officers, know the great power for good which those ladies exercise in the hospital; and that benefit is not only extended to the patients, but to the subordinates, the nurses of the hospital, who work under those ladies. These worthy young women, who are perhaps of less gentle birth and breeding than their superiors, owing to the force of excellent example, are no less gentlewomen in the best sense of the word than the ladies above them.

The implicit function of the lady volunteers was to render the kindness of the ideal middle-class mother to the patients, and to knock off the rough edges of the paid nurses, thereby making them more fitted for their role within the hospital, and as ambassadors for the HSC.[28] However, this was not enough for some of these pillars of the hospital community. By the mid-1860s, perhaps inspired by the success of the general nursing graduates of the Nightingale School of Nursing, several of them were agitating for a greater say in the running of the hospital, in spite of the fact that they were independent of the all-male medical committee. To these women, a gentle reminder of their place in the grand scheme of things was administered by a speaker at the hospital's annual fund-raising dinner:[29]

> [The lady volunteers] are doing a work, both external and internal in the hospital, which we could not afford to dispense with. They assert a voluntary position; they assert woman's rights in the most emphatic way. I hold that it is a woman's right to be kind to man, and above all to her little ones; and I am sure that it is the right that they would most earnestly vindicate for themselves. We all of us feel that women occupy a position sacred to humanity – a position on which we need not expatiate in complimentary terms, because all our hearts are ready to acknowledge it.

The message could not be more clear. HSC needed their labours, but the male establishment did not want them to occupy any official management role within the institution. In its nursing management structure, however, HSC was unusual; as most of the other children's hospitals established after 1852 had ladies' committees with serious responsibilities. They inspected the wards, supervised the matron and had control over the hiring, firing and disciplining of the nursing staff.[30] The matrons and lady superintendents of the children's hospitals in Edinburgh and Liverpool operated under their supervision until the 1890s, by which time matrons tended to be trained nurses, and began to demand autonomy from the ladies' committees, and access to the boards of management.[31] As has been mentioned, HSC had a ladies' committee (with very limited responsibilities) for only three years (1860–3), after which date the lady superintendent took overall charge of nursing matters and the domestic economy of the hospital.[32]

In 1879, the Bishop of Winchester gave the chairman's speech at the annual dinner, and dwelt on the debt that the HSC owed their volunteers. He emphasised the disinterestedness of the ladies' motives, for, where no payment was extracted, no accusation of greed could be made.[33] Given the paucity of the paid nurses' wages, this compliment seems like an insult to them, but it does beg the question: what was the motivation of these women?

Working with the children might be seen as domestic visiting without the dangers of encountering the poor in their own homes, with their accompanying distressing sights and smells. There was no opportunity for interaction between the visitors and the parents, preventing requests for money, but also giving no arena for any sophisticated exploration of the reality of urban poverty in Victorian London. The mothers were rarely present at the same time as the lady volunteers, thus giving the latter free rein to educate the children in middle-class manners and mores away from the doubtful influence of the parents. In the words of Seth Koven, this voluntary labour, untainted by commercialism, had a powerful sub-text:[34]

> It channelled middle-class women's activism into a traditionally female area of expertise, while providing mechanisms by which middle-class women could impose their domestic ideals on working-class women and children [...] 'Lady' social welfare workers invariably represented the exercise of their authority as demonstrations of their motherly love for impoverished children and their sisterly solicitude for unfortunate or feckless working-class women.

The work provided an opportunity to 'be mother' to middle-class women whose children were grown up, or who had lost their children, or to those who, husbandless, were unlikely ever to experience motherhood first hand.[35] The hospital provided a safe and socially acceptable environment for occupying their time, and offered the opportunity to meet women of their own class, and those of higher social standing. It gave respectability, and a certain seriousness of purpose, to educated women, for whom getting a paid job was out of the question, and for whom social delicacies banned them from fulfilling similar functions in adult hospitals.[36] The work could also be seen as educational, in that the example of the ladies would provide templates of domestic hygiene and childcare to nurses and mothers, and would (it was hoped) create a demand for higher standards of mothering in the children.

The Nurses

Until the Great War, all doctors at HSC were male (although an American physician, Dr Emily Morgan, was allowed to observe hospital practice in the 1890s), and until the last quarter of the twentieth century, all nurses were female. In the hospital family, the doctors were the patriarchs, and the nurses were their handmaidens. The lady superintendent, perhaps like a mother-in-law, wielded power over the running of the hospital with little responsibility to the medical officers, but she was a distant figure to the patients. It was the ward nurses who fitted the requirement of one medic, who described the nurse as not only his right hand, but his alter ego.[37]

Like the working father, the doctors were seen by the children at a specific hour of the day, and for a limited time. Like the Victorian mother, the nurses (who worked in a specific ward and rarely moved from it) were on call and dedicated to the twenty-four hour care of the patients. Nursing in a children's hospital was different to that undertaken in an adult institution. Many patients were too young to articulate their symptoms or to ask for help when they needed it. There were no adults in the next bed to call out for the nurse, or to provide informal nursing care. The doctors themselves were learning much about childhood conditions, and were not always able to make swift diagnoses.[38] It was up to the nurse in the children's wards to keep her charges under constant scrutiny and to interpret their needs accordingly. She it was who reported on progress to both the medical officers and the parents. The nurses were the lynchpins of the whole organisation:[39]

> Reliance on nurses allowed hospitals to develop, families to trust the care of their members to people other than family, physicians to admit patients for medical interventions and surgeons to perform extensive operations, and all of them to go home at night, comfortable in the knowledge that a competent expert would be there to comfort the patient, interpret symptoms and signs, make valid judgements, and take appropriate action.

The training philosophy of the hospital regarding the nursing of sick children was simply expressed by Catherine Wood, lady superintendent of the convalescent home from 1869, and of the main hospital from 1878 to 1888; 'What we have to aim at is the development of the individual nurse by the individual child'.[40] Each nurse had a certain number of children (ideally eight, but no more than ten) allocated to her care, depending on her experience and the nature of the patients' diseases. The nurse had the entire care of her patients; she did everything for them, and was expected to know everything about them, 'as though she were their mother; and this she is, for the time being'.[41] Great emphasis was placed on regularity of habits, and it was the nurses who had responsibility for instilling table manners into their patients, and instructing them in that most middle-class of obsessions, the daily post-breakfast bowel movement. Probationers worked on each ward for at least six months, and were given charge of one child, usually, 'some miserable babe, neglected and forsaken by its mother'.[42] They were taught how to hold, feed, clothe and wash the child, and, in the improvement of 'their' babies, were introduced to the nursing system that pertained throughout the institution:[43]

> We want each nurse to gather her little ones into her arms with the resolve that she will spend and be spent for them. They are hers, and for a time they will look to her for a mother's love and a mother's care.

Sick children's nurses were regarded as vital to the efficient running of the institution, but were also seen as inherently 'difficult', requiring to be both controlled, and trained in acceptable social mores.[44] The nurses were responsible for keeping the wards clean, for cooking patients' meals, for feeding, cleaning and observing the children. Their cleaning duties were a vital part of their work; the constant battle against dirt was part of the educative process, and the means through which order might come out of chaos.[45] The children's nurse performed the same domestic tasks in relation to housework and child-care as the patient's mother, but she did so in a quiet, regulated, and ordered manner. The embodiment of the constantly-cleansed hospital as the ideal home was expressed by John Simon in his report to the Privy Council in 1868:[46]

> That which makes the healthiest house likewise makes the healthiest hospital, – the same fastidious and universal cleanliness, the same never-ceasing vigilance

against the thousand forms in which dirt may disguise itself, in air and soil and water, in walls and floors and ceilings, in dress and bedding and furniture, in pots and pans and pails [...] for the establishment which has to be kept in such exquisite perfection of cleanliness is an establishment which never rests from fouling itself.

While lady superintendents came from the leisured classes, HSC nurses in the mid-nineteenth century were either respectable young working-class women, usually from the country, or middle-class trainees, whose fees ensured a shorter training period and good prospects of advancement within the voluntary hospital system. Whatever their origins, hospital training mean that, in Alison Bashford's phrase, Victorian hospital nurses were 'culturally recoded [...] as middle-class'.[47] Urban working-class women, from whose ranks came the patients' mothers, were not considered suitable HSC nursing material:[48]

It is a mistake to suppose that the most sympathetic and skillful [sic] for the poor are to be found among their own class. Any one who has seen much of their homes will have observed that the majority of the poor are congenitally deficient in, and only acquire after much training, those habits of cleanliness, delicacy, order, and restraint so needful in the nursing of the sick; and that long familiarity has produced a certain insensitiveness to suffering, disease, and dirt in those around them.

Thus, working-class trainees were seen to be inherently incapable of cleanliness, order and kindness, yahoos among women, and unfit for the task of caring for the sick children of their own class. This view stems from middle-class domestic visitation, and a lack of understanding amongst the management and visitors of the care networks that existed among those coping with fragile economic uncertainty.[49] The philosophy also undermined one of the stated aims of the institution, namely, that of training patients to demand high standards of hygiene, order and cleanliness. If, as a matter of genetic inheritance, the poor were 'congenitally deficient' in what the well-off considered good habits, then what was the point in trying to inculcate middle-class mores into their sick children?

It was up to the nurses to keep the hospital as hygienic as possible, in addition to dispensing medication and working to the medical officers' orders. This meant hours and hours of cleaning. They had little time to spend amusing or coaxing the children, although it is clear that they would have welcomed the opportunity to carry out the less physically demanding aspects of nursing sick children. In 1860 Louisa Twining arranged to send some of the girls from her Industrial Home to HSC to be trained. She recorded that the nurses spoke of their work as being wearying and monotonous, and how they longed for some variety in their daily routines.[50] It is likely that they would have liked to have had the time to play with the patients, or read to them, or just sit and cuddle them. Their heavy physical work-load, however, precluded them from doing this. Given the nature of the work they performed, it might be argued that the nurses resembled domestic servants rather than mother-substitutes, but the qualities that the hospital management looked for in a nurse were not exclusively those of a housemaid.[51] All nurses employed at HSC had to be able to read and write easily, and to possess attributes of kindness verging on the saintly:[52]

> It shall be the duty of every Nurse, not merely to watch the children with care, and to tend them with kindness, but also by all means to keep them cheerful and contented; and while impatience, ill-temper, or anger towards the Patients will be followed by dismissal, the mere inability to make children happy will of itself be regarded as a sufficient cause for not retaining a Nurse in the service of the Hospital.

If a nurse was found to have struck a child, she was dismissed without a reference. In this, she was expected to emulate the manners of the middle-class mother and not those of the patients' domestic background, where corporal punishment administered by adult family members and neighbours was the norm.[53] A similar fate befell those nurses who accepted tokens of gratitude from patients' families. This may have been necessary to prevent any accusation of bribery and favouritism, but it also frustrated any bonds of friendship growing between the nurses and the families, and denied the parents the pleasure of expressing their gratitude in what, to them, would have been the normal fashion. These paragons also had to put up with the medical officers' expectations that they were there only to serve the doctors' demands. They were 'new nurses', as far away from the popular Dickensian image of drunkard slovenly old women, as it was possible to be:[54]

> The new nurse was a sanitised version of the old nurse, a middle-class figure of efficiency, neatness and whiteness. in that ordering, cleansing, purifying and moralising the domestic hand came to be so firmly the cultured territory of middle-class women, the new 'lady nurses' and 'lady superintendents' were crucial in the process by which hospitals were modernised and sanitised.

The nurse occupied a peculiar position within the hospital: she was at once the servant of her medical masters, and the principal agency through which the hospital cared for its patients. She was paid a pittance, and expected to subject herself to numerous rules and regulations that controlled her conduct both inside and outside of the institution. The fact of her being paid put her at a moral disadvantage in relation to the lady superintendent, the volunteers and the paying probationers, and ensured that she would never herself become part of the hospital management. She was the guarantee of respectability of the hospital, the proof to mothers and supporters alike that the patients were being looked after well in the best place possible. In the words of Robinson and Elkan:[55]

> [The nurse was] a social catalyst in care, across-class and cultural conduit into the lives and social spaces of groups otherwise beyond the reach of agents of social authority.

By the 1880s, as elsewhere, training for sick children's nurses was formalised at the HSC.[56] In future, the nurses would see themselves increasingly as professionals, with responsibility for the principal care of the patients. While deference to the male medical staff remained de rigueur, confidence in their own abilities and status lead to an increasingly sceptical attitude towards the lady visitors. The nurses began to define themselves in the light of their qualifications and elevating position in society. They were no longer well-trained domestic servants, dressed and addressed as such, but a visible and vocal speciality who took pride in the high levels of care they gave their patients. As in other hospitals, they 'bartered temporary workplace exploitation and devaluation for the enduring status and prestige their identity as nurses gave them in their communities'.[57]

The Mothers of the Patients

The mothers of the patients at HSC have been left till last because they were at the bottom of the hospital hierarchy; below that of the lady visitors, the lady volunteers, and the nurses. They may have given birth to the patients, but the fact of them surrendering their children to the hospital effectively meant that they had given up (albeit temporarily) their parental rights. Charles West had planned his campaign to open a children's hospital in Britain very carefully, as there were not only objections to the establishment of such an institution on moral grounds (feckless parents would abuse such a charity), but there was a long cherished belief in Britain that the mother was the best nurse for a child.[58] If a children's hospital, with beds for in-patients, was successful, this would challenge the view that mother – even a poor one – knows what is best for her child, and, once challenged, the state and the voluntary sector could be expected to intervene further in the child-parent relationship.

Children's hospitals had a contradictory view of the parents of the patients. On the one hand, without parental consent there would be no patients, and it was important to 'sell' the hospital's services to the families. This was no mean feat for the HSC; London poor housewives had well-established networks of local support in times of family sickness, and removing a sick child to this new institution could upset the delicate balance of neighbourhood dependence.[59] In order to induce them to proffer their children to the hospital for treatment, it had to offer a level of care and range of services that made the transaction worthwhile.

Subscribers to children's hospitals were wooed with tales of parents as decent hard-working people who could not afford to pay for the medical care of their children, and thus, worthy of assistance. On the other hand, their neglect or vicious behaviour was seen as the cause of their children's sickness. The General Hospital and Dispensary for Children, Manchester claimed its justification was:[60]

> In counteracting the thousand nameless and nameless evils which attend bad feeding and bad nursing, or the neglect and vices of the parents; and which either nip in the bud the precious lives of these 'little ones', or cause them to grow up sickly and diseased men and women – their lives too often a burden to themselves and others!

Almost invariably it was the child's mother who accompanied the would-be patient to see the admitting registrar or the medical officer in the Outpatients' Department. She it was who made the decision to submit the child to the HSC's scrutiny, and, by association, her own mothering of that child. The casenotes, here as elsewhere, record the first impressions of the physician of the child and its family, and cover such territory as the pregnancy record of the mother, the method of weaning of the child, and the sobriety and health of the mother. The mothers presented as acceptable a picture of respectability as possible. Surviving photographs of mothers and their children in the waiting room show prematurely aged women, dressed in their best clothes and hats, holding children who were dressed (and indeed, overdressed) in emulation of their better-off counterparts. While it is clear that most of the clothes are old or second-hand, or borrowed from neighbours, there is not a ragamuffin in sight, and the children and their mothers are turned out as well as the family budget allowed. It is also significant that, of nearly 80,000 Victorian and Edwardian children on the in-patient database, fewer than one hundred are described as suffering from neglect or ill-treatment.[61] This first meeting in Out-Patients was frequently the only one that the mother would have with the male hospital hierarchy; thereafter her negotiations with the institution would be conducted with other women.

In the earliest days of the hospital's life, certain maternal responsibilities were still expected to be fulfilled, for example, mothers of in-patients were charged with undertaking their child's laundry. Every in – patient was supplied with slippers and a wrapper by the HSC, but parents were expected to supply decent clothing for all but the eruptive fever cases, and to take away the dirty clothing and linen for washing. Measles and scarlet fever cases were put in fever wards, separated from rest of hospital, and in these cases the HSC supplied all clothing, and returned their own clothes, disinfected, when they left.[62] As the hospital grew, however, and the dangers of risking the export (or import) of infection through the clothes and bedding became appreciated, this task was gradually assumed by the hospital itself. Once the mothers were no longer required as washerwomen, it was relatively simple to employ the fear of infection as the reason for their increased exclusion from the wards.[63]

The limited facilities for infectious cases before and after the hospital's expansion in the 1870s were used to restrict visitors, including the parents of the patients. In the absence of their birth mothers, the nurses were encouraged to act *in loco matris*. Dedicated to the care of their patients, reference to the child's home life was not encouraged, but, rather, the daily routine of the ward was established as the 'normal' life of the child. It would be almost a century after the establishment of HSC before Rene Spitz and John Bowlby's work provided insight into the psychological effects of the stress caused by separating the child patient from all that they knew and loved.[64] Instead, the fact that children became upset after visits from family members was used as an excuse for denying regular contact with relatives, as it was seen to be harmful to the well-being and recovery of the patient.

Visiting hours for parents were strictly controlled. From 1880, mothers were allowed to visit on Thursday afternoons, Sunday thereafter being known as 'fathers' day'.[65] The grief of the children on their parents' departing was dealt with by a different ward routine on visiting days; as soon as the visitors had gone, the children's tea was brought in, with extra treacle or sugar on the bread.[66] Risk of infection and disruption to the other patients were used as the reasons for excluding the patients' siblings from visiting. This rule was particularly harsh given the traditional role of older and sisters (and also, to a lesser degree, brothers) in childcare among working-class families. As a family grew, older sisters in London took over the watching of younger siblings, and the bonds between the so-called 'little mothers' and their charges were strong. Given the average length of stay at the HSC (usually three to four weeks), whether the patient was an older

child or 'her' baby, this long separation must have been difficult for
them to endure. There is no record of these so-called 'little mothers'
being prominent in the daily life of the HSC, but they were a familiar
sight at the Out-Patients' department of the Children's Hospital in
Hackney:[67]

> Sometimes one of these tiny little 'grown-ups' will walk into the hospital
> holding by the hand a child [...] and she will busy herself keeping the little one
> quiet, soothing her, or scolding her, just like a mother, while the doctor is find-
> ing out what is the matter.

The frequency of parental visits was determined on the other side by
family circumstances. Having a large family could mean that mothers
were unable to attend each week, and parents living at some distance
from the hospital could find it impossible to see their child throughout
its hospital stay. Mothers found ways round this – often relatives
living in London or family friends were commissioned to visit the
child – and mothers coming up to London especially to see their
children could insist on more relaxed visiting hours. HSC did make one
short-lived experiment in childcare that acknowledged the difficulties
of poor working mothers in London. In the late 1850s, it opened a
model children's nursery, which, for a small payment, looked after
local children under the age of five. The children were cared for according to the current best practice, and mothers were not only assured
of their child's safety and comfort, but also given the opportunity to
learn from the nurses in charge of the crèche.[68]

The hospital sent weekly postcards to parents outside London
with a brief report on the patient's progress, although this system did
not always work; the mother of Daisy Ricketts from Wootton Basset
wrote to the hospital about the difficulties of visiting on a Sunday, as
there were no trains on that day. She added, 'On Wednesday next the
Duchess of Beaufort will be here hunting and will want to know how
the child is and I am sorry to tell her I cannot get any news [...]'.[69]
Thus, it would seem, the Board of Management and the lady volunteers were not the only ones with exalted contacts.

When a child was dying, mothers were sent for, and admission to
the ward allowed at any hour of the day or night, but, apart from

mothers who were breast-feeding patients, this was the only time when unlimited access to their children was allowed. To the disapproval of the HSC, parental judgement on the efficacy of treatment or family circumstances dictated the removal of a patient before the medical staff was ready. Dying or unrelievable patients afforded the parents the most understandable ultimate expression of their own rights over the fate of their children, but, on occasions, the fact that the mothers could not bear to be parted from the children was sufficient to lead them to reject what the hospital had to offer. The patient database reveals that 800 patients were removed by families between 1852 and 1899, often against medical advice. Where reasons were given, the principal impetus for taking the patient away was that the patient and his or her family could no longer bear to be parted. A high proportion were also taken away when it was clear the hospital had nothing more to offer by way of cure or relief. In these circumstances, it was clearly preferable to have the child home to die, or to make arrangements for the invalid child more suitable to the health of the family as a whole, than to surrender all control of the patient to the HSC.[70]

The medical establishment was not shy about excluding a mother if it felt that her visits impeded recovery. Charles West admitted a child who had been unable to walk for seven months, in spite of his conviction that the girl was malingering:[71]

> 'Put her down', I said to her mother, 'and let me see her stand', 'Oh sir! She has not put a foot to the ground for seven months'. The order was repeated, the child obeyed the unwonted tone of command, and stood. 'Now walk!' – again a remonstrance, but she walked.

She was first persuaded to stand and then walk in the hospital, but when it was observed that she regressed after each maternal visit, her mother's attendances on the wards were restricted. Once the child was walking normally, she was not sent home immediately, but sent to the country, away from her mother's influence.[72]

One of the avowed aims of the hospital was to educate the poor in the best practice of childcare and household management. This is illustrated in the Earl of Carnaervon's speech at the hospital annual dinner on 21 February:[73]

No doubt it may be said that those children found in the hospital a vast improvement on their own poor squalid homes of dirt and disorder; but I believe that when they leave the Hospital, they go away not only with their diseases cured, but with the moral frame of their minds improved and invigorated, and there is no telling how far the discipline to which they have been subjected in the Hospital, the kindly gentle influences to which they have been exposed bear fruit in the comfort and happiness of those squalid homes to which they often return.

When the hospital opened, it was important for its success that it gained the trust and acceptance of poor families, and, to that end, parental rights were observed. However, as the nursing establishment grew, the nurturing role of the mothers was gradually reduced, until they became hospital visitors, with fewer rights of access than the ladies for whom HSC was part of their social round. Sunday afternoon, the one on which lady visitors were not allowed, was until 1880 the best chance mothers and fathers had of seeing their hospitalised children. There was little opportunity for the ladies and the mothers to meet, and thus little chance for the women supporters to gain first-hand knowledge of the difficulties of raising a family in poverty in the great metropolis.

From the beginning, the HSC management believed that the home circumstances of the children were often the root cause of their patients' infirmities.[74] The apparent strictness and censure meted out to the mothers arguably stemmed from a sense that their lack of mothering skills was partly to blame for their offspring's illness. Prince Christian tacitly expressed this view at the annual fund-raising dinner in 1876:[75]

It should be remembered that, besides the cure and relief of bodily suffering, these children are treated with the greatest kindness and attention. Living in large, airy rooms, everything around them is conducted with cleanliness, regularity and order – a life to which a great proportion of the inmates have hitherto, I fear have been strangers.

The majority of the children were brought to the hospital out-patients' department by these mothers, who were supposedly strangers to cleanliness and kindness.[76] By autumn 1869, demand was so high that new regulations were introduced requiring new applicants to have the recommendation of a doctor, minister of religion, scripture-reader or city missionary. The recommended form of wording on the certificate was; 'I certify that the bearer is too poor to pay for medical attendance, and is a proper object for charity.'[77] A mother's opinion that her child needed treatment was no longer sufficient; in future, a male figure of authority – not necessarily medically experienced – had to be approached to filter out the frivolous or hopeless cases. It would stand to reason that such pillars of the community would favour parents already known to them, and that those who rejected the services of the city missionary or who drank, smoked or frequented the pawn shop may find themselves disadvantaged in their attempts to obtain medical care for their children. The initial vision of the hospital entailed the child's experience of the institution as being a civilising force within the home, it did not describe its ideal patients as coming from those working-class families which were already deemed to be respectable according to the lights of Victorian evangelism:[78]

> The untutored little Bohemian becomes transformed into a civilised and well-behaved member of society [...] The child goes back into its native wilds and becomes an example to other children, a lasting illustration of an excellent lesson to parents.

Parents were subjected to a strict set of rules themselves. They were forbidden from bringing food in for the children, apart from sponge cakes, and were expected to behave with propriety at the child's bedside.[79] The hospital was strict about punctuality, but did not always make it easy for the mothers to comply. One prominent local resident wrote to the authorities complaining that the posts at the entrance to the hospital were too narrow to allow prams to pass through, resulting in wheels coming off and the occupants being tipped onto the pavement.[80]

Waiting times in Out-Patients for mothers could stretch to many hours, causing havoc to family routines and childcare arrangements. It was not unusual for a mother to wait seven or eight hours in out-patients, and still not see a doctor.[81] Parents could complain to the patient's sponsor (if there was one), whose continued support was important to the hospital. In these cases, apologies were generally sent to the family, but, in its desire to treat the patient as an individual, the hospital could have been accused of insensitivity to the child's home and family circumstances, and a disregard of the claims of affection of the other family members, and the feelings of the parents. A case in point was the use of post mortems to study childhood diseases. Although it was written in the rules and regulations that the hospital would carry out this procedure, the lack of contact with parents meant that. Occasionally, parental consent was not sought beforehand. By the beginning of the twentieth century, the Society for the Protection of Hospital Patients was beginning to take an interest in the use of hospital patients in medical research, and addressed the Prince of Wales at the Children's Welfare Exhibition at Olympia on the subject, deploring:[82]

> The widespread habit and tendency [...] to the effect that medical men claim and exercise an absolute license to experiment at their will upon patients in hospitals both in regard to drugs and to surgery, for the purpose purely of scientific observation, for hypothetical scientific results, without any reference to the improvement of the health of the particular patients in question.

The bad publicity this created in the press, and the distress to families and staff, resulted in a change of policy in 1911, and, from thence forward, written consent was required in each case. It would take another forty years for the medical establishment to be shown that the separation of a child from his or her home, even to the best children's hospital facility that could be created, caused inordinate distress to that child. It took another few decades for the principle of close parental involvement in the treatment of the hospitalised child to be accepted.

Conclusion

Within the world of the Victorian children's hospital, women of all classes had clearly defined functions. The female upper-classes raised funds, interested their husbands in the institution, and visited the wards as part of their social rounds. Their daughters occasionally became lady superintendents, whose social superiority enabled them to govern the nursing establishment, and negotiate their territory with the male management and medical committees. In this, they provided the three elements identified by Koven and Michel in the Victorian maternalisation of society: care, nurturance and morality.[83] Their work was firmly in the tradition of the personal social work that was deemed an acceptable occupation for the Victorian woman who had no need to seek paid employment.[84]

For most of the second half of the nineteenth century, nurses were the work horses of the establishment, and treated by the lady visitors and the lady superintendents much as domestic servants. They were expected to maintain middle-class standards of cleanliness, obedience to their superiors, to work long hours for little pay, and to subject their leisure hours and conduct to scrutiny and censure. Although subservient to most of the other adults connected with the institution, the nurses were trained to be mother-substitutes to their patients. Through constant vigilance of a small number of patients, for whom she was entirely responsible, the nurse fulfilled the role of the ideal mother. By the time the child left her charge, it was not only well, but educated in habits that were deemed essential for an orderly society. The nurse, as mother substitute, gave her patients expectations of what a good home and a good mother might be, and, the hospital hoped, provided an example to the patients' mothers of what they themselves might achieve in their own homes.

The mothers of the patients had the lowliest women's role in these institutions. Restricted to one short afternoon's visit a week, and allowed freer access to their children only when they were dying, the patient's mothers were kept away from the hospital 'home' as they were perceived as one of the causes of the child's sickness. The hospitals were middle-class institutions with middle-class values, and there was no room in them for a working-class mother. Until she had been educated by the other hospital women in 'correct' child management, and by the demands of a child who had experienced and been cured by this, her status in the hospital hierarchy would remain low.

Notes

1   This is in contrast to many children's hospitals in North America, which were the brainchildren of resolutely Christian women. See M. Braithwaite, *Sick Kids: the Story of the Hospital for Sick Children in Toronto* (Toronto, 1974) and J. Golden (ed.), *Infant Asylums and Children's Hospitals: Medical Dilemmas and Developments 1850–1920* (New York and London, 1989), introduction.

2   See A. White Franklin, 'Children's Hospitals', in F.N.L. Poynter (ed.), *The Evolution of Hospitals in Britain* (London, 1964), pp.103–23.

3   Board of Governors of the United Bristol Hospitals, *The Bristol Royal Hospital for Sick Children* (Bristol, 1968), Dr Charles Wilson, *On the Expediency of Founding a Hospital for the Diseases of Children in Edinburgh* (Edinburgh, 1859), D.A. Williamson, *Ninety Years of Service: a History of Southampton Children's Hospital 1884–1974* (Southampton, 1990).

4   Hospitals were not unique in the charitable world in being dominated by male supporters. See R.J. Morris, 'Voluntary Societies and British Urban Elites, 1780–1850: An Analysis', *Historical Journal*, 26 (1983), pp.95–118.

5   Quoted in 'Paediatrics Past', *Nursing Times*, 9 December 1981.

6   For women's negotiation of power in welfare work, see J. Lewis, 'Gender, the Family and Women's Agency in the Building of Welfare States: The British Case', *Social History*, 29 (1994), pp.37–55.

7   The inaugural meeting to launch the hospital had more women in the audience than men, but, significantly, not one of them was mentioned by name in the press reports of the meeting. *Morning Chronicle*, 19 March 1851.

8   Great Ormond Street Hospital Archive, GOS/8/1 February 1859.

9   This may have had to do with the powerless role of the first matrons, who, at HSC, was more of a housekeeper than a head of nursing staff.

10   *The Englishwoman's Journal*, April 1860, p.120.

11   This division of labour in the philanthropic world is dealt with in detail in F. Prochaska, *Women and Philanthropy in Nineteenth-Century England* (Oxford, 1980).

12   In 1888, this activity blossomed into a major social event, when a ladies' committee (headed by Princess Frederica and composed entirely of titled ladies) organised a two-day Doll Show in aid of the hospital. Great Ormond Street Hospital Archive, GOS/8/1/ref. 71.

13   For a fuller exploration of the role of visitors at the hospital see A. Tanner, 'Care, Nurturance and Morality: The Role of Visitors in a Victorian Children's Hospital', in G. Mooney and J. Reinarz (eds), *Permeable Walls: Historical Perspectives on Hospital and Asylum Visiting* (Amsterdam, forthcoming).

14   *Twentieth Annual Report of the HSC, 1872.*

15 For the royal family's involvement with the hospital see F. Prochaska, *Royal Bounty: the Making of a Welfare Monarchy* (New Haven and London, 1995), pp.124 and 193.

16 *HSC Annual Reports, 1853–75.*

17 Great Ormond Street Hospital Archive, GOS/7/1/2, 30 October 1861.

18 The Hospital, especially after the 1860s, trained more nurses than it could employ, and private nursing service was one of the few opportunities open to trained sick children's nurses.

19 John Walter, MP and proprietor of *The Times*, was chairman of the committee of management for some years. He suggested that HSC should treat children from the upper and middle-classes as well as the poor, emphasising the moral benefit to be gained from children from all classes being together in times of sickness. Great Ormond Street Hospital Archive, GOS/8/1, 22 March 1876.

20 Ada Bois was an untypical nurse in many respects; she was a talented artist of independent spirit, as witnessed by her marrying clandestinely while still a trainee nurse at HSC.

21 The social climbing of Adrian Hope was remarked upon by one of the senior physicians: 'Well known in Society, it was an education to see him slightly bending and walking backwards with a tray of toys before Royalty'. 'Reminiscences of Dr Frederick Poynton', Great Ormond Street Hospital Archive, ref. GOS/8/156.

22 See I. Bradley, *The Call to Seriousness: the Evangelical Impact on the Victorians* (London, 1976).

23 The Gatty family's literary heredity was considerable. Mrs Gatty's eldest daughter, Juliana Horatia Ewing, exceeded her mother's fame as a children's author, and maintained the family's connection with the Hospital. C. Maxwell, *Mrs Gatty and Mrs Ewing* (London, 1949), and S. Drain, 'Margaret Gatty' (1809–73), and 'Juliana Horatia Ewing' (1841–85), *Oxford Dictionary of National Biography* (Oxford, 2004).

24 Great Ormond Street Hospital Archive Management Committee Minutes, GOS/1/2/10, 7 January 1869.

25 Great Ormond Street Hospital Archive, GOS/8. Cromwell House Correspondence, no date.

26 The first unpaid lady superintendent, with a responsibility to the board of management, was appointed in 1862. Catherine Wood, lady superintendent from 1878, and the woman charged with establishment a training school for sick children's nurses at HSC, began her association with the hospital as a child visitor. J. Kosky, *Mutual Friends: Charles Dickens and Great Ormond Street Children's Hospital* (London, 1989), pp.57–8.

27 Great Ormond Street Hospital Archive, GOS/8/1. Letters and press cuttings, vol. 1, part 2.

28 The volunteer middle-class nurse was a feature of London hospitals, many of them trained by semi-religious nursing sisterhoods, such as the St John's House

sisterhood, which had the monopoly of nursing at the highly Anglican King's College Hospital. J. Moore, *A Zeal for Responsibility: The Struggle for Professional Nursing in Victorian England, 1868–83* (Athens and London, 1988).

29   Great Ormond Street Hospital Archive, GOS/8/1, report of the Anniversary Festival, 1880, speech by Sir James Paget, Bt, FRS, chairman. By 1880, these women worked in the outpatient department, dressing wounds and putting on splints. They gave classes in household management to the mothers, and visited children at home.

30   The visiting committee at HSC, until the end of the nineteenth century, was made up of members of the management committee and male supporters of the hospital.

31   E.M.R. Lomax, *Small and Special: The Development of Hospitals for Children in Victorian Britain* (*Medical History*, Supplement, 16, London, 1996), pp.64–5.

32   The Manchester General Hospital and Dispensary for Sick Children used its ladies' committee in an unusual way; members visited children who had been discharged from the hospital and reported on their progress. Lomax, *Small and Special*, p.92.

33   Great Ormond Street Hospital Archive, GOS/8/1, letters and press cuttings, vol. 1, part 2. Ref. 71: 'Report of the Proceedings at the Twenty-Seventh Anniversary Festival, Held at Willis's Rooms, St James's, Thursday February 20th 1879'.

34   'Borderlands: Women, Voluntary Action, and Child Welfare in Britain, 1840–1914', in S. Koven and S. Michel (eds), *Mothers of a New World: Maternalist Politics and the Origins of Welfare States* (New York and London, 1993), pp.98, 124.

35   See A. Summers, 'A Home from Home: Women's Philanthropic Work in the Nineteenth Century', in S. Burman (ed.), *Fit Work for Women* (London, 1979), pp.33–63. D. Epstein Nord, '"Neither Pairs nor Odd": Female Community in Late Nineteenth-Century London', *Signs*, 15.4 (1990), pp.733–54.

36   See K. McCarthy, 'Parallel Power Structures: Women and the Voluntary Sphere' in K. McCarthy (ed.), *Lady Bountiful Revisited: Women, Philanthropy, and Power* (New Brunswick, 1990).

37   'Nursing Institutions and Hospitals', *The Hospital*, 26 February 1887, p.375.

38   L. Pollock, *A Lasting Relationship: Parents and Children over Three Centuries* (London, 1987), p.93.

39   E.D. Baer, 'Women and the Politics of Career Development in the Case of Nursing', in J. Robinson and R. Elkan (eds), *Nursing History and the Politics of Welfare* (London, 1977), p.246.

40   C. Wood, 'The Training of Nurses for Sick Children', *Nursing Record*, 6 December 1888, p.507.

41   C. Wood, 'The Nursing of Sick Children', *The Nursing Record*, 23 August 1888, p.269.

42   *Ibid.*

43   Wood, 'The Training of Nurses', p.508.

44   Regulations for nurses covered not only duties and behaviour while on duty, but restricted movement outside the hospital and controlled the behaviour of these young women in the nurses' home. Food was not allowed in rooms, they were not allowed to congregate in each other's rooms, no pictures were allowed on the walls of their rooms, loud talking and loitering on the staircases were forbidden, and they had to be in bed with lights out by 10.30 in the evening. Great Ormond Street Hospital Archive, GOS/5/2/49. Rules for Day Nurses, 25 July 1897.

45   A. Bashford, *Purity and Pollution: Gender, Embodiment and Victorian Medicine*, Studies in Gender History (Basingstoke, 1998), p.19.

46   J. Simon, *Sixth Report of the Medical Officer of the Privy Council (1863)*, reprinted in *Public Health Reports*, 2 (London, 1887), pp.148–9.

47   Bashford, *Purity and Pollution*, p.22.

48   Warrington Haward, assistant surgeon at HSC. *Contemporary Review, 1879.* The surgeon's wife was a regular – and highly critical – visitor to the Hospital.

49   A. Davin, *Growing Up Poor: Home, School and Street in London, 1870–1914* (London, 1996).

50   Great Ormond Street Hospital Archive, Lady Visitors' Book, 20 November 1860.

51   Alison Bashford argues that, in general voluntary hospitals, nurses were women who would otherwise have been superior domestic servants. *Purity and Pollution*, p.22. This is only true in part for the HSC, where qualities of kindness and empathy with the children were regarded as of equal importance with good health and the ability to work hard.

52   Great Ormond Street Hospital Archive, GOS/8/1, letters and press cuttings, vol. 1. p.95. The threat of dismissal was serious; in August 1869 a nurse was sacked for putting the wrong linament on a child and causing much pain. Great Ormond Street Hospital Archive, GOS/1/2/11, Management Committee Minutes, 25 August 1869.

53   E. Ross, 'Survival Networks: Women's Neighbourhood Sharing in London before World War One', *History Workshop*, 15 (1983), pp.4–27, 12–13.

54   Bashford, *Purity and Pollution*, p.xv.

55   J. Robinson and R. Elkan (eds), *Nursing History and the Politics of Welfare* (London, 1977), Introduction, p.3.

56   In 1866, there were 111 Metropolitan nursing staff, by 1883–4 it had risen to 784, and by 1901 it had reached 1, 246. B. Abel-Smith, *A History of the Nursing Profession* (London, 1960), p.51.

57   P. d'Antonio, 'Rethinking the Rewriting of Nursing History', <http://www.nursing.upenn.edu/history/chronicle/s98/antonio.htm>.

58   E.R. Lomax, 'Advances in Paediatrics and in Infant Care in Nineteenth Century England' (unpublished PhD thesis, University of California, 1972), ch. 3.

59   See Ross, 'Survival Networks', pp.4–27, and Davin, *Growing Up Poor*.

60   *Thirty-Third Annual Report of the General Hospital and Dispensary* (Manchester, 1862), p.62, quoted in Lomax, *Small and Special*, p.33.

61   Great Ormond Street Hospital Historic In-Patient Database, currently accessed through the Centre for Local History Studies, Kingston University.

62   R.A. Clavering, 'Dr Charles West and the Founding of the Children's Hospital in Great Ormond Street' (1956), MS in Great Ormond Street Archive, p.37.

63   The exclusion of parents from the wards on the grounds of fear of infection was not challenged until the late 1940s, when the British Paediatric Association conducted a study of cross-infection in hospitals that showed that there was no correlation between cross-infection and adult visitors. A.G. Watkins and E. Lewis-Faning, 'Incidence of Cross-Infection in Children's Wards', *British Medical Journal*, 2 (1949), pp.616–19, 718.

64   Central Health Services Council, Ministry of Health, *Report of the Committee on the Welfare of Children in Hospital* (HMSO, 1959). See also L. Shillers and J. Nixon, '"I Want My Mummy": Changes in the Care of Children in Hospital', *Collegian*, 5.2 (April 1998), and J. Young, 'Changing Attitudes Towards Families of Hospitalised Children from 1935 to 1975: a Case Study', *Journal of Advanced Nursing*, 17.12 (December 1992), pp.422–9.

65   James Greenwood, 'Tiny Tim in Hospital', Pamphlet, 1880. At least the parents were permitted to see their children properly shod, at the Royal Hospital for Sick Children in Glasgow, they had to take their boots off and visit the wards in their stockinged feet until 1909. E. Robertson, *The Yorkhill Story: the History of the Royal Hospital for Sick Children, Glasgow*, Board of Management for Yorkhill and Associated Hospitals (Glasgow, 1972), p.33.

66   *Daily Telegraph*, 11 July 1872.

67   J.B. 'Our Lodgers', *Children*, 2, April 1897, p.54, quoted in Davin, *Growing Up Poor*, p.89.

68   Great Ormond Street Hospital Archive, Correspondence Registers, GOS/8/1, February 1859.

69   Great Ormond Street Hospital Archive, GOS/8/163, Correspondence Registers for 1910.

70   For a fuller examination of parents removing their children from the institution, see A. Tanner, 'Choice and the Children's Hospital: Great Ormond Street Hospital Patients and their Families, 1855–1900', in A. Borsay and P. Shapeley (eds), *Reconfiguring the Recipient: Historical Perspectives on the Negotiation of Medicine, Charity and Mutual Aid* (Aldershot, forthcoming).

71   C. West, 'On the Mental Peculiarities and Mental Disorders of Childhood', *Medical Times and Gazette*, 1 (1860), pp.133–7.

72   E.M.R. Lomax, 'A Mid-Nineteenth Century British Pediatrician's Interpretations of the Mental Peculiarities and Disorders of Childhood', *Clio Medica*, 17.4 (1982–3), pp.223–333.

73   Great Ormond Street Hospital Archive, GOS/8/1, letters and press cuttings, vol. 1, part 2, 1877, fol. 67d.

74   The fact that many children, once cured or relieved at HSC, would return immediately to the very conditions that had made them sick in the first place was not lost on the hospital authorities. In 1869, it opened Cromwell House, a convalescent home in Highgate, north London, and even before that date, a fund, paid for out of penny donations from patients' families, sent children who were being discharged from Great Ormond Street to spend a month at the seaside. 'The Country Branch Hospital and Convalescent Home, the Bank, Highgate', *The London Mirror*, 7 August 1869. Favoured places were Margate, Eastbourne, Torquay and Brighton. Cromwell House opened 29 July 1869, and had room for 56 convalescents, as well as chronic medical and surgical cases who needed to be built up before undergoing further treatment. *Eighteenth Annual Report of the HSC, 1870.*

75   *The London Mirror*, 1 April 1876.

76   Not surprisingly, the majority of out-patients were local children. Between 1852 and 1855, the out-patient distribution included 4,517 from St Pancras, 1,411 from St Andrew Holborn, 2,349 from St George the Martyr and St George Bloomsbury, and 1,875 from Clerkenwell. Great Ormond Street Hospital Archive, Correspondence Registers, GOS/8/1.

77   Great Ormond Street Hospital Archive, GOS/1/6/5, Medical Committee minutes, 22 September 1869.

78   *The Day*, April 1867.

79   This was not just in the case of the HSC; see Ruth Hawker's study of the Exeter Hospital, 'For the Good of the Patient', in C. Maggs (ed.), *Nursing History: the State of the Art* (London, 1987), pp.143–51.

80   Great Ormond Street Hospital Archive, GOS/8/163, Correspondence Register, 17 July 1885.

81   *Ibid.*, 1 October 1910.

82   Great Ormond Street Hospital Archive, GOS/6/161, Correspondence Register.

83   Koven and Michel, *Mothers of a New World*, p.4.

84   J. Lewis, *Women and Social Action in Victorian and Edwardian England* (Stanford and Aldershot, 1991).

Part Two: The Visual Impact

CAROLE RAWCLIFFE

Chapter 6: 'A Word from Our Sponsor':
Advertising the Patron in the Medieval Hospital

One of the most visually compelling torments of Hell catalogued in Dante's *Divine Comedy* may be found Canto XVII, which describes the seventh circle of the pit. Here, beneath the scorpion tail of the monster Geryon, the scorched bodies of aristocrats deformed by their passion for filthy lucre writhe in agony. Burnt beyond recognition in the blistering heat, these lost souls can still be identified by the coats of arms prominently displayed on the moneybags hanging, as a badge of dishonour, around their necks.[1] Not only have they debased their noble lineages through greed and usury, but they have also, implicitly, failed to display the generosity and Christian compassion without which riches on earth lead inexorably to suffering after death.

The fate of Dives, the wealthy sybarite condemned to everlasting damnation because of his disregard for the sick poor, presented an even more terrible warning, this time from Christ himself (Luke 16, vv. 19–31). Medieval preachers dwelt with relish upon the torments in store for those who lived selfishly with no thought for others. In the words of one homilist, writing in English rather than Latin for the guidance of lay readers, the parable was directed unequivocally 'agens riche men that [...] han no pitee of pore folk'. Far from indulging themselves, he argued, they should [2]

> haue grete drede that it falle not to hem as dide to the riche glotoun of whom God speketh in the gospel, that eet euery day deliciousliche and plentyuousliche and leet the pore mesel [Lazarus the leper] dye at his gate; but at the deth the dees [dice] weren y-chaunged. For the mesel was borne with aungeles in-to paradis, and the couetous gloton was not y-biried in halewed erthe, for he was acursed bi the autorite of God, but in stynkyng helle [...] in that endeles brennyng fier that may not be queynt [extinguished].

Was it possible to shed the spiritual millstone of wealth while still enjoying its tangible benefits? Lazarus, the wretched and diseased beggar, so despised in this life, held the key to paradise, where, at last, the tables would be turned and the earthly hierarchy of 'good lordship' spectacularly reversed.

The obvious solution was to found or support a hospital, which would not only meet a real social need, but also establish a lasting reserve of spiritual credit for the patron. Put crudely, charitable institutions gave medieval benefactors a unique opportunity to kill two birds with one stone: in return for charity to the sick poor of Christ they could purchase a place in heaven, rendered additionally secure through intercessionary prayers and masses offered both in their own lifetimes and for the welfare of their souls after death. Such concerns were manifest from the earliest days of hospital endowment. Herbert de Losinga (d.1119), bishop of Norwich, and founder of the city's first leper house, reminded his congregations of their obligation to perform the Comfortable Works incumbent upon all devout Christians: [3]

> Know ye, brethren, that the Church's poor are themselves among the saints [...] make them your friends, as the Lord saith, that when you shall fall they may receive you into everlasting dwellings. The holy poor are lean with hunger, and shiver with cold, but hereafter in heaven they shall be kings, and in the presence of God shall sit in judgement upon your crimes and those of all the wicked.

From 1349 onwards, successive outbreaks of plague, and the terrifying prospect of *mors improvisa* concentrated the minds of potential benefactors even further. Hospitals, caught between the pincers of falling rents and rising wages, did all they could to attract new sources of patronage in the face of intense competition from other religious houses. Ambitious building schemes offered the rich and powerful a suitable backdrop against which to advertise their munificence, while the provision of elaborate rituals and liturgy satisfied the growing desire for funerary spectacle. Theological developments, whereby the geography of the afterlife, and most notably of purgatory, was mapped with cartographical precision, further encouraged endowments, enabling donors to augment their celestial capital. [4]

Richard Whittington (d.1424), one of the leading merchant-financiers of later medieval England, clearly smelt the sulphur and burning pitch of purgatory, if not of hell. It is unclear if his massive loans to the crown and leading members of the aristocracy were usurious in the strict sense of the word, but he was taking no chances. Three times mayor of London, he also possessed a strong sense of civic pride, which found expression in numerous projects for urban improvement, including an almshouse.[5] Yet, as the executors who drew up the long and detailed statutes of his new foundation explained, his principal concerns revolved around the state of his soul:[6]

> the fervent desire and besy intension of a prudent, wise and devoute man shold be to cast before, and make secure the state and thende of his short lyff, with dedes of mercy and pite; and namely to provide for such pouer persones whiche grevous penurie and cruelle fortune have oppressed, and be not of power to gete their lyvyng either by craft or by eny other bodily labour: wherby, that at the day of the last jugement he may take his part with hem that shalle be saved [...]

In return for their physical support, the bedesmen were to follow a taxing daily round of prayer, meditation and church services dedicated to Whittington's memory. We do not know how the almshouse was decorated, but it seems more than likely that the inmates were surrounded by visual reminders of their benefactor. A fifteenth-century copy of the statutes owned by the Mercers' Company, which ran the almshouse, depicts him on his deathbed, attended by a group of grateful bedesmen, clutching their rosaries in preparation for the task ahead.[7] Whittington's posthumous largesse extended to other London hospitals, including St Bartholomew's, Smithfield, whose master was one of his executors and diverted over £174 from the estate for pious works there. These comprised a stained glass window depicting the Seven Comfortable Works so necessary for salvation and an impressive new gatehouse. Not surprisingly, Whittington's coat of arms was prominently displayed on the stonework, being the first thing a visitor would encounter on his or her arrival.[8]

Whittington's choice of glazing scheme seems especially appropriate, as hospitals like Bartholomew's offered the patron a unique opportunity to perform these Works vicariously. He or she had simply to provide the resources, in cash or kind, for others to clothe, nourish, accommodate, succour and bury the sick poor. The contemporary belief that ostentatious displays of charity robbed alms deeds of their power none the less demanded a degree of restraint in the matter of self-promotion.[9] It is easy to dismiss the frieze commissioned in 1514 by Leonardo Buonafede, master of the Ospedale del Ceppo, Pistoia, for the new loggia he had built as little more than as a blatant advertisement of his investment (Fig. 6.1). Executed by Giovanni della Robbia in brilliant colour, a series of seven panels depicts Buonafede centre stage ministering personally to Christ and his representatives on earth.[10] Yet, along with the desire for respect, admiration and gratitude, which he no doubt hoped to inspire, goes a powerful message about the work of the hospital, the obligations of the rich towards the poor, and a need, explored below, to establish close iconographic proximity to the divine.

Because of the vagaries of the northern climate, England's larger medieval hospitals boasted gatehouses rather than loggia, but these, too, were impressive structures. The heraldic emblems of founders and leading benefactors, and carved or painted inscriptions recording their names, often appeared beside statues of the patron saint. Most were destroyed at the Dissolution, but enough evidence has survived to suggest that some were very imposing indeed.[11] Because of the threat represented by Scottish raiding parties and other marauders, St Giles's, Kepier, maintained stout defences. The arms of Bishop Bury (d.1345), who built the gateway with its vaulted entrance, and Edmund Howard, master during the early 1340s, presented a stern reminder to potential assailants that the house lay under the protection of the prince bishop of Durham himself.[12] Although the Savoy palace had been sacked by rebels in 1381, the magnificent hospital built on the site by Henry VII and his executors needed no such fortifications. The great gateway, which bore an inscription recording Henry's generosity to the poor, gave easy access to the precinct. The hundred paupers admitted by the matron and master each evening then proceeded towards the 'middle tower', where a display of royal arms and Tudor badges (the rose and portcullis) left the illiterate in no doubt as to the identity of their benefactor.[13] As we shall see, the interior of the hospital presented an even more aggressive display of

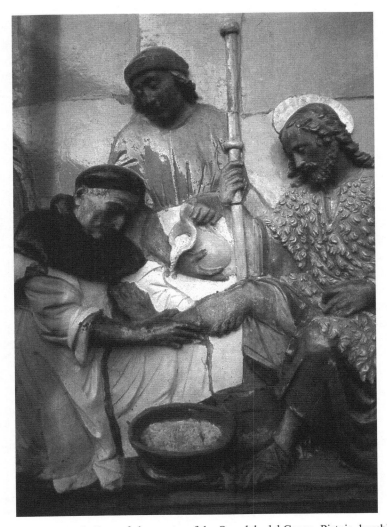

Figure 6.1 Leonardo Buonafede, master of the Ospedale del Ceppo, Pistoia, humbly washes the feet of Christ, who appears as a weary pilgrim in search of hospitality. This striking frieze, which Buonafede commissioned in 1514 for the loggia he had just added to the hospital, depicts each of the Seven Comfortable Works in sequence, with Buonafede himself as principal donor. As well as advertising his personal devotion to the sick poor and munificence as a patron, the façade reflects the combination of charity and reciprocity that underpinned all medieval hospitals.
(School of World Art Studies Picture Library, University of East Anglia)

Tudor propaganda, which served to dispel any misgivings about the future of an initially insecure dynasty and counteract King Henry's notorious reputation for meanness.

One of his mother's kinsmen, the ambitious and mercenary Cardinal Beaufort, had also spent his last years planning, or more accurately redesigning, a hospital. The 'house of noble poverty' which he attached to the twelfth-century foundation of St Cross, Winchester, was conceived on a scale commensurate with his wealth, power and, quite possibly, apprehension at the fate awaiting him after death. He was, after all, said to have acquired his great fortune through usury. The massive three-storey gatehouse was completed just before his last visit in 1446–7, when he may well have contemplated his own stone effigy, kneeling in prayer in one of the three niches at the top.[14] His arms and those of the crown (he was great-uncle to Henry VI, for whom his thirty-five almsmen were also to pray) were carved in the spandrels of the outer gateway, where poor travellers queued each day for hospitality. The most treasured of his earthly possessions, the cardinal's hat which had cost so much political manoeuvring to acquire, appears in the moulding above, and, significantly, in the stained glass of the adjacent hall.[15] In the words of his most recent biographer, Beaufort 'had full confidence in the hierarchies of this world and their ability to influence those of the next', a belief which found expression in this ambitious architectural venture.[16]

At its most basic, the purchase of intercessionary prayers could be reduced to a straightforward monetary transaction. As Nicolas Rolin (1380–1461), chancellor to the duke of Burgundy, and builder of the Hôtel-Dieu in Beaune, recognised, a shrewd investment in the physical and spiritual welfare of the sick poor secured the *salus*, or eternal health, of the rich. Suffused with the language of commerce, the preamble to his foundation charter of 1443 describes a project undertaken 'in the interest of my salvation, so that by a happy transaction I may trade celestial merchandise against the earthly goods which I owe to divine bounty, and thus render the perishable eternal'.[17] But were matters quite so simple? For all but the elect, a speedy passage through purgatory required *post mortem* commemoration, as well as evidence of a charitable life. How best could the medieval benefactor achieve a *lasting* memorial? The inscription of names in hospital martyrologies and obit rolls, the compilation of cartularies recording donations made in return for perpetual intercession, and the frequent recitation of statutes, specifically framed by founders to provide spiritual services, perpetuated the memory of generations of medieval philanthropists.[18]

Stone inscriptions, prominently displayed, offered a more permanent and conspicuous memorial than parchment. The great gateway of one of Europe's most imposing hospitals, built on the citadel of Rhodes by the Knights of St John, is surmounted by a testimonial to the generosity of its first patron. Beneath the arms of the Grand Master, Antoine de Fluvian (1421–37), is a marble plaque recording his gift of 10,000 crowns, which made the enterprise possible. On the painted doors below (now removed) and throughout the building visitors could admire the heraldic devices of other knights, whose largesse brought Fluvian's scheme to completion.[19] Fewer people may have attended the chapel of the leper house dedicated to St Mary Magdalen outside Bath, but here, too, a master sought commemoration. An inscription in the porch, in English rather than Latin, solicits prayers for the soul of Prior John Cantlow, who repaired the dilapidated buildings in the 1490s:[20]

> Thys chapelle florysschyd with formosyte spectabyll
> In the honowre of Magdalen prior Cantlow hathe edyfyd,
> Desyring yow to pray for hym with yowre prayers delectabyll,
> That suche wyll inhabyt hym in hevyn ther evyr to abyd.

But was the written record, however durable, enough? Images offered a more permanent *aide mémoire*, easily understood by literate and illiterate alike. They served, moreover, not only to inspire gratitude in the beholder, but also to proclaim the patron's sense of civic responsibility. The casual viewer would be more easily impressed by his or her careful stewardship of wealth for the greater good, by the antiquity of a noble line or by the new found wealth of an ambitious *arriviste*, anxious to leave a mark in society.[21]

One such *arriviste* was Chancellor Rolin, whose magnificent hospital is as much an expression of earthly power as it is of the desire for celestial reward, although, if Louis XI was right, he had beggared so many people through extortion that it was his moral duty to care for them in adversity.[22] And Rolin did, indeed, fear the eternal torments of hell, so vividly depicted in the magnificent Last Judgement, commissioned by him from the Flemish artist, Roger van der Weyden, for the hospital in the 1440s. In their closed state, which is how the patients in the *salle des pauvres* would normally have seen them, the central panels of the altarpiece contain portraits of Rolin and his third wife, Guigone de Salins, with angels displaying their respective coats of arms on shields (Fig. 6.2). These arms, along with other heraldic trappings, appeared throughout the hospital, disseminating the very same message. A striking touch of verisimilitude is achieved by painting the couple in vibrant colour, while the healing saints before whom they kneel appear as statues in grisaille.[23] It would have been harder for viewers to detect the likenesses of various benefactors among the celestial company on either side of Christ, when the altarpiece was open, but the fact that some of the intercessionary saints bear the features of Pope Eugenius IV, the duke and duchess of Burgundy, Rolin and his wives and children is an established local tradition widely accepted by art historians today.[24]

In many institutions it was the senior staff who provided painters, sculptors and carvers with commissions in which they themselves were depicted next to their patron saints. One of the most famous examples of hospital art in pre-Reformation northern Europe, the towering retable executed by Mathis Grünewald for the Antonines at Isenheim in about 1515, was designed to frame an unfinished carved wooden shrine. This had been ordered by a previous master (d.1490), easily identifiable as the small wooden donor figure at the feet of St Augustine, whose order the house followed.[25] The sisters and brothers of St John's hospital, Bruges, were equally fortunate to secure the services of Hans Memling, who produced, *inter alios*, a spectacular new reliquary (1489) for the remains of St Ursula and her companions already in their possession and an altarpiece depicting the mystic marriage of St Katherine to Christ (1479). Both of these works, which were intended for the richly appointed and newly extended hospital chapel, contain portraits of the staff who commissioned them, including the prioress, Agnes Casembrood.[26] A more intimate triptych, painted in 1479 by the same artist for one of the side altars, was

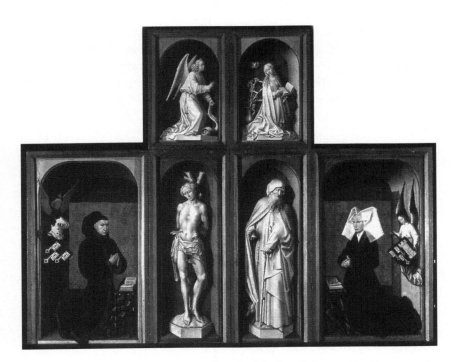

Figure 6.2 In its closed state, the great triptych of the Last Judgement by Roger van der Weyden (1440s) depicts the founder of the Hôtel Dieu, Beaune, Nicolas de Rolin, and his wife, Guigone de Salins. They are recognisable by their coats of arms, prominently displayed throughout the entire hospital. Their proximity to the Annunciation (above), when Christ became flesh, and to the healing saints Anthony (right) and Sebastian (left) enhances the power of this image, which would have been clearly visible to the patients in the *salle des pauvres*. (Photograph by I.J. Michot, Beaune)

favoured by Jan Floreins, a brother (and future master) of the hospital, who appears kneeling, to the right of the central panel, as a pious spectator of the Adoration of the Magi. Significantly, in its closed state, the frame of his altarpiece displays the coat of arms of Floreins's most illustrious kinsmen, the lords of Rijst.[27]

It is worth pausing at this stage to reflect upon the power of the carved or painted image upon the medieval mind. During the later middle ages, the proliferation of high quality religious art had a striking impact upon devotional practices at all levels of society. For the sophisticated and literate, depictions of saints and sacred symbols constituted a valuable aid to spiritual development. They could, moreover, be used to provide moral guidance and a basic education for the young or unlettered, while, at the same time, inspiring intense devotion and underscoring the authority, wealth and majesty of the Church. But, as critics from both within and without the ecclesiastical establishment so often complained, veneration of the subject represented in stone or paint easily gave way to worship of the icon itself. The thousands of pilgrims who travelled across Europe to visit statues of the Virgin, miraculous crucifixes and other celebrated images did not always make this important theological distinction.[28] Close proximity to a disconcertingly lifelike saint, or, even better, Christ and his mother, gave the hospital patron a spiritual aura of his or her own. He or she could bask in the reflected glory of a celestial hierarchy of good lordship which, implicitly, shed its light upon the patients, their carers and other benefactors, too. The emphasis placed upon spiritual health in the medieval hospital meant, moreover, that religious iconography played a crucial part in the therapeutic process.[29] To commission images which inspired, soothed, enlightened or comforted was itself a charitable work, further augmenting the store of merit accruing to the men and women commemorated in them.

So far as we know, no English hospital possessed works to rival those still to be seen in Bruges or Beaune, although the wholesale destruction of religious iconography and hospital records at the Dissolution now makes it impossible to tell. Surviving documentary evidence reveals, however, that even quite modest houses were profusely decorated: at the most basic level, lengths of 'stenyd' or painted canvas (rather like stage scenery) were hung in wards and infirmary chapels, and wall painting must have been common. Traces survive, for example, at the Commandery, Worcester, which boasted a Last Judgement, at St Mark's, Bristol, where a complex and theologically sophisticated iconographic programme was executed, and at *leprosaria* at Harbledown, outside Canterbury, and Wimborne in Dorset.[30] That they once displayed the arms and portraits of patrons seems more than likely, as does the incorporation of these images in the liturgy of intercession and commemoration. Benefactors of the Saffron Walden almshouse in Essex were remembered in daily prayers which called down blessings upon them. 'May their names be written in the book of life with the just and chosen', ran the invocation, 'and in the day of tremendous judgement they shall come finally together among the sons of God'.[31] Such a striking eschatological image, which draws upon scenes of the Last Judgement described in the Book of Revelation, lent itself especially well to iconography.

It is tempting to speculate that the artists who decorated this almshouse and the chapels of other English hospitals and *maisons Dieu* deployed the type of schema adopted in the 1320s at the Heilig Geist Spital in Lübeck. Here Christ appears in Majesty, the book of life open in his left hand, the emblems of the four Evangelists at his head and feet (Fig. 6.3). In a semicircle around him are twelve coats of arms and twelve medallions (a suitably apostolic number) bearing the names and portraits of benefactors. Each roundel is encircled with the legend '+ *orate pro eo*', and, in the case of one Englebert Kruse, the further appeal, '+ *miserere mei Deus secum magnam misericordiam tuam*'.[32] Before its restoration, a late thirteenth-century wall painting of Christ in Majesty, surrounded by similar emblems, in the hall of St Thomas's hospital, Canterbury, was surmounted by a partially visible coat of arms; and although scenes from the life of Becket appear, appropriately enough, to have been depicted below, there is every likelihood that archiepiscopal and other influential connexions were advertised here as well.[33]

Dominating an altar in the north-eastern corner of the hospital church, the Lübeck fresco served the same purpose as the *tabula* which stood over the high altar at the Sherburn leper hospital, County Durham, from 1434 onwards. Bearing the names of Bishops Le Puiset and Kellaw, it prompted the officiating priest to commend them

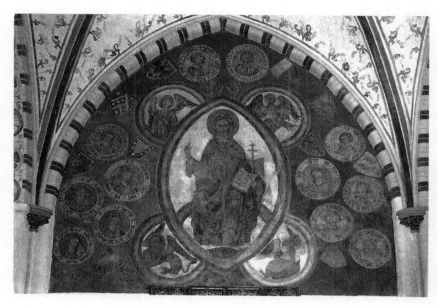

Figure 6.3 The north-east wall of the church of the Heilig Geist Spital, Lübeck, is dominated by a painting of Christ in Majesty, surrounded by portraits of twelve of the principal benefactors and their coats of arms (*c*. 1320). Such imagery, replete with apostolic overtones, served as a reminder of the scale of their generosity, as well as their anxiety about the life to come. Each roundel bears the name of the donor, together with an appeal for intercessionary prayer. (Photograph by Carole Rawcliffe)

especially to God every time he celebrated Mass (and to remind his congregation of their obligations, too).[34] At the *maison Dieu* in Hull erected by the alderman, John Gregg, and his wife, in 1414, there hung 'two antient tables', one bearing the regulations and the other pictures of the couple alongside their redeemer, to whom the house was dedicated. During Queen Elizabeth's reign the portraits were defaced, and the ordinances rewritten not only to forbid recourse to images but also to remove any reference to the arduous round of suffrages previously required of the almsfolk by their benefactors.[35] Examples such as these help us to understand why so many English hospitals fell victim to the sweeping doctrinal changes of the sixteenth century. As Cardinal William Allen was to argue with such vigour, the patrons 'of all noble foundacions [...] euer sithe the first daie of oure happy calling to Christes faithe' had insisted 'that theire worke of almose and deuotion was for this one especiall respect, to be prayde and songe for, as they call it, after theire deathes'.[36]

Nor was this type of memorial confined to single individuals. As we have already seen in the case of Whittington's almshouse, many European hospitals were managed by mercantile and craft guilds, which paid handsomely for collective commemoration. At the London hospital of St Thomas Acon, the Mercers invested heavily in the construction of a guild chapel, whose lavish decor reflected the commercial success and political influence of one of the City's most powerful companies. Two crests and four retables (two small, two large) were commissioned from a local painter in 1449, along with appropriate hangings. The overall effect must have been sumptuous.[37] In a far homelier, but no less telling, juxtaposition of images, the bakers and shoemakers of Obernai, near Strasbourg, commissioned two panels of a new retable (1508) for the hospital of Saint Erhard. Presumably on their instructions, the artist, Hans Hag, painted their arms next to pictures of saints giving bread, clothing and money to the poor. The message can hardly have escaped the sick, barefoot and hungry paupers, for whom the hospital had been founded two centuries before.[38]

The decorative scheme at Gregg's almshouse may well have been known to Alice Chaucer, duchess of Suffolk, who arranged in 1462 for the Carthusians of Hull to acquire 'two stone images' of herself and the duke bearing jugs and dishes as a symbol of their generosity to the poor. It was before these statues of their earthly benefactors that the monks were to distribute meals to two poor almsfolk every day.[39] Herself something of a *parvenue*, whose family, like that of her third husband, hailed from the purple of commerce, Alice was as anxious to assert her aristocratic connexions as she was to advertise her Christian compassion. She was buried in a tomb of regal proportions in the almshouse which she and the duke built at Ewelme, in Oxfordshire (Fig. 6.4). As a condition of entry, the bedesmen were obliged to pray beside it every day for the founders' salvation, the magnificent display of heraldry above contrasting sharply with the harrowing effigy of the duchess's cadaver which would have been visible to them as they knelt at their devotions.[40] If they did not always command the financial resources of the de la Poles, the founders and patrons who sought burial in their hospitals none the less demanded the best memorial possible. In death, as in life, humility fought an unequal contest with pride. A fine tomb or incised brass proclaimed the rank, wealth and munificence of the departed, while serving as a focus for intercessionary prayers.

Some patrons were remarkably specific on this score. John Clapham, master and generous benefactor of Knolles's almshouse, Pontefract, demanded in his will of 1494 that two of the choristers whom he had undertaken to support should recite the *de profundis* and *collecta fidelium* each day for the benefit of his parents' souls while actually standing upon his tomb slab ('*super tumulum meum stantes*') in the chancel.[41] Burial near an altar where the Mass was celebrated, and where they could thus enjoy close physical proximity to the redemptive body and blood of Christ, was an understandable preoccupation of many benefactors. It was for 'the singuler comforth and gostly releff' of his sinful soul that Thomas, seventh earl of Ormonde, requested burial beneath the Easter sepulchre in the church of the hospital of St Thomas Acon, to which he and his family had long proved generous patrons. The earl clearly hoped to derive spiritual benefit from the most solemn liturgy of the ecclesiastical year, and testamentary bequests in the order of at least £126 ensured that his wishes would be carried out.[42]

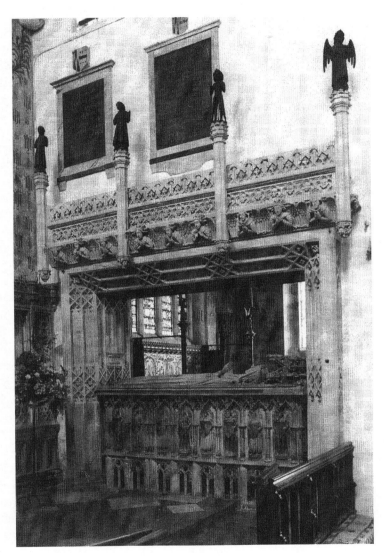

Figure 6.4 The spectacular alabaster tomb of the founder, Alice Chaucer, duchess of Suffolk, is the most prominent feature of the church of God's House at Ewelme, Oxfordshire. It provided a focus for the prayers of the almsmen, who were required to intercede here daily for the salvation of their patron. Erected in 1470–75, it represents a notable investment in personal commemoration, not least because of its emphasis upon her aristocratic and royal connections. (National Monuments Record)

The open ward hospitals of medieval Europe were designed specifically so that patients could see, or at least hear, the celebration of the Eucharist. The basic plan (subject to considerations of space and topography) comprised a chapel at the east end, often, as we have already seen, profusely decorated with religious and heraldic imagery. Tombs or memorial slabs placed strategically before the high altar thus became a pronounced architectural feature in their own right and served to focus the devotions of clergy and patients. Following the example of her saintly brother-in-law, Louis IX, and moved by 'a desire to merit the reward the Evangelist has promised us', the widowed Marguerite de Bourgogne, queen of Sicily (d.1308), founded the Hôpital des Fontenilles at Tonnerre, where she herself retired to nurse the sick poor. At the end of the barrel-vaulted infirmary (almost 100 metres long) she constructed an imposing and lofty polygonal apse, with side chapels, the structure as a whole offering a unique opportunity for personal commemoration. All but a few fragments of the 'vast ensemble of stained glass' have been destroyed, but we know that the portraits and arms of Marguerite and her late husband dominated the overwhelmingly secular glazing programme of the fifty or so windows. Her tomb, surmounted by a bronze effigy strikingly at odds with her epitaph as *'humilitatis speculum'* (mirror of humility), stood at the base of the high altar steps, and was thus the focal point of daily worship.[43] The tomb of Guigone de Salins (d.1470), who had fought to retain the patronage of the Hôtel Dieu, Beaune, after her husband's death and had eventually taken the veil as a sister there, occupied a similar position before the great altarpiece of the Last Judgement. There, in effigy, she appeared in widow's weeds, beside her late husband in full armour.[44]

In England, the tombs, chantry chapels and memorials of patrons proliferated at such a rate that some of the larger urban hospitals, such as St Mary's Bishopsgate, London, were obliged to move the patients elsewhere to cope with the demand for space.[45] Like many benefactors, the influential Yorkshire landowner, Sir Henry Pleasington (d.1452), who rented lodgings in the precinct of St Mary's, sought burial in a suitably prominent position next to the high altar, in a tomb chest decorated with his family's arms.[46] Betraying less ancestral pride but a similar concern for commemoration, the Londoner,

Thomas Acton (d.1489), another tenant and generous supporter of the hospital, asked that a tomb slab depicting his and his wife's shrouded bodies should be set next to the wall, beneath a marble relief[47]

> with two images graven in the latter: one of the Trinity and the other of Our Lady of The Assumption; and I myself, like death, kneeling with eight sons on one side before the Trinity, and my wife kneeling likewise with eight daughters on the other side before Our Lady of The Assumption.

The transformation of England's larger hospitals into liturgical centres for the Christian departed necessarily involved the acquisition of substantial collections of plate, illuminated service books and vestments, some of which are described in the surviving records, but almost all of which were lost during the doctrinal upheavals of the sixteenth century. The best documented instance of such investment concerns the massive outlay recorded between 1383 and 1407 by John Campeden, friend of the reforming bishop of Winchester, William Wykeham, and master of the hospital of St Cross.[48] He was buried beneath a fine memorial brass in the crossing of the hospital church which he had greatly enlarged and refurbished to provide a worthy setting for the commemoration of the dead, including, of course, himself.[49] Both he and Wykeham relied upon the generosity of others to augment the hospital's store of liturgical equipment, but less fortunate houses were totally dependent upon such patronage. Many gifts displayed the arms, monograms and mottoes of donors who wished to associate themselves with and further embellish the ritual of the Mass. As late as 1528 Henry Plumstede left a vestment of white damask embroidered with his initials to St Mary's hospital, Yarmouth, hoping, no doubt, that each time the letters became fully visible to the congregation at the elevation of the Host, his soul would progress a little faster through purgatory.[50]

Patrons used a variety of media, including stained glass, to establish personal connections with the incarnate body of Christ, the Physician of their souls. Among the most striking English examples is the juxtaposition of the rebus of William Browne (d.1489), a wealthy wool merchant and founder of the eponymous almshouse in Stamford, with Marian and Christological imagery of remarkable subtlety (Fig.

6.5). Glass was an extremely popular, although sadly perishable, vehicle for commemoration, and Browne was clearly not unusual in exploiting its potential for heraldic display throughout his foundation. It also admitted light, the *lux aeternam* invoked in the requiem masses sung and said daily in charitable institutions across Europe. The gradual of the Lady Mass in the Sarum Rite (widely followed in English hospitals) compared the Virgin to a pane of glass, the *fenestra caeli*, through which the Holy Ghost passed as a sunbeam at the moment of Christ's Conception. One of the panels in the chapel of Browne's almshouse depicts this moment; and, although the complex iconographic scheme deployed throughout the building has suffered too much damage and rearrangement to permit any convincing interpretation, there can be no doubt that, like the duchess of Suffolk, Browne and his relatives envisaged it as a soteriological exercise for their own personal benefit. How far did his almsmen understand the theological implications of what they saw? Did they, perhaps, confuse the stork which Browne adopted as a device (his wife came from the Stokke family) with the dove of the Holy Ghost fluttering in the chapel windows? Never one to do good by stealth, Browne could at least reassure himself that future generations would remember his bounty.[51]

Protestant iconoclasm was not, however, the only threat to the survival of painted glass. The refurbishment of the chapel of the hospital of the Holy Trinity, York, in the 1490s gave rise to what might be termed a 'glazing war' between successive masters, as each sought to outdo the other. The struggle to secure a lasting – and more imposing – memorial reached a climax in 1501, when John Gillot apparently replaced one of his rival's windows altogether, in a gesture which, at the very least, aimed to establish his superior wealth and status. Since the hospital was run by the city's most prosperous guild, the battle for commemoration may have been waged with particular intensity, but is unlikely to have been unique.[52]

The richer the patron, the better placed he or she was to call the tune. At the Florentine hospital of Santa Maria Nuova, founded in the late thirteenth century by the mercantile dynasty of Portinari, the display of arms or insignia belonging to any other 'person, organisa-

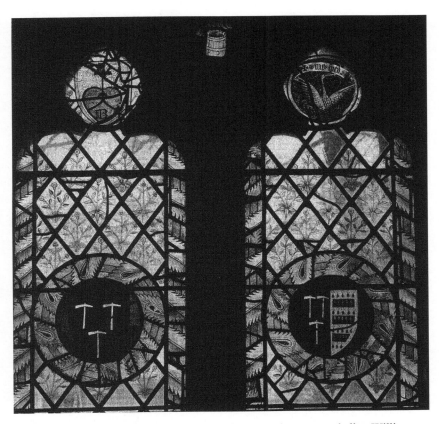

Figure 6.5 Early sixteenth-century stained glass in the entrance hall to William Browne's almshouse, Stamford, displays the founder's coat of arms (bottom left), along with those of the Stokke and Elmes families (bottom right), to whom he was related by marriage. In roundels above, an image of the Sacred Heart (left) is juxtaposed with the rebus of the stork (Stokke) and the legend 'Christ me sped[e]', leaving the viewer in no doubt as to the identity of the patron or his piety. Thomas Stokke, Browne's brother-in-law, ran the hospital after his death in 1489, and was no less anxious to secure a lasting memorial. (National Monuments Record)

tion, guild or corporation' was expressly prohibited in the statutes. Exceptions were sometimes made for those who were rich enough to purchase visual commemoration, but one suspects the charge was high.[53] It is worth noting that the great retable of the *Adoration of the Magi* by Hugo van der Goes, which dominated the hospital church from 1483 onwards, is generally known as the *Portinari Altarpiece*, after the patron, Tommaso Portinari, who appears along with his family in the side panels.[54] Santa Maria Nuova served as a model for the Savoy, which, as we have seen, was planned on a far more ambitious scale than any of its English medieval precursors. The hospital positively blossomed with Tudor roses, which climbed riotously over the masonry, erupted on bedspreads, clung to the poor men's uniforms and even bloomed on the nurses' bosoms. The stained glass, which must have been magnificent, depicted the Last Judgement and the Crucifixion as well as numerous saints, Henry's arms appearing prominently not only in the windows but also held aloft by a host of carved wooden angels. The glazed lantern over the crossing of the cruciform dormitory was surmounted by 'a grete Crowne Imperiall of ij fote and xviij ynches' supported by heraldic beasts, which proclaimed Henry's patronage across the rooftops of London. One did not even have to visit the hospital to be impressed by his generosity, as its seal, used to authenticate all legal documents and administrative records, bore the stamp of the Tudor rose and Beaufort portcullis.[55]

The combination of writing and image made seals a particularly useful vehicle for the transmission of a variety of sacred and secular messages, not least because they helped 'to bridge the gap between the literate and the non-literate'.[56] As might be expected, hospital seals often incorporated the arms or badge of the founder, sometimes alongside a depiction of the patron saint. Wealthy London hospitals, such as St Mary's Bishopsgate (Brune), and St Mary's Cripplegate (Elsing), followed this practice, as did the leper house at Burton Lazars, Leicestershire (Mowbray), the Ewelme almshouse (de la Pole and Chaucer) and the pilgrim hospital at Billingsford in rural Norfolk (Beck). The seal of the Trinity hospital, York, reflected the maritime interests of its patrons, the Merchant Adventurers, with a striking depiction of the ships which kept it financially afloat.[57] Like the heraldic devices worn by brethren and staff, hospital seals were, above all, a statement of authority and corporate identity, signalling to the outside world that the user or wearer enjoyed powerful protection. In lay society, badges proclaimed the ties of allegiance and mutual dependence between lord and retainer, often in a quasi-military context. The staff of St Mark's hospital, Bristol, who sported the badge of the founder, William Gaunt (three white geese, or 'gaunts' against a red background) on their outer clothing at all times, were, in a very real sense, his liveried servants, fighting a spiritual battle for his soul in return for their board and lodging. As they distributed bread each day to indigent paupers outside the hospital gateway (which undoubtedly bore the same image), they left passers-by in no doubt that Bristol's open-handed elite would be spared the fate of Dives.[58]

Yet Gaunt did not enjoy a monopoly of advertising space. Older foundations, like St Mark's, were profusely decorated with the arms and images of a motley and constantly expanding crowd of benefactors. The wholesale destruction of the fabric as well as the contents of most English hospitals makes it easy to forget how ubiquitous this practice was, and, indeed, the extent to which they were tied into a complex network of earthly as well as spiritual 'good lordship'. Given the number of predators, both lay and religious, with designs upon the assets of vulnerable institutions, the search for protection is understandable. It began at the top, with the monarchy. A royal connection bestowed tremendous *cachet* upon provincial hospitals such as St Giles's, Norwich, which enlisted Richard II's support in 1383 for the completion of its costly rebuilding programme. In return, the new chancel, designed to provide more space for burials and the elaborate liturgical spectacle which patrons now demanded, was roofed with 252 stencilled panels bearing the arms of Richard's queen, Anne of Bohemia (the church of the Savoy had a mere 138, displaying Tudor and Lancastrian heraldic badges, carved in pear-wood). His generosity almost certainly prompted other donations, but the benefits were not entirely one-sided. As well as reminding every priest and chorister to pray for the queen's soul each time he raised his eyes to heaven, this imposing eyrie of Imperial eagles broadcast Richard's marriage into the house of Habsburg, which he was keen to advertise.[59] The hospital could, meanwhile, bask in the warm glow of royal approval.

In the same fashion, patrons of lesser rank seized the opportunity to make the most of their own links with the crown. The courtier, Sir Robert Poyntz (d.1520), decorated the fan-vaulted ceiling of his chantry chapel at St Mark's hospital, Bristol, not only with his family's arms, but those of Henry VIII, Catherine of Aragon, whose vice-chamberlain and chancellor he had been, and of his wife, who was the illegitimate niece of Edward IV's queen, Elizabeth Wood-ville.[60] Wishing to honour the memory of his own royal patron, the Lady Margaret Beaufort, mother of Henry VII, Thomas Denman (d.1500–1) left jewellery, plate and vestments bearing her various badges to the Bethlehem hospital, London, of which he had been master, and where he asked to be buried.[61] The elaborately engraved vessels used in the Mass offered donors, such as the above-mentioned John Clapham, a particular opportunity to shine, literally as well as figuratively. Once again, they could achieve symbolic proximity to the body and blood of Christ, while impressing the assembled congregation with their munificence. Since the Mass, with its promise of spiritual as well as physical healing, stood at the very heart of hospital life, it might indeed be argued that the gift of an emblazoned chalice or pyx was the supreme act of patronage, relegating all others to second place. A collecting plate or almsdish, such as that presented to St John's hospital, Sandwich, in about 1418 by one Christina Pikefysch, likewise placed the donor at the centre of another important ritual. Displaying her image (complete with purse), and calling down Christ's blessing upon her soul, the silver dish effectively made all acts of charity to the hospital her own.[62]

Any historian attempting to disentangle, let alone rank, the motives of medieval benefactors is, in the final resort, bent upon an anachronistic and essentially fruitless task. Just as earthly and spiritual therapeutics merged together seamlessly in the hospital infirmary, so the search for salvation was conducted according to the codes and values of a quasi-feudal and intensely hierarchical society, in which the material trappings of wealth and power assumed overriding importance. No corporate institution could afford to ignore these rules, and it is ironic that the most successful English hospitals were the ones to suffer particular depredations at the hands of Protestant iconoclasts. Less worthy – but even less tangible – considerations of personal ambition, hubris and vulgar display must also be taken into account. Snobbery and one-upmanship can always be concealed under a veneer of civic responsibility and pious intent. In this respect, many medieval hospitals can hardly have differed from the Ospedale Maggiore, Genoa, which the penal reformer, John Howard, visited in 1786. The benefactors, he observed, [63]

> are distinguished by the different postures and attitudes in which their statues are placed, in the wards, and on the staircase, according to the different sums which they have contributed. Many are placed standing; but an hundred thousand crowns entitles to a chair [...] I was well informed that some have hurt their families through the ambition of having their statues placed in this hospital.

They were heirs to an enduring tradition.

Notes

1   Dante Alighieri, *Hell*, trans. S. Ellis (London, 1994), pp.101–4.

2   W. Nelson Francis (ed.), *The Book of Vices and Virtues*, Early English Text Society, original series, 217 (1942), p.204.

3   E.M. Goulburn and H. Symonds (eds), *The Life, Letters and Sermons of Bishop Herbert de Losinga*, 2 vols (Oxford, 1878), 2, pp.242–7.

4   Discussed at greater length in C. Rawcliffe, *Medicine for the Soul: The Life, Death and Resurrection of a Medieval English Hospital* (Stroud, 1999), ch. 4.

5   J. Roskell, L. Clark and C. Rawcliffe, *The History of Parliament: The House of Commons 1386–1421*, 4 vols (Stroud, 1992), 4, pp.846–9.

6   J. Imray, *The Charity of Richard Whittington* (London, 1968), p.109.

7   Reproduced in Imray, *Charity of Richard Whittington*, facing p.56.

8   N. Kerling (ed.), *Cartulary of St Bartholomew's Hospital* (London, 1973), pp.175–6.

9   See, for example, N. Zemon Davis, *The Gift in Sixteenth-Century France* (Oxford, 2000), pp.23–6.

10   F.G.A. Amendola, *Il Fregio robbiano dell'Ospedale del Ceppo a Pistoia* (Pistoia, 1982), figs 57–68, 54–6, 69–70.

11   The practice, bereft of its intercessionary function, continued in Protestant England. The external decoration of Tudor and Stuart almshouses proclaimed the social consciences and civic virtues of founders, together with their pride in

old lineage or new money. Indeed, as portraiture and the use of emblems developed during the Renaissance, some institutions boasted elaborate displays of
monograms, effigies, mottoes and heraldic imagery: E. Prescott, *The English
Medieval Hospital 1050–1640* (Melksham, 1992), pp.85, 94–8, 109–10, 115–
19, 124, 126, 128, 130–2, 148–50, 153–4, 156, 162–6.

12   D.M. Meade, *Kepier Hospital* (Durham, 1995), pp.21–3.

13   H.M. Colvin (ed.), *The King's Works, III, 1485–1660* (London, 1975), pp.196–
206.

14   K.B. McFarlane, *England in the Fifteenth Century* (London, 1981), pp.115–37;
G.L. Harriss, *Cardinal Beaufort: A Study in Lancastrian Ascendancy and
Decline* (Oxford, 1988), pp.370–1. One of the now empty niches would prob-
ably have contained a statue of the hospital's original founder, Bishop Henry de
Blois, and the other a cross: W.T. Warren, *Official Guide to St Cross Hospital*,
5th edn (Winchester, n.d.), pp.18, 42.

15   G. Goldin, *Works of Mercy: A Picture History of Hospitals* (Boston Mills,
1994), pp.112–13; McFarlane, *England in the Fifteenth Century*, pp.79–113.
His almsmen wore striking gowns in cardinal red, with a badge displaying the
controversial hat: N. Orme and M. Webster, *The English Hospital 1070–1570*
(New Haven and London, 1995), pp.125–6.

16   Harriss, *Cardinal Beaufort*, p.381.

17   A. Perier, *Nicolas Rolin 1380–1461* (Paris, 1904), p.370; E. Bavard and
J.B. Boudrot, *L'Hôtel Dieu de Beaune* (Beaune, 1881), pp.7–8.

18   C. Rawcliffe, 'Passports to Paradise: How English Medieval Hospitals and
Almshouses Kept their Archives', *Archives*, 27 (2002), pp.2–22.

19   E. Kollias, *The Knights of Rhodes: The Palace and the City* (Athens, 2003),
pp.120–6.

20   J. Manco, *The Spirit of Care: The Eighth-Hundred-Year Story of St John's
Hospital, Bath* (Bath, 1998), pp.46–7.

21   C. Richmond, 'Religion', in R. Horrox (ed.), *Fifteenth Century Attitudes*
(Cambridge, 1984), pp.183–201, at p.198, thus categorises Thomas, Lord
Burgh's imposing almshouse at Gainsborough.

22   N. Veronee-Verhaegen, *L'Hôtel-Dieu de Beaune*, Les Primitifs Flamands, 13
(Brussels, 1973), p.63.

23   *Ibid.*, pp.46–50, 58–9, 61, plates I, II, CXLV–LXI. See also P. Jugie and
D. Sécula, 'L'Hôtel-Dieu de Beaune revisité', in F.O. Touati (ed.), *Archéologie
et architecture hospitalières de l'antiquité tardive à l'aube des temps modernes*
(Paris, 2004), pp.231–57.

24   Veronee-Verhaegen, *Les Primitifs Flamands, XIII*, pp.38–40, 74.

25   A. Hayum, *The Isenheim Altarpiece: God's Medicine and the Painter's Vision*
(Princeton, 1987), plate 1 and pp.15–16. The masters of medieval hospitals
must often have been depicted in the chapels where they had worshipped. At St
Giles's, Norwich, John Hecker (d.*c*.1532) commissioned a set of exquisitely

carved bench-ends, one bearing his initials, another depicting him at prayer: Rawcliffe, *Medicine for the Soul*, p.131, plates 33–4.

26   D. de Vos, *Hans Memling* (Bruges, 1994), pp.72–9, 138–46. In its closed state, the altarpiece, which stood on the high altar, depicted two hospital sisters on one wing and two brothers on the other with their patron saints.

27   De Vos, *Memling*, pp.80–3.

28   See generally, C. Dupeux, P. Jezler and J. Wirth (eds), *Iconoclasme: vie et mort de l'image médiévale* (Berne, 2001); and for pilgrims, D. Webb, *Pilgrimage in Medieval England* (London, 2000), pp.147–52, 242–8.

29   See, for example, J. Henderson, 'Healing the Body and Saving the Soul: Hospitals in Renaissance Florence', *Renaissance Studies*, 15 (2001), pp.188–216; C. Rawcliffe, 'Medicine for the Soul: The Medieval English Hospital and the Quest for Spiritual Health', in J.R. Hinnells and R. Porter (eds), *Religion, Health and Suffering* (London, 1999), pp.316–18.

30   M. Gill and H. Howard, 'Glimpses of Glory: Paintings from St Mark's Hospital, Bristol', in L. Keen (ed.), *Almost the Richest City: Bristol in the Middle Ages* (Bristol Archaeological Association Conference Transactions, 19, 1997), pp.97–106; Rawcliffe, *Medicine for the Soul*, p. 104; P.H. Newman, 'Notes on the Preservation of some Ancient Wall-Paintings', *Proceedings of the Society of Antiquaries*, 20 (1903–5), pp.41, 46. 'Stenyd' cloths are harder to document, but in 1499 the London hospital of St Anthony owned several: Archives of St George's Chapel, Windsor, MS XV.37.23. Three years later, the steward bought 'iij dosyn hokes grette and smalle to faste the wyre with to hange the clothys of saint antonis lyffe and the tabulls [painted wooden panels] in the chyrche': MS XV.37.25.

31   F.W. Steer, 'The Statutes of Saffron Walden Almshouses', *Transactions of the Essex Archaeological Society*, n.s., 25 (1955–60), pp.465–6. See C. Rawcliffe, 'Written in the Book of Life: Building the Libraries of Medieval English Hospitals and Almshouses', *The Library*, 7th ser., 3 (2002), pp.12–29, for a discussion of this imagery.

32   G. Schaumann, 'Das Heiligen-Geist-Hospital', in *Die Bau- und Kunstdenkmäler der Freien und Hansestadt* (Lübeck, 1906), pp.465–6; U. Pietsch, 'Die Wandmalereien in Heiligen-Geist-Hospial zu Lübeck', *Archäologie in Lübeck* (Lübeck, 1980), pp.74–5.

33   E.W. Tristram, *English Medieval Wall Painting: The Thirteenth Century*, 2 vols (Oxford, 1950), 1, pp.520–1; 2, plates 118–21, supplementary plate 49.

34   G. Allan, *Collections Relating [to] Sherburn Hospital in the County Palatinate of Durham* (1771, privately printed), unpaginated, sub 'Bishop Langley's Statutes'. The elicitation of prayers (sometimes in English) for leading benefactors during mass was common in hospital chapels: see, Rawcliffe, *Medicine for the Soul*, p.110; R.R. Sharpe (ed.), *Calendar of Wills Proved and Enrolled In the Court of Husting, London, 2, 1358–1688* (London, 1890), p.508.

35   W. Page (ed.), *Victoria History of the County of York*, 3 (London, 1913), pp.312–13.

36   William Allen, *A Defense and Declaration of the Catholike Churchies Doctrine Touching Purgatory* (John Latius, Antwerp, 1565), fos 132r–32v.

37   J. Watney, *Some Account of the Hospital of St Thomas Acon* (London, 1892), pp.37–8.

38   Dupeux, Jezler and Wirth, *Iconoclasme*, p.202.

39   J.A.A. Goodall, *God's House at Ewelme* (Aldershot, 2001), pp.273–7.

40   Goodall, *God's House*, pp.175–97, and pp.234–7 for the prayers.

41   J. Raine (ed.), *Testamenta Eboracum*, 4 (Surtees Society, 53, 1869), pp.93–4.

42   TNA, London, PROB 11/18 [old style PCC, Holder 8].

43   M.P. Lillich, *The Queen of Sicily and Gothic Glass in Mussy and Tonnerre* (*Transactions of the American Philosophical Society*, 88.3, 1998), pp.68–95, 112. Although somewhat fanciful, M. Viollet-le-Duc, *Dictionaire raisonné de l'architecture française*, 10 vols (Paris, 1868), 6, pp.109–11, provides a useful guide to the layout of this hospital. See also, Goldin, *Works of Mercy*, pp.34–5, and eadem and J.D. Thompson, *The Hospital: A Social and Architectural History* (London and New York, 1975), pp.22–3.

44   Perier, *Nicolas Rolin*, p.378; Bavard and Boudrot, *L'Hôtel Dieu*, pp.83–94.

45   C. Thomas, B. Sloane and C. Phillpotts, *Excavations at the Priory and Hospital of St Mary Spital, London* (Museum of London Archaeology Service, 1997), pp.45, 65–6, 80, 82–3, 94–5, 119–22.

46   Roskell, Clark and Rawcliffe, *House of Commons 1386–1421*, 4, pp.86–8; TNA, PROB 11/1/17 [old style PCC, 17 Rous]. Such requests were common in smaller hospitals, too. See, for example, Manco, *The Spirit of Care*, p.24.

47   This spot appears to have become the site of a family chantry: Thomas, Sloane and Phillpotts, *Hospital of St Mary Spital*, pp.79, 80, 123.

48   The total outlay of £1,980 is itemised in British Library, Additional MS 39976, fos 80r–91r. See Rawcliffe, 'Building the Libraries', pp.150–1, for the use of books to advertise patronage.

49   Prescott, *English Medieval Hospital*, pp.30–3.

50   TNA, PROB 11/22 [old style PCC, Porche 33].

51   *Royal Commission on Historical Monuments: The Town of Stamford* (London, 1977), pp.37–42, plates 36–7, 39; R. Marks, *Stained Glass in England during the Middle Ages* (London, 1993), pp.85, 102, figs 82, 170; A. Breeze, 'The Blessed Virgin and the Sunbeam through Glass', *Celtica*, 23 (1999), pp.19–29.

52   K. Giles, *An Archaeology of Social Identity: Guildhalls in York, c. 1350–1630*, British Archaeological Reports, British Series, 315 (2000), p.71.

53   K. Park and J. Henderson, '"The First Hospital among Christians": The Ospedale di Santa Maria Nuova in Early Sixteenth-Century Florence', *Medical History*, 35 (1991), p.185.

54   F. Winkler, *Das Werk des Hugo Van der Goes* (Berlin, 1964), pp.23–36, plates 12–21; Henderson, 'Healing the Body', pp.199–203.

55   Colvin, *King's Works*, 3, pp.204, 206; R. Somerville, *The Savoy* (London, 1960), pp.15–16, 18, 30–1, 33.

56   M.T. Clanchy, *From Memory to Written Record: England 1066–1307* (Oxford, 1999), pp.308–17.

57   W. de G. Birch, *Catalogue of Seals in the Department of Manuscripts in the British Museum*, 6 vols (London, 1887–1900), 1, respectively nos 3541, 3542, 2789, 3120, 2625, 4408.

58   Ross, *Cartulary of St Mark's*, pp.8–9. For the political aspects of the medieval badge, see N. Saul, 'The Commons and the Abolition of Badges', *Parliamentary History*, 9 (1990), pp.302–15. See also note 13, above.

59   N. Saul, *Richard II* (London, 1997), pp.83–95; Rawcliffe, *Medicine for the Soul*, pp.115–19, plate 28, and ch. 5, passim, for a full discussion of the importance of political patronage to the medieval hospital. It is interesting to note the steps taken in about 1430 by the hospital of the Holy Spirit, Dijon, to commemorate its foundation by Eudes, duke of Burgundy in 1204, and to consolidate its close connection with Duke Philip the Good. A profusely illuminated *charte de fondation* shows the latter visiting the wards with his wife and courtiers: J-P. Lecat, *Le siècle de la Toison d'Or* (Paris, 1986), p.34.

60   Prescott, *English Medieval Hospital*, pp.36–9; *The Oxford Dictionary of National Biography*, 60 vols (Oxford, 2004), 45, pp.195–6.

61   Canterbury Chapter Library, Cathedral Priory Register F, fos 25r–25v.

62   Orme and Webster, *English Hospital*, p.57.

63   J. Howard, *An Account of the Principal Lazarettos in Europe* (London, 1791), p.57.

CHRISTINE STEVENSON

Chapter 7: Prints 'proper to shew to Gentlemen': Representing the British Hospital, *c.* 1700–50

In 1749, the Earl of Chesterfield wrote to his son, then aged seventeen and visiting Berlin.[1] As was his custom, the Earl advised the boy on how to derive greater advantage from his travels than other young men did:

> For instance, if they see a public building, as a college, an hospital, an arsenal, etc., they content themselves with the first *coup d'oeil*, and neither take the time nor trouble of informing themselves of the material parts of them, which are the constitution, the rules, and the order and economy in the inside.[2]

This is one way to look at hospitals: at a glance. Their fabrics do not, in themselves, deserve much more attention than that, because hospitals' real, 'material parts' are, paradoxically, the immaterial ones: the rules, the economy.

Chesterfield also warned his son that gentlemen who took too much interest in architecture risked sinking to the level of workmen or (worse) to that of the 'virtuosi'.[3] Yet for many British gentlefolk some knowledge of construction was no shame, and might even be a mark of distinction. In 1755, for example, when the Middlesex Hospital in London was seeking an architect, one of its governors wrote to the Earl of Northumberland, the hospital's President, and asked for his advice; because, as he explained, the members of the Middlesex's building committee were 'not builders', that is, not experienced patrons.[4]

The present essay surveys a body of work that has received little attention:[5] printed pictures of British hospitals that were more or less directly employed in efforts to raise funds and other support in the first half of the eighteenth century. It advances two hypotheses. The first is, that these charities, and their audiences, ascribed significance to the forms as well as to the contents of the prints; that the graphic conventions were themselves meaningful to (say) the members of the Middlesex building committee. The second is that the pictures could convey information about the hospitals' architecture that narrative texts did not, or could not. (By 'narrative' texts I mean records like sermons, institutional histories, and governors' minutes, as opposed to the letterpress in tables or images.) This is not to make a semiotic claim, merely a statement of fact: the dearth of references in the written record from before 1770 or so confirms that whatever medical instrumentality the English then attributed to the architecture, they did not write about it, at least not directly. (The Scots were notably more forthcoming.)[6] Thereafter we do find the first articulations of the links between architectural means and medical ends and, specifically, of architecture's potential for doing two contradictory things: promoting air circulation while thwarting aerial contagion. The texts' earlier lack of specificity can be attributed to the civil hospitals' defensiveness – for they were by no means the logical or inevitable response to sickness among the poor – and to the efficacy of the images.

Forms of Representation

Prints showing new public buildings – buildings, that is, sponsored by corporate but secular patrons – were not published in England before 1660. The genre's emergence was encouraged by the prevalence of architectural metaphors in Restoration rhetoric, as well as by new, and tangible, construction, particularly in London, Oxford, and Cambridge. Even so, it is hard to find references to the uses of such pictures any more specific than Charles II's phrase, 'usefull Ornaments'.[7] More suggestive of the proprietary pleasure that images of buildings can give is the Duchess of Beaufort's comment, from 1699, about a print (Fig. 7.1) that she had commissioned from Johannes Kip (it would be published by him and Leonard Knyff). The Duchess wrote

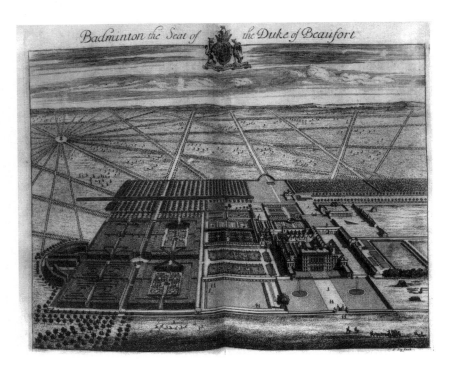

Figure 7.1 Prospect (*c.* 1699) of Badminton, Gloucs., drawn by Leonard Knyff, engraved by Jan Kip, and published in their *Britannia Illustrata* of 1707. (Photo: Conway Library, Courtauld Institute of Art)

that she would use this and Kip's other view of Badminton as gifts showing 'what a noble place my deare Lord', the recently deceased first Duke of Beaufort, 'has left'.[8]

It was also during Charles II's reign that engravings showing un-realised projects were first circulated to raise funds for construction: the earliest example, from 1664, is seemingly, and surprisingly, the Tangier Mole, part of the new colony's harbour defence.[9] Christopher Wren remarked four years later that 'a fair building may easier be car-ried on by contribution, with time, than a sordid one'.[10] Prints allowed more, and more dispersed, potential contributors to appreciate the 'fairness', or not, of what was being proposed than could a three-dimensional model, the traditional medium for publicly displaying an architectural project. They were first used to charitable ends when, in 1700, the committee planning the construction of the Royal Hospital at Greenwich, for old and disabled sailors, having already tried a model, ordered that sets of engravings be sent to 'such of the Sub-scribers as have paid their Subscriptions'.[11] Subscribers could legitimately take the kind of pride in Greenwich that the Duchess of Beaufort took in Badminton; anticipation of that pride might even encourage their delinquent fellows to pay their arrears.

The print reproduced here as Fig. 7.1 is a prospect, or bird's-eye view; this was the commonest type of topographical representation in any medium around 1700. Prospects display certain things very well, among them Badminton's astonishing box hedges and internal court-yards. Neither the pattern of the hedges nor the form of the courts would be comprehensible from the lower, 'perspective' view – that is, one taken from more or less ground level – which was the other regu-lar format. None the less, the depiction of architecture itself is not a major aim of the Badminton engraving, from which we learn less about the buildings than about the surroundings and attributes that fix their meanings, their functions.[12] Though it positions us much closer to the building, the same could be said of the view (Fig. 7.2), probably also by Kip, of St Thomas' Hospital in London, as it was rebuilt in the years around 1700 and published in John Strype's 1720 edition of Stow's *Survey of London* (the engraving itself was probably made years earlier).[13] A courtyard plan seems to demand a prospect; St

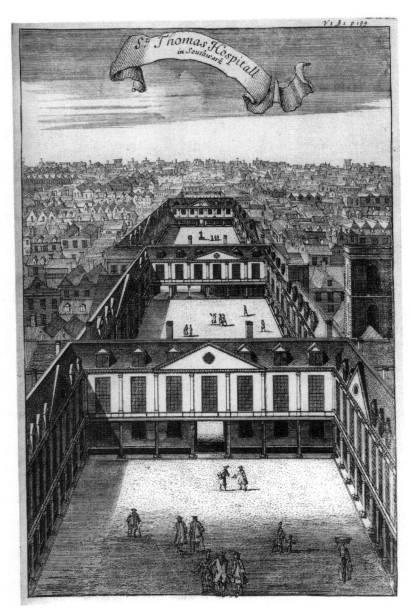

Figure 7.2 Prospect of St Thomas's Hospital, London, as published in John Strype's 1720 edition of John Stow's *Survey of London*. (Photo: Wellcome Library, London)

Thomas's form would be hard to understand if our vantage point were lower down.

A prospect view also shows the full extent of a property, and with it the extent of stewardship. Badminton is the centre 'from which [...] orderliness radiate[s] outwards to merge [...] with the wilderness of hills and woods'.[14] Uncultivated, formless land appears at the very top of the picture, where the estate's avenues finally end. Badminton is an imposition on nature, but also an improvement on it; the Duchess of Beaufort might have laughed at the later eighteenth century's fondness for highly contrived 'artlessness' in a park. St Thomas' is similarly represented as both an imposition and an improvement on its environment, but here the wild, formless surroundings are not natural, but urban. The city presses close to a building that is turned entirely inwards, its display towards its courtyards,[15] and not to the world outside.

As an institution, St Thomas' was centuries old. It was not one of the voluntary hospitals that began to be founded, and built, in England and Scotland in the eighteenth century, the adjective signifying that they were supported by free and personal volition and not, for example, by the terms of some ancient legacy. Innovative imagery was not the prerogative of the new foundations: it was St Bartholomew's in London, another ancient and 'royal' hospital, which in 1729, with the help of the enterprising architect James Gibbs, inaugurated its rebuilding by publishing a print. Sent to each of St Bartholomew's hundreds of governors in an attempt to widen interest in and financial support for the rebuilding, the engraving can no longer be identified with certainty, but it resembled, and may have been, that reproduced here as Fig. 7.3. Yet it was the voluntary foundations which soon constituted the great majority of hospitals, and hence hospital buildings, and it was voluntary hospitals that in the late 1740s began to be described as struggling in the market-place that was the London charitable world. It was construction and competition that encouraged the prints' publication.

St George's Hospital in London, founded 1733, was the second of the English voluntary hospitals; the perspective (Fig. 7.4) was drawn by Isaac Ware, who was also St George's architect. His assign-

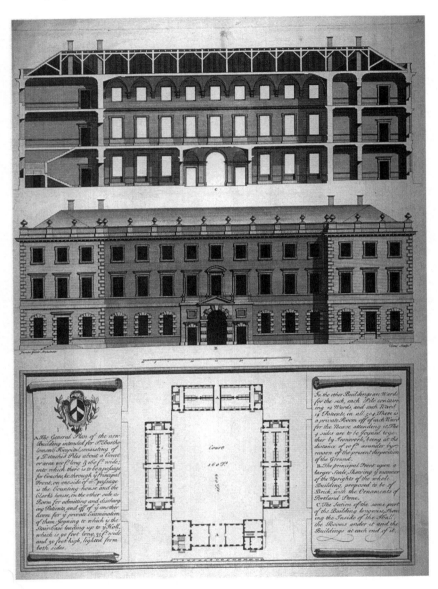

Figure 7.3 Section, elevation, and plan of St Bartholomew's Hospital, London.
(Photo: Guildhall Library, City of London)

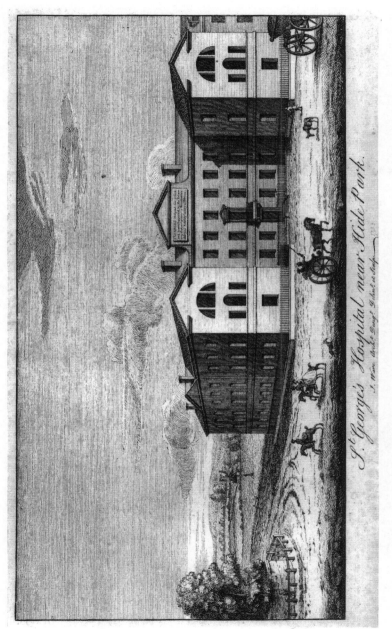

Figure 7.4 Perspectival view (1733) of St George's Hospital, London, drawn and engraved by its architect, Isaac Ware.
(Photo © Copyright The Trustees of the British Museum)

ment was to adapt and expand a thirty-year-old villa in outer-suburban London, on the road called Knightsbridge. The picture emphasises this suburbanism with the inclusion of the equestrians and the happy hound; it makes a good contrast with that of St Thomas' in other respects, too. Ware chose a perspective, a (slightly elevated) ground-level view because he did not need to show enclosure, the space gained and defended from the city. In general, closed courtyards like St Thomas's were being abandoned at civilian (as opposed to naval) hospitals. The new, extended arrangements were enabled, in turn, by the use of cheaper sites on the outskirts of towns. On its site St George's wards could freely stretch out, and the building be admired (as the men in the carriage are doing) from the height of a human eye, not a bird's.

Perspectives and prospects do resemble one another in two general ways. Both locate buildings in their social and topographical contexts by indicating passers-by, trees, roads, other buildings, horizon lines and so on. And neither demanded from their early eighteenth-century viewers much expertise, much experience of architectural visual conventions of the sort then seen only in foreign treatises and relatively expensive native productions like *Vitruvius Britannicus* (1715–25) or Gibbs's *Book of Architecture* (1728). Though the prospect view might seem inherently elitist, implying as it does the privileged standpoint,[16] as a form of representation it was widely available, being used in printed maps, for example, too.[17] On the other hand, one did not often come across cross-sections, orthogonal elevations (that is, diagrammatic, non-perspectival elevations of the sort seen in the middle of Fig. 7.3), or architectural plans. These are representational conventions specific to the art or science of architecture, conventions that leave prints purged of landscape, of 'all traces of the local and contingent'.[18]

The formal stringency of the St Bartholomew's print (Fig. 7.3) is therefore worth remarking; Gibbs used the specialised conventions also seen in his book. The *Book of Architecture* is prefaced by a list of distinguished subscribers' names and an introduction explaining Gibbs's hope that its designs for great houses would be useful for what he called 'Persons of Quality', and especially persons whose estates were so remote that they must act as their own architect and instruct the workmen.[19] Needless to say, not all the book's readers, or even subscribers, would build themselves palaces in the backwoods, but they did not object to the imputation, nor to the related imputation that they had no trouble deciphering sectional views of buildings for the workmen's benefit.[20] The art historian Ernst Gombrich (who made productive use of Freud's 'reality principle') might have said that Gibbs was placing demands on his readers' interpretative skills by using forms of depiction for which experience of other kinds of pictures, like maps, would not have prepared them.[21] Moreover, Gibbs was doing so in the full expectation that the demands would be experienced as pleasurable, since intellectually, and socially, flattering and offering psychic compensation in proportion to the difficulty. Today's advertisers are very familiar with the principle, but pictures of hospitals are even more interesting than, say, Guinness advertisements in this connection, because the hospitals explicitly represented their memberships as cutting across political and religious divides, and, implicitly, across class differences. Any man of good character, for example, who could afford a £50 donation might be elected a governor of St Bartholomew's, which prided itself that in this way the baker and the clothier sat in its grand Court room alongside the greatest in the land.[22]

At least five of the earliest provincial hospital foundations published their plans, or had them published, which is a disproportionate number compared to other building types. Among them were the first voluntary hospital outside London, the (Hampshire) County Hospital in Winchester, founded 1736, and the Liverpool Infirmary, a purpose-built structure from sometime in the mid-1740s.[23] The latter includes a particularly informative key to the three floor plans, which indicates, for example, vents that will carry off 'scents' from the latrines, and ward functions: ward 'F' on the top floor holds female venereal-disease patients. We read, too, that the operating theatre beside this ward has a skylight. In these technicalities are two additional points of interest. First, though it would be twenty years before the first prescriptive or general discussion of hospital architecture was published in English (Edward Foster's *Essay on Hospitals* (Dublin, 1768)), the Liverpool picture implies a consensus on the desirability of, for example, overhead lighting in operating rooms. Second, it seems to be assuming an audience that will understand that operating rooms need skylights – or at least an audience that will be flattered by this assumption.

Some hospital governors thought that such plans should form part of their publicity and we can conclude that this was for the reason just discussed: they implicitly flatter the viewer by presenting him or her with a kind of representation otherwise largely confined to books like Gibbs's. Yet plans like Liverpool's also convey highly specific information about how separation, services, and human and air circulation work in buildings, and more besides. Many hospitals were planned to be built in parts, as the money came in, and clear graphic indications of the relative locations of entrances, stairs, and partition walls could reassure governors of the feasibility, as well as the prudence, of this mode of proceeding.

Hospital plans continue to be published occasionally (most notably in 1751, when the widely-read *Gentleman's Magazine* illustrated the London Hospital's proposed new building);[24] and small orthogonal elevations continue to appear as the head-pieces to hospitals' annual reports. By and large, however, the prospect does not yield to the diagrammatic forms of representation, for two reasons. As a comparison of William Adam's and Paul Sandby's views (Figs 7.5 and 7.6) of the Royal Infirmary in Edinburgh shows, perspectives are much better at indicating the long ward-wings that distinguished most of the voluntary hospitals: the architect Adam's view is simply confusing without his plan. The other reason for sticking with anecdotal representation was that visual incident reinforced an important new message about hospitals' suburban locations (compare Figs 7.3 and 7.7). Roads and church spires suggest a convenient proximity to the city, while herders and huntsmen evoke airy salubriousness.

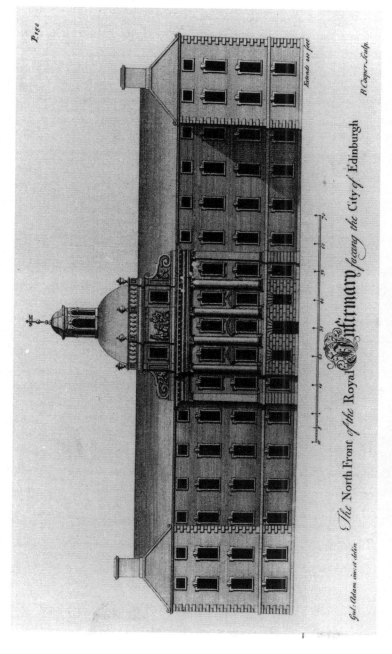

Figure 7.5 Engraved elevation (1739) of the Royal Infirmary, Edinburgh, drawn by its architect, William Adam, and published in his posthumous *Vitruvius Scoticus* (c. 1812).

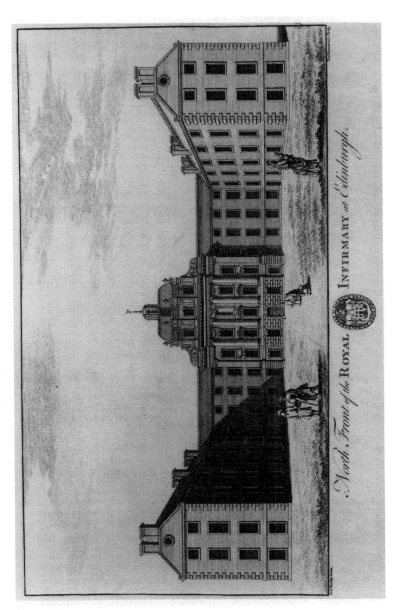

Figure 7.6 Perspectival view (1749) of the Royal Infirmary, Edinburgh, drawn by Paul Sandby and engraved by Paul Fourdrinier. (Photo: Wellcome Library, London)

Christine Stevenson

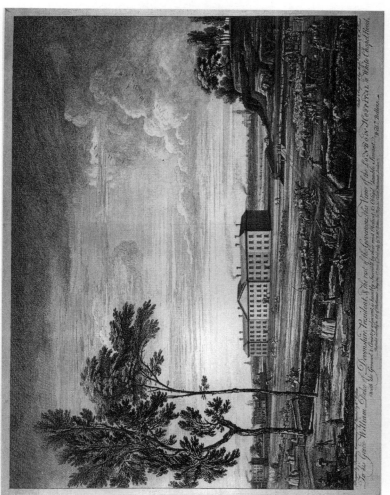

Figure 7.7 Engraving after William Bellers' painting (1752) of the London Hospital.
(Photo: Guildhall Library, City of London)

Airiness

For St Bartholomew's, Gibbs planned four detached wings around a square, three of them with wards set back-to-back on either side of the carriageways through each wing (Fig. 7.4).[25] The architect himself explained that the overall configuration, which was without precedent, was to reduce the risk in case of fire; and we can infer that it was also intended to maximise air circulation, because of the Governors' complaint, recorded in their minutes, that the old precinct had become a hodge-podge whose cramped confusion was obstructing the 'free Course of the Air for the benefitt of the poor', that is, the patients. What is not mentioned in any text is the way in which this arrangement could if necessary lend itself to a practice the hospital was certainly adopting by mid-century: that of using the gaps between the wings to isolate what after their admissions turned out to be cases of contagious illnesses like smallpox, which St Bartholomew's, like other civil hospitals, generally tried to exclude. Yet this capacity was surely evident to anyone able to read ground plans, if only because (as Margaret Pelling has suggested, writing about smallpox)[26] sick members of ordinary private households were regularly isolated, so regularly that the practice helped to direct early modern perceptions of what constituted a good house – it was, among other things, one allowing such segregations, or privacies.

And segregation was being discussed in 1723, when the St Bartholomew's rebuilding committee was first convened, because England had recently been terrified by what would be Western Europe's last great plague epidemic, the Marseilles outbreak of 1719–20. The epidemic had also sparked a political crisis at the end of 1721, when Walpole's Parliamentary opponents seized the opportunity to link the new Quarantine Act with what Paul Slack has pithily summarised as 'standing armies, corrupt absolutism, and other foreign monstrosities'.[27] Dr Richard Mead, who advised on the framing of the Act, was a member of the St Bartholomew's rebuilding committee. In Mead's *Short discourse concerning pestilential contagion*, published in 1720 and then in many subsequent editions, we read that the afflicted should be taken three or four miles out of town, and there put into what he called '*clean* and *airy* Habitations', pesthouses.[28] One could reasonably predict, however, that in case of an epidemic some victims would accidentally be admitted to London's general hospitals, among them St Bartholomew's, and that they would need immediate and effective isolation before they infected others. Yet any claim that Gibbs's design for the new St Bartholomew's made it capable of particularly effective isolation was best left implicit,[29] because what Mead called the pestilential contagion was not only terrifying, it was political.

Though airiness features in the texts published by the early voluntary foundations, they are not explicit about how this quality was to be achieved on the wards. St George's Hospital (Fig. 7.4) was founded after a dispute at the Westminster Infirmary, the first of the voluntary hospitals; disaffected governors and medical men broke away in the autumn of 1733. Their (ostensible) reason for the split was that the Westminster was refusing to move from its relatively central London site, which, though convenient for the officers, threatened the health of their charges. St George's, by contrast, would (we read in the pamphlets it published) provide accommodation that was airy, spacious, and healthful. The texts do not explain why airiness is desirable, but they hardly needed to. Everyone then knew that fresh air in gentle motion is as healthy as stinking and stagnant atmospheres are pathogenic.[30] The assumption had directed advice for house-builders published in English, like every other language, for the previous two hundred years[31] and, even more convincingly, it had also inspired a fair number of lawsuits in London.[32]

As St George's explained, its 'country air', 'would be more effectual than Physick in the Cure of many Distempers, especially such as mostly affect the Poor who live in close and confin'd Places within the great Cities',[33] the kind of places shown outside the hospital in the St Thomas' print (Fig. 7.2). As far as the texts are concerned, then, simple relocation would effect the airiness, but this is not an explanation to convince anyone with much experience of houses. It is Ware's print (Fig. 7.4) which makes clear that the large windows on the cleanly-separated ward-wings will open these wards up to the healthy air of Hyde Park Corner.

Like St George's, the Winchester hospital publicly committed itself to moving the sick poor from what it called the 'Closeness or Unwholsomness' of their homes and into the hospital's 'free Air'.[34] At a time when no medical or surgical procedure was too specialised to be conducted in a private house, this was a critical justification for hospitals' very existence, at least hospitals serving a resident population. They were cleaner and airier than the houses of many poor. For some potential supporters this promise was surely reinforced by the Winchester's many windows, carefully marked on the plans, but the Winchester's records have nothing to say about windows, and indeed very little about the house.

Not every silence in the texts is a silence about the plague; memories of the Marseilles outbreak faded. Yet it was by no means self-evident that hospitals offered significant advantages over the existing system of domiciliary relief for the sick poor – hence the Winchester's emphasis on unwholesome dwellings – and, as unnaturally dense accumulations of the sick, hospitals might even be medically inadvisable. The Winchester Infirmary explained to potential backers, in print, that it presented no public-health threat to the town, even though it was next to the Cathedral. Though subsequent foundations did not feel the same obligation to defend their very presence – they were in more suburban locations and in any case, as became apparent, they presented little threat to healthy populations, at least not before mid-century – it would be more than thirty years before the texts reached a level of specificity comparable to the images'. Yet we cannot entirely account for this difference by granting hospital promoters' natural reluctance to engage with the potential problems of cross-infection, for example, in so many words. We must also allow the possibility that the imagery worked. It made the hospitals look attractively useful, a usefulness that extended (for those who cared to look hard enough) to their capability of segregating, as well as airing, their inhabitants where necessary.

Using Pictures

Like James Gibbs, the architect William Adam planned to publish his own works and accordingly had the plans and elevation (Fig. 7.5) of his Royal Infirmary in Edinburgh (begun in 1738) engraved. He donated copies of the prints to the hospital's Managers, who arranged for their sale by local booksellers as well as for their presentation to prospective donors: at least, they were still being used this way a decade later, when the Infirmary obtained the services of a fund-raiser in London, Adam Anderson.

Anderson was generally pessimistic when he agreed to act on the hospital's behalf,

> by reason of so many *new* Charity-*Projects* […] which are lately set up, & which, tho' merely *local* (& *some* of 'em not rational) do greatly interfere with much better calculated Designs […] such as yours![35]

London had gone mad for hospitals: this was the story, and it was soon widely told.[36] Men and women of fashion and influence were, supposedly, casting their old charities aside when attractive new ones came along. This perception of competition undoubtedly helped to raise promotional thresholds and, possibly, to refine notions of what forms of representation are more 'real', or unmediated, than others. Like statistics and other tabulated forms of data, notably lists of patients (whose privacy was not a priority), engravings had become highly desirable adjuncts to the printed, narrative texts – sermons, annual reports, and institutional histories – that the charitable public had come to expect.

Anderson's first target was Colonel William Sotheby, a gentleman with charitable funds at his disposal as the executor of an estate. Anderson showed Adam's prints to Sotheby and asked for more copies from Edinburgh, 'together with any other papers that it may be proper to shew to Gentlemen'. But Sotheby had become convinced that the Infirmary had few patients in it because the poor were frightened of the place, and Anderson had to take time to persuade him otherwise.[37] This episode inspired the production of the first printed version of the Infirmary's *History and Statutes*:[38] it is probably significant that Sotheby seems to have been loaned an old manuscript in the first instance. Meanwhile the topographical artist Paul Sandby donated a perspective view (Fig. 7.6), which Anderson had engraved by the expert Paul Fourdrinier, along with up-to-date plans.[39] As mentioned earlier, the perspective format allows us to see the Infirmary's generous capacity. It also permits the inclusion of human figures, including the sick poor whom Sotheby had worried were staying away. Three years later, Anderson was, he reported, still giving to 'Gentlemen Books & plans' of the Infirmary as part of his struggle against what he called Londoners' 'frolicksome Disposition for new Charities'.[40]

One of these charities was certainly the London Hospital, then planning a new building for itself. The print reproduced as Fig. 7.7 here was sold as part of the publicity and fund-raising for the project. Again, we see healthful suburbanism; the artist, William Bellers, has perhaps even overdone the cows and the sheep. Even the composition is derived from the Grand (landscape painting) Style,[41] with its framing devices. None the less the print aspires to a documentary quality: even the far-distant church tower on the right, beyond the old bulwark (itself both a framing device and a landmark, part of London's Civil War defences) can be identified as that of Nicholas Hawksmoor's St George in the East.

The gentlemen, and ladies, to whom Anderson referred may have been frolicsome, but they knew what they wanted. With printed pictures whose formats, as well as contents, carried significance for viewers, the charities demonstrated the healthfulness and convenience of their buildings, or planned buildings. Only in the early 1770s did medical commentators and the institutions' own publications begin attempting comparable levels of specificity. Thereafter architectural means and medical ends were correlated with increasing precision at the English and Scottish civil hospitals, a development directed, in part, by contemporary developments in Paris and at England's great naval hospitals.

The hospital's rise was not unchallenged. More than twenty dispensaries, charitable institutions that offered medical advice, medicines, and food to the poor,[42] but not beds, were founded in London between 1769 and the end of the century, and many more in the provinces. Some of their promoters pointed out that unlike hospitals, dispensaries did not have to divert any of their charitable funds from the care of the poor to the care of bricks and mortar. The *Plan of the Surr[e]y Dispensary* thus argued in 1777 that 'The immense sums expended on building and supporting great houses are more usefully employed in relieving a number of objects from the distresses of sickness.'[43] Moreover, many of the inmates of London's 'noble hospitals',[44]

> from the nature of their disorders, became worse, by being *pent up* in close wards and impure air; without mentioning the contagion incident to hospitals, which frequently infected most of those who were confined therein.

Far from protecting its inmates from urban stinks and congestion, as the engraving of St Thomas's illustrates, or removing them entirely to suburban safety, as Ware showed St George's doing, here is the hospital actually intensifying, by confinement, the dangers of the city. Though some dispensaries did construct buildings for their work,[45] pictures of them were, tellingly, never printed.[46] Chesterfield's view that a building is, or should be, merely the envelope for organisational substance had not lost its adherents.

Notes

1   I am grateful to the University of Reading's Research Travel Grant Sub-Committee for funding my travel to Verona, where I presented the paper upon which the present essay is based.

2   'You will, I hope, go deeper, and make your way into the substance of things.' B. Dobrée (ed.), *The Letters of Philip Dormer Stanhope, 4th Earl of Chesterfield*, 6 vols (London, 1932, facs. edn, New York, 1968), 4: *1748–1751*, p.1298: letter 1618, dated 24 January 1749 (o.s.).

3   *Ibid.*, 1419–20 (letter 1665; 17 October [o.s.] 1749). This was, at least, his implication; compare *ibid.*, 1335 (letter 1635; 27 April [o.s.] 1749); 1377 (letter 1652, 7 August [o.s.] 1749); 1409 (letter 1661; 27 September [o.s.] 1749).

4   P. Leach, *James Paine* (London, 1988), pp.194–5 quotes the letter, on which
     see also E. Wilson, *The History of the Middlesex Hospital during the first cen-
     tury of its existence, compiled from the hospital records* (London, 1845), p.20.
     This deference annoyed other governors.

5   Aside from scattered discussions of individual prints, though a useful exception
     is B. Allen, 'Engravings for Charity', *Journal of the Royal Society of Arts*, 134
     (1986), pp.646–9.

6   At least, those at the Edinburgh Infirmary, on which see C. Stevenson,
     '*Æsculapius Scoticus*', *Georgian Group Journal*, 6 (1996), pp.53–62.

7   K.S. Van Eerde, *John Ogilby and the Taste of his Times* (Folkestone, 1976),
     p.141: in February 1682, Charles 'recommended to the Vice Chancellors of the
     universities of Oxford and Cambridge that they procure copies of [John Ogilby
     and William Morgan's] [...] great new map of London and place them in public
     rooms "as usefull Ornaments."'

8   'I have had Mr Knyff here, who is doing three drafts [...] my designs when
     these are all done is to have some of them bound in books & given them to
     show what a noble place my deare Lord has left.' Quoted by J. Harris and
     G. Jackson-Stops in the Introduction to L. Knyff and J. Kip, *Britannia Illustrata*
     (1707), repr. edn (Bungay, 1984), n.p.

9   L. Jardine, *Ingenious Pursuits: Building the Scientific Revolution* (London,
     1999), pp.209–10. Followed by, in 1676, the new Library at Trinity College,
     Cambridge, and the astronomical observatory at Greenwich: *ibid.*, pp.211–12;
     D. McKitterick, 'Introduction', in D. McKitterick (ed.), *The Making of the
     Wren Library, Trinity College, Cambridge* (Cambridge, 1995), pp.1–27, on
     pp.7–8.

10   In a letter from Oxford, transcribed, with modernised spelling, in J. Elmes,
     Memoirs of the Life and Works of Sir Christopher Wren [...] (London, 1823),
     pp.237–9, quotation on 238.

11   Quoted C. Stevenson, *Medicine and Magnificence: British Hospital and Asylum
     Architecture 1660–1815* (New Haven and London, 2000), p.77; two of the
     prints are reproduced *ibid.*, pp.74, 77 and a copy of the third on 78.

12   J. Steegman, *The Artist and the Country House* (London and New York,
     [1949]), p.12: 'the house-portraitist devoted himself less to the house than to its
     surroundings, attributes and setting. We know more from his picture about the
     house's position in the social scale of houses than we do about its real
     architectural character.'

13   See n.14, below.

14   Steegman, *The Artist*, p.17.

15   Even the frontispiece (1682) with its statues was moved inside and re-erected
     over the entrance to Edward (that shown in the middle) Square in 1724. That
     was after the print (Fig. 7.2) was published, but it was outdated in 1720, too:
     Strype's volume was many years in preparation.

16   The prospect had been the naturalised form of estate portraiture, and maybe the natural one too. 'In their capacity as landowners, the gentry were considered natural statesmen, able to grasp as from a height the nation as a whole, to see the entire picture in contrast to the partial view of those of lowlier status and more specialised occupations.' S. Daniels, 'Goodly Prospects: English Estate Portraiture, 1670–1730', in N. Alfrey and S. Daniels (eds), *Mapping the Landscape: Essays on Art and Cartography* (Nottingham, 1990), pp.9–12, on 9.

17   *Ibid.*, p.10.

18   N. Savage, 'Introduction', in R. Middleton et al., *The Mark J. Millard Architectural Collection, 2, British Books, Seventeenth through Nineteenth Centuries* (Washington and New York, 1998), pp.ix–xii, on x.

19   J. Gibbs, *A Book of Architecture, Containing Designs of Buildings and Ornaments* (1728), repr. edn (New York, 1968), p.1.

20   Gibbs certainly assumed that his readers would understand what a 'section' and 'geometrical plan' are: *ibid.*, p.v.

21   See E.H. Gombrich's 'Psycho-analysis and the History of Art', in *Meditations on a Hobby Horse and other Essays on the Theory of Art* (London, 1963), pp.30–44.

22   '*[L]es plus grands seigneurs*', as a French visitor, Jacques Tenon, put it later in the century: quoted Stevenson, *Medicine and Magnificence*, p.108, as part of a chapter that examines this myth of inclusivity in relation to hospital construction.

23   The Winchester and Liverpool prints are reproduced in Stevenson, *Medicine and Magnificence*, pp.136, 139. The other early foundations which published their plans are those in Edinburgh (1738), Bath (1738), Bristol (1742), and possibly Exeter (for which see the plan reproduced in H. Richardson et al., *English Hospitals 1660–1948: A Survey of their Architecture and Design* (Swindon, 1998), p.22.

24   Reproduced Stevenson, *Medicine and Magnificence*, p.143. At its peak the *Magazine* had 10,000 purchasers and many more readers for each number: R. Porter, 'Lay Medical Knowledge in the Eighteenth Century: the Case of the *Gentleman's Magazine*', *Medical History*, 29 (1985), pp.138–68, on 141.

25   The internal arrangements of the ward wings as constructed differed from those shown in Fig. 7.4. On what follows see Stevenson, *Medicine and Magnificence*, pp.129–32.

26   M. Pelling, 'Skirting the City? Disease, Social Change and Divided Households in the Seventeenth-Century Metropolis', in M.S.R. Jenner and P. Griffiths (eds), *Londinopolis: Essays in the Cultural and Social History of Early Modern London* (Manchester, 2000), pp.154–75, on pp.165–6.

27   Paul Slack, *The Impact of Plague in Tudor and Stuart England* (London, 1985), p.332.

28   R. Mead, *A Short Discourse concerning Pestilential Contagion, and the Methods to be Used to Prevent It* (London, 1720), pp.38–9.

29   Compare D. Chandler, *Semiotics: the Basics* (London and New York, 2002), p.47: 'contemporary visual advertisements are a powerful example of how images may be used to make implicit claims which advertisers prefer not to make more openly in words' – because they might sound offensive, or just plain silly.

30   A. Wear, *Knowledge and Practice in English Medicine, 1550–1680* (Cambridge, 2000), ch. 4, 'Preventative Medicine: Healthy Lifestyles and Healthy Environments'.

31   E.g. R. Morris, *An Essay upon Harmony. As it relates Chiefly to Situation and Building* (1739), repr. edn (New York, 1982), pp.iv–v.

32   See, for example, those described in E. McKellar, *The Birth of Modern London: the Development and Design of the City 1660–1720* (Manchester, 1999), pp.26, 28, 75, 195, 209, 211.

33   *An Account of the Occasion and Manner of Erecting an Hospital at Lanesborough-House [...] Published [...] February the 6th, 1733[/4]* ([London], 1734).

34   Stevenson, *Medicine and Magnificence*, p.137.

35   Emphases in the original: Lothian Health Services Archive, Special Collections, Edinburgh University Library (LHB), LHB 1/72/2 (8.), Anderson to George Drummond (5 November 1748).

36   [J. Gwynn], *An Essay on Design [...]* (London, 1749), p.78; T. Smollett, *The Adventures of Ferdinand Count Fathom* (1753), ed. P.-G. Boucé (London, 1990), pp.328–9; S. Johnson in *The Idler* 4 (Saturday 6 May 1758), repr. (London, 1761), 22; B. Croxson, 'The Foundation and Evolution of the Middlesex Hospital's Lying-In Service, 1745–1786', *Social History of Medicine*, 14 (2001), pp.27–57, on 28–9.

37   LHB 1/72/2 (8.) and (10.), Anderson to Drummond (5 November and 17 November 1748).

38   LHB 1/72/3 (5.) (taken from the summary).

39   The managers told Anderson to order as many copies of the plans as he needed, plus 200 for their use: LHB 1/1/3, pp.18–19 (7 August 1749).

40   LHB 1/72/8 (2.), Anderson to Gavin Hamilton (21 March 1752).

41   D. Solkin, *Richard Wilson: the Landscape of Reaction*, exh. cat. (London, 1982), pp.149–50, referring to Wilson's painting of St George's.

42   B. Croxson, 'The Public and Private Faces of Eighteenth-Century London Dispensary Charity', *Medical History* 41 (1997), pp.127–49, on 138.

43   *A plan of the Surr[e]y Dispensary [...] for the relief of the poor inhabitants of Southwark [...] at their own habitations. Instituted in [...] 1777* (London, 1777), pp.8–9; compare D. Andrew, *Philanthropy and Police: London Charity in the Eighteenth Century* (Princeton, NJ, 1989), p.134. The argument was not specious; a couple of the new London hospitals may indeed have been too eager to build new wards that in the event stayed empty. D. Owen, *English Philanthropy, 1660–1960* (Cambridge, Mass., 1964), pp.44, 48–50; A.E. Clark-

Kennedy, *The London: A Study in the Voluntary Hospital System*, 1, *The First Hundred Years 1740–1840* (London, 1962), pp.169–73, 181–2.

44   *A plan of the Surr[e]y Dispensary*, 7 (my emphasis); compare George Armstrong as quoted by U. Tröhler, 'The Doctor as Naturalist: the Idea and Practice of Clinical Teaching and Research in British Policlinics 1770–1850', *Clio Medica* 21 (1989 (for 1987–8)), pp.21–34, on 27.

45   R. Kilpatrick, '"Living in the Light": Dispensaries, Philanthropy and Medical Reform in Late-Eighteenth-Century London', in A. Cunningham and R. French (eds), *The Medical Enlightenment of the Eighteenth Century* (Cambridge, 1990), pp.254–80, on 256.

46   None of twenty-one dispensaries Croxson lists ('The public and private') appear in the index to B. Adams's authoritative *London Illustrated 1604–1851: A Survey and Index of Topographical Books and their Plates* (London, 1983), and a search on the Guildhall Collage and the Wellcome Library iconographic databases yields no image of a dispensary from 1815 or earlier.

ANNMARIE ADAMS

Chapter 8: 'That was Then, This is Now': Hospital Architecture in the Age(s) of Revolution, 1970–2001

Hospitals built in the last thirty years or so are easy to identify.[1] Two images (Figs 8.1 and 8.2) of the Hospital for Sick Children in Toronto of 1951 and of 1990 articulate this difference.[2] Although both buildings are essentially brick and glass towers, the 1990s perspective by Zeidler Roberts Architects reveals important changes in the intentions of the hospital four decades later. Here the institution's circulation system is expressed by an all-glass spine; the brick seems to be literally hanging off the frame of the building, rather than acting as a supportive structure; varying window sizes and treatments reveal functional zoning; and perhaps most notably, a covered walkway defines the hospital's entrance and acknowledges the scale of the individual patient.

Seasoned architectural aficionados may also note that the building's ziggurat-like massing recalls both the stepped monuments of Mesopotamia, and the debates over the height restrictions of tall buildings in New York of the 1930s, references not-so-obviously related to healthcare. And the hospital's main public space looks like an urban shopping mall. What happened between the 1950s and the 1990s is postmodernism.

In the field of architecture in general, the tenets of postmodernism are well known. Postmodern buildings are often neo-conservative, feature high-tech virtuosity, references to everyday landscapes, and are sometimes even humorous. Postmodern characteristics are less well articulated in medicine, although David B. Morris of the University of New Mexico has suggested that a bio-cultural (rather than bio-

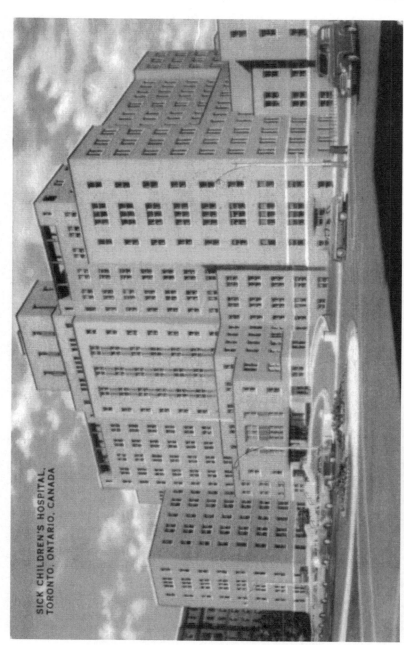

Figure 8.1 Postcard of Hospital for Sick Children, Toronto. (Collection Annmarie Adams)

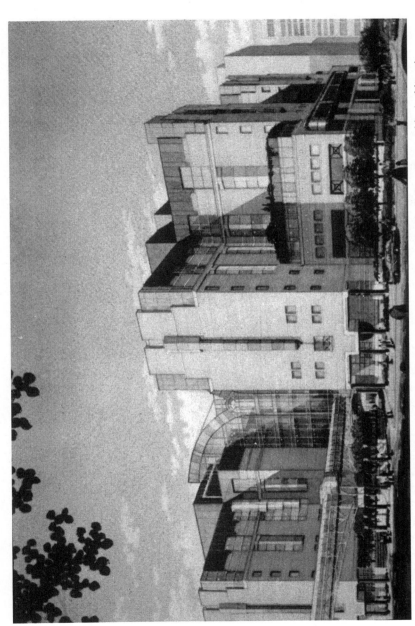

Figure 8.2 Perspective rendering, Hospital for Sick Children, Toronto. (Zeidler Roberts Partnership Architects)

medical) model of illness is emerging as an essential part of postmodernism.[3]

Although Morris makes no references to healthcare architecture per se, he notes that the term postmodernism was first used to describe architecture in a series of influential books by architectural theorist Charles Jencks in the 1970s. In *The Language of Post-modern Architecture* (New York, 1977) Jencks pinpointed the death of modern architecture as having occurred on 15 July, 1972, at 3:32 pm in St Louis, with the demolition of the Pruitt-Igoe housing project built in 1952. Symbolic of a growing critique of modern architecture, the demolition of the public housing tower ushered in a new 'after-modernism' era, in which buildings engaged multiple, simultaneous codes of expression.

Among the most profound and under-studied postmodern places are the Disney parks. Disneyland in Anaheim, California, of 1955, and Disney World in Orlando, Florida, which opened in 1971, illustrate many of Jencks' original points about the movement. They are variegated, witty, messy, picturesque, and orderly. In the case of the Disney parks, a clear sense of separation from other realms also serves to underline their postmodernity. Boundaries, gates, and an expensive admission ticket add to a sense of disconnectedness for visitors, compounded recently through the extensive use of cell phones and video cameras by visitors. Although we are visitors, we are not really. Our real experience of postmodern architecture occurs later, when we look at images of buildings in an environment of our choice: the private home.

This paper has three objectives: (1) to explore recent hospital architecture in terms of a broader understanding of the twentieth-century hospital; (2) to illustrate that postmodern hospital design is actually more reactionary than revolutionary. Most of the ideals postulated by hospital planners today that is – for example, increased provision for outpatients, flexibility, accessibility, and comfort – echo nearly verbatim the notions put forth during the 1920s and 1930s, and even earlier. And (3), to argue that, in general and not unrelated to the second point, change in hospital architecture is more culturally than medically driven or determined. Hospitals look like shopping malls, that is, because many public buildings now look like shopping malls, not because of a medical imperative to design them this way.

An approach which engages the methods of architectural history to explore the present also offers a unique opportunity to sketch out a tripartite explanatory model of the development of hospital architecture in the twentieth century. This diagram (Fig. 8.3) illustrates: modern (1916–39), Modern (1945–80), and postmodern (1980–present) hospital architecture. It contrasts with classic architectural surveys, notably John D. Thompson and Grace Goldin's 1975 book, *The Hospital: A Social and Architectural History*, which leap directly from pavilion-plan buildings like Johns Hopkins Hospital of 1888 to skyscraper mega-hospitals of the 1930s.

Evidence to support this argument that the postmodern hospital is a renaissance of earlier ideas is visual evidence drawn from hospitals – past and present, real and proposed – associated with my own institution, McGill University in Montreal, Quebec. Since 1994, five of McGill University's teaching hospitals have voluntarily merged into a single institution: the McGill University Health Centre (MUHC). The MUHC is currently planning to abandon four of its historic urban hospitals, and to open a purpose-built facility on a polluted former railway yard at some distance from Montreal's city centre in 2011.[4] The 1,579.5 million dollar project is known locally as the superhospital, despite the best efforts of its planners to shake the nomenclature. The Université de Montreal, a French-speaking university, is planning an equally ambitious French-speaking facility to open simultaneously, also involving the reconfiguration of three historic hospitals.[5]

In 1997, MUHC consultants reported that although the Royal Victoria Hospital is eminently unsuitable for re-use as a hospital, it would make good condominiums, especially if all the buildings constructed after World War II were to be removed.[6] This demolition mostly entails postwar Modern towers, but also includes the $29 million 1994 emergency, ICU and birthing centre (the condition of the buildings is apparently irrelevant). This scenario is a good illustration of the sequence, denounce-demonise-demolish, which often precedes the destruction of hospitals.

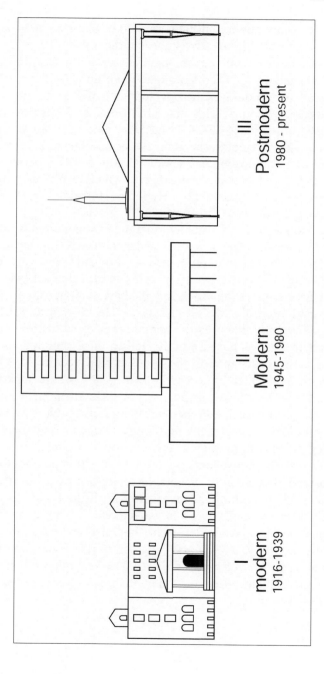

Figure 8.3 Conceptual diagram of twentieth-century general hospital types. (Drawing by David Theodore)

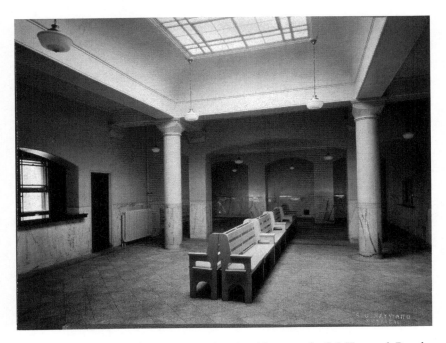

Figure 8.4 Photograph of women outpatients' waiting room by S.J. Hayward, Royal
Victoria Montreal Maternity Hospital,
Montreal. (Collection Royal Victoria Hospital)

Many new medical facilities constructed in the last thirty years or so, like the new addition to the Hospital for Sick Children in Toronto, claim to be more flexible, accessible, humanly scaled, comforting, and homelike than those constructed between 1945 and 1970. They also identify themselves as healthcare facilities, rather than hospitals. Healthcare facilities planners assert that these architectural reforms come from the so-called revolution in the delivery of medical care which has taken place since about 1980, whereby treatment is now patient- rather than physician-centered, and new technologies have resulted in a huge increase in day surgeries and outpatient services. In Quebec this change is known popularly as the *virage ambulatoire*. Stephen Verderber and David J. Fine's book, *Healthcare Architecture in an Era of Radical Transformation*, suggests that the hospice movement (begun in UK in 1967) and the move to managed care in the United States is largely responsible for such changes.[7] Most of these architectural ideas, however, are not so new. Hospital architecture evolves as part of a larger cultural discourse rather than mostly as a result of medical change or innovation. In the interest of brevity, this can be illustrated through five popular misconceptions about contemporary hospital architecture.

Ambulatory Care

Outpatients' departments are not a new idea. Hospital administrators today constantly state this: 'older hospitals do not accommodate outpatients.' It was, in fact, one of the most significant new parts of older hospitals in the 1920s. A survey of 500 non-teaching hospitals conducted by the journal *Modern Hospital* in 1926 revealed that 34 had new outpatient buildings, 85 had new buildings projected, 76 had some new construction finished, 83 had assigned more space to the outpatient department without construction, and 87 planned improvements to the outpatients department, not yet undertaken.[8]

The provision for outpatients countered that for private patients in every possible way. The floor plans of general urban hospitals, such as Montreal's Royal Victoria Hospital (opened 1893), illustrate how wealthy patients experienced a flowing, oblique, uninterrupted experience in the hospital, while outpatients' (and other poor patients') experience was much more jarring and interrupted. Private patients' departments were typically located at some distance from the main hospitals, while outpatients were often in the basements of older hospitals. So while paying patients literally traveled upwards to their quarters, poorer patients descended. And not surprisingly, while private patients were offered privacy and seclusion, outpatients departments were nearly always congested. This is perhaps most evident in the ubiquitous bench seating, whereby families would huddle next to each other without any separation. Architect Edward Stevens' outpatients' departments, such as he designed for the Royal Victoria Hospital, were among the most dignified of the interwar era (Fig. 8.4).

Flexibility

A second common misconception is that hospital architects of the past never thought about flexibility. Architects of pavilion-plan hospitals, as we know from Jeremy Taylor's superb 1999 book, *The Architect and the Pavilion Hospital*, were obsessed with the typology's potential for infinite expansion, and with the fact that the open-plan spaces of the Nightingale wards were infinitely malleable.[9] And in an uncannily postmodern way, much of the furniture designed for hospitals in the 1920s and 1930s was double coded. A table, for example, designed by the Canadian department store Eaton's served multiple purposes simultaneously (Fig. 8.5). The table design also shows this obsession with smooth, flowing movement, like the micro-levelling elevators used in hospitals of this era.

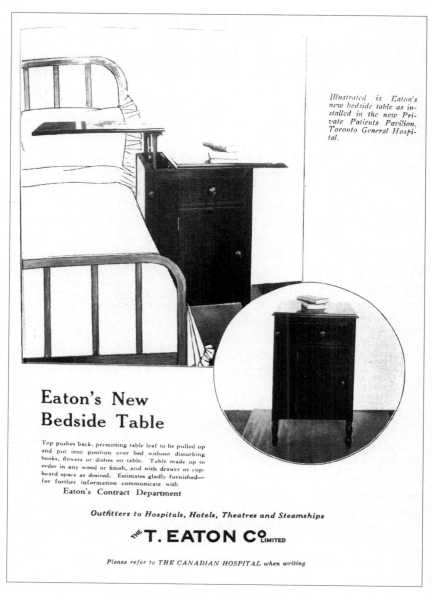

Figure 8.5 Advertisement of bedside table,
Canadian Hospital, 7, No. 7 (July 1930), p.29

Accessibility

Postmodern hospital planners are insistent that healthcare facilities should be more accessible. This echoes the concerns of interwar architects, who carefully sited their buildings for easy access, by public transportation, pedestrians, and automobiles simultaneously. The gateway at Stevens' 1916 Ross Memorial Pavilion (part of the Royal Victoria Hospital) and his Ottawa Civic Hospital of 1924, show how hospital design anticipated the arrival of patients and physicians by automobile.

Concealed Technology

Hospital planners today want both patient rooms and circulation spaces to look comforting and homelike, rather than hard-edged and high-tech. Nowhere is this as evident as in the design of children's hospitals, which nowadays typically include references to zoos or transportation systems (balloons, trains, planes). This is very postmodern; the application of architectural 'style' as a thin veneer on a modern frame.

The Disney parks illustrate this same notion. At Disney World the facades along Main Street USA are fake and everybody knows it. This neo-traditional picture is only possible through high technology, hence the proximity of Tomorrowland to Main Street.

Hospital architecture of the 1920s, too, concealed plenty of medical technology outside the patient's immediate environment. At Ross Memorial Hospital, among Canada's first private patients' pavilions, the elevator, fans, and ventilation equipment were housed in the hospital's monumental central tower, which overlooked the patients' entrance (Fig. 8.6). A typical patient room of the same period included wiring for telephone and special night-lights that allowed nurses to illuminate the rooms at night without using ceiling lights. A call system

Annmarie Adams

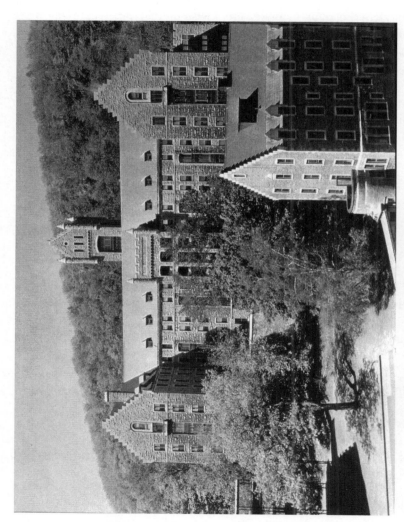

Figure 8.6 Ross Memorial Pavilion, Royal Victoria Hospital, Montreal. (Collection Royal Victoria Hospital)

similar to those found in many hospitals today comprised a system of lights over the doors of rooms indicating the location of doctors and nurses. Instrument cabinets, refrigerators, blanket warmers and drying closets were built right into patient room walls; and each floor had receptacles for electro-cardiograph.

Residentialism

Details of what the superhospital site will look like are sketchy. Few architectural images have been produced by the MUHC, however, they have described what the new superhospital will resemble. When the project was first announced, former MUHC director Hugh Scott and former MUHC planning director Nicolas Steinmetz boasted that the hospital would look like a university campus, with an arrangement of interconnected low-rise pavilions integrated in a landscape of parks, walkways and playgrounds, an absurd suggestion, given the enormous scale of the proposed institution.[10] Perhaps they were imagining something like the Freeport Health Care Village (first phase 1986–9) in Kitchener, Ontario, by the NORR Partnership with McMurrich and Oxley Architects. The Kitchener hospital is significant for its decentralised plan, clustered buildings, courtyard plaza and use of brick.

This new 'residentialism,' as Verderber and Fine have called it, intended to counter the hospital architecture of the intervening period in 1945–70, was very different than both the preceding and succeeding eras. These mostly stark, undecorated towers expressed both a faith in medical progress and a more democratic stance as a public institution than hospitals before or after them. Modern hospitals looked like Modern office buildings, just as interwar and postmodern hospitals look like hotels and malls respectively.

How have contemporary planners missed the foreshadowing of their own needs in the buildings of the 1920s? While I once believed that planners, anxious to justify their own new projects, simply overlooked the buildings of the past, I now believe that the interwar buildings themselves are to blame.

Conclusion

Although many hospitals of the 1920s looked quite conservative, they were actually modern in their spatial attitudes, structure, endorsement of aseptic medical practice, anticipation of expansion and change, sanctioning of expert knowledge, and appeal to new patrons.[11] This is why stage 1 of the tripartite model is called 'modern.' But because architectural historians have tended to read elevations, rather than plans of hospitals, these building have generally been omitted from studies of the building type and have been seen, mistakenly, as simple reverberations of the nineteenth-century model.

Today's hospital planners, unfortunately, also don't look beyond the mere image of these hospitals. A historic building which resembles a 'Scottish castle' is to them old-looking and therefore bad. How can futuristic research take place within an institution which appears medieval, even if the interior has been continuously updated for eight decades? At the same time, however – and here's where postmodernism comes in – they build new places to look and function like less threatening institutions, just the way eighteenth-century industrialists built factories to look like churches and schools by including clock towers.

Medical change does not necessarily inspire new architectural forms. This is an assumption which runs throughout the literature in the history of the hospitals as social institutions. Part of the problem comes from the fact that hospital architecture is only used to illustrate the history of medicine, rather than as evidence. When the story is solely derived from medical milestones and medical men, buildings are passive.

Architecture changes architecture – sometimes inspired by changes in other fields like medicine – but hospital architecture is not a passive illustration of medical history. Contemporary hospitals are much more closely derived from contemporary architectural ideas than medical ones; if it were the other way around, we would likely see houses, hotels, and malls that look like hospitals.

The larger problem comes from a head-on collision of architectural and medical reasoning. While architectural reasoning is based on case studies and precedent (like law), modern medicine is founded on a notion of progress. The assumption is always that the next step (or next building) will be better than the last, as if design is the final stage of a scientific experiment. Hospital planners derive their sense of confidence from this model of progress, and their educations from the model of precedent. Such collisions, juxtapositions, and untidy explanations make up our postmodern world.

Notes

1   Ideas for this paper are drawn from several research initiatives, most notably 'Medicine by Design: A Hospital for the Twenty-First Century', funded by the Canadian Institutes of Health Research (CIHR), and my forthcoming book, *Medicine by Design: The Architect and the Modern Hospital, 1893–1943* (Minneapolis, 2007). I have benefited in both projects from the assistance of David Theodore.

2   For a more detailed analysis of the evolution of children's hospitals, see A. Adams and D. Theodore, 'Designing for "the Little Convalescents": Children's Hospitals in Toronto and Montreal, 1875–2006', *Canadian Bulletin of Medical History* 19.1 (2002), pp.201–43.

3   See D.B. Morris, 'How to Speak Postmodern: Medicine, Illness, and Cultural Change', *Hastings Center Report*, 30, no. 6 (November–December 2000), pp.7–16; and D.B. Morris, *Illness and Culture in the Postmodern Age* (Berkeley, 1998).

4   A. Derfel, 'At Last, Superhospitals Get Go-Ahead', *The Gazette* (8 April 2006), A1.

5   On the CHUM, see M. Turenne, 'L'hôpital de 850 millions', *L'Actualité*, 25, no. 20 (15 December 2000); J. Heinrich, 'French Superhospital due by 2003', *The Gazette* (17 October 1998), A1; and A. Derfel, 'CHUM's "Hospital of the Century" Unveiled', *The Gazette* (20 December 2001), A3. On the MUHC, see

C. Adolph, 'Dawn of the Superhospital', *The Gazette* (14 May 1994), B1–B2; A. Derfel, 'Superhospital's Costs Rising', *The Gazette* (24 April 2002), A1, A6

6   Lecavalier-Lalonde and Saïa et Barbarese, 'Evaluation of Potential for Reuse of Existing Sites, Working Document #3, Heritage Evaluation of the Sites' (McGill University Health Centre Planning Group, November 1997). See especially the plan that shows the authors' evaluation of the heritage value of each building on page RVH10.

7   S. Verderber and D.J. Fine, *Healthcare Architecture in an Era of Radical Transformation* (New Haven, 2000), pp.84–6.

8   M.M. Davis, 'Planning Buildings for Out-patient Service', *Modern Hospital*, 26.3 (March 1926), pp.219–27.

9   Jeremy Taylor, *The Architect and the Pavilion Hospital: Dialogue and Design Creativity in England 1850–1914* (London, 1997).

10   See McGill University Health Centre Report on Planning Activities Related to the Creation of a New Facility (3 April 1998), p.38, and the quotes from former McGill University board chairman Alex Paterson in M. Lalonde, 'Super-Hospital Idea Clears a Big Hurdle: Panel Warms to Union of 5 Big Institutions', *The Gazette* (8 June 1993), A1; and A. Derfel, 'Super-hospital Site Set', *The Gazette* (23 October 1998), A2.

11   A. Adams, 'Modernism and Medicine: The Hospitals of Stevens and Lee, 1916–1932', *Journal of the Society of Architectural Historians*, 58, no. 1 (March 1999), pp.42–6.

Part Three: The Impact on Rural Landscape

MAX SATCHELL

Chapter 9: Towards a Landscape History of the Rural Hospital in England, 1100–1300

Most studies of the hospitals of the medieval West have concentrated on those in or on the margins of urban places, the location of the majority of such institutions.[1] This paper attempts to begin redressing this imbalance by focussing on the rural hospitals of one country (England) over a limited time-span (1100–1300). To date no work has taken the English rural hospital as its primary focus and burgeoning interest in rural welfare has been largely conceived and researched in terms of other forms of relief.[2] Attempts to redefine historical and archaeological approaches to the medieval hospital and its landscape have also been notably silent concerning rural hospitals.[3]

Rural hospitals were numerous in the twelfth and thirteenth centuries. Even if a very broad definition of a medieval town is adopted, about one in nine hospitals can be classified as rural.[4] This figure is dependent on classifying as urban all hospitals named after towns (about two-thirds of some 600 hospitals under discussion here) as well as all of the remainder sited within a radius of 3 miles (4.8 km) from a town. This ensures that all hospitals reviewed in this paper can be solidly classified as rural, because a distance of three miles is far greater than the distances of all those hospitals with tangible urban associations, whether through having townsfolk as founders, benefactors or patrons, or more simply in sharing the name of a town.[5] The ratio of rural to urban hospitals would also have been greater in the twelfth and thirteenth centuries. This is because the capacity of hospitals to become extinct before leaving an enduring trace in the documentary record was greater for rural than urban hospitals. The figures concerning hospitals also make no allowance for those which were founded in rural areas that subsequently became urbanised.

The reticence of document-led historians concerning rural hospitals is understandable given their great loss of muniments. Before 1300 the chief source materials for studying rural hospitals are charters, most of which simply record grants of lands or rents. Over half of rural hospitals have lost all their charters. Most that survive are only extant as transcripts, not as originals. Few hospitals can muster even five transcripts, and holdings greater than five are virtually unknown.[6] The loss of documents is largely a product of the generally early dissolution of rural hospitals with many of them having ceased to exist by or before the end of the fourteenth century.[7]

The emphasis of hospital studies on towns has meant that virtually every aspect of rural hospitals remains either unknown or under-investigated. This is a not unimportant omission given the significant numbers of rural hospitals that were evidently once in existence. While the loss of documents largely frustrates conventional historical analysis, much can be inferred from the selective application of those interdisciplinary techniques that fall under the variable and ill-defined terms of landscape archaeology or landscape history. This approach is by no means novel. Work on urban hospital landscapes has already been mentioned. This study has also benefited from some simple applications of Geographical Information Systems (GIS) software, which has no claims to novelty either, but remains underutilised in medieval studies, and makes it possible to compare the distribution of hospitals to be accurately compared against large datasets of other features.[8] Constraints of space and the number of maps determine that what follows represents only a preliminary outline of some key themes concerning rural hospitals in medieval England.

Rural hospitals were unevenly distributed across England (see Fig. 9.1). They are virtually unrepresented in the southwest. If a line is drawn stretching from Southampton to Gloucester, all but four of the rural hospitals considered in this study lay to the east of it. Rural hospitals occur in some numbers in East Anglia, especially in and around the Fens, in the North of England east of the Pennines, and in a cluster within the London Gap, the area around London devoid of towns. If the distribution of rural hospitals is analysed in relation to town density, an exercise inevitably speculative as it is grounded on incomplete data, rural hospitals generally occur in greatest numbers in

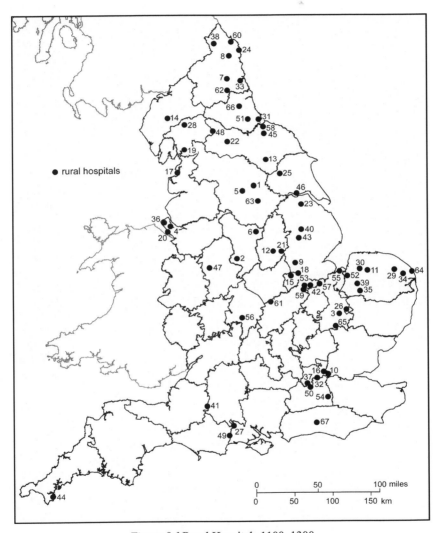

Figure 9.1 Rural Hospitals 1100–1300

Key to Figure 9.1

No.	Name	Type	No.	Name	Type
1	Aberford	NLH	35	Ickburgh	LH
2	Alkmonton	LH	36	Irby Mill	LH
3	Anglesey	NLH	37	Kempton	NLH
4	Bebington	LH	38	Kirknewton	NLH
5	Beeston	NLH	39	Langewade	LH
6	Beightonfields	LH	40	Langworth	LH
7	Bolam	NLH	41	Maiden Bradley	LH
8	Bolton	LH	42	Marholm	NLH
9	Boothby Pagnell	LH	43	Mere	NLH
10	Bow Bridge	LH	44	*Nancledgy*	LH
11	*Boycodeswade*	NLH	45	Newton-in-Cleveland	LH
12	*Bradebusk*	LH	46	North Ferriby	NLH
13	Brandsby	NLH	47	Ranton	NLH
14	Caldbeck	NLH	48	Reycross	NLH
15	Castle Bytham	NLH	49	Rushton	NLH
16	Clayhanger	NLH	50	Sandown	NLH
17	Cockersand	NLH	51	Sedgefield	NLH
18	Cottesmore	NLH	52	Setchey	LH
19	Crosscrake	LH	53	Southorpe	NLH
20	Denhall	NLH	54	Tandridge	NLH
21	East stoke	LH	55	Terrington	LH
22	Ellerton	NLH	56	Thelsford	NLH
23	Elsham	NLH	57	Thorney	NLH
24	Embleton	NLH	58	Upsall	LH
25	Fangfoss	NLH	59	Wansford	LH
26	Fordham	NLH	60	Warenford	LH
27	Fordingbridge	NLH	61	Welford Bridge	LH
28	*Gilduswad*	LH	62	Welton	NLH
29	Great Hautbois	NLH	63	Wentbridge	LH
30	Great Massingham	NLH	64	West Somerton	LH
31	Greatham	NLH	65	Whittlesford Bridge	NLH
32	Hammersmith	LH	66	Witton Gilbert	LH
33	Hartford Bridge	NLH	67	Wyndham	NLH
34	Horning	NLH			

LH = leper hospital; NLH = non-leper hospital

those areas that had lower densities of small towns in the later Middle Ages. In the less-urbanised eastern counties north of the Humber, for example, about a third of all hospitals were rural. Conversely in the southwest and parts of the Midlands, where towns had a much higher density, counties had few or even no known rural hospitals.[9]

Distribution in part reflects various sorts of rural feature that might generate a hospital. In seven instances distribution was apparently influenced by the desire of rural monastic communities (or their lay founders) to have hospitals sited near their precincts.[10] In the instance of the hospital of Horning, this is attributable to the monastic community itself as foundation can be credited to Daniel, abbot of St Benet of Hulme, *c.* 1150–53.[11] Such relationships are usually only implicit through the proximity of rural hospitals to monasteries, but were not universal across the religious orders. Of the eight rural hospitals sited near monastic houses, five were located near houses of canons (three Augustinian, one Gilbertine, one Premonstratensian). Such topographical associations may on occasion be coincidental as with the leper-house of *Bradebusk*, which lay near Thurgarton Priory. In this instance the foundation of the leper-house can be attributed to the Heriz family, who retained patronage of the leper-house and had no substantive connection with the priory.[12] This pattern is in stark contrast to towns where many Benedictine houses had strong associations with hospitals. Though the monastic church had some association with rural hospitals, the role of bishops has been exaggerated. Claims concerning the role of bishops in the foundation of rural hospitals are based on a passage in a *vita* of St Hugh of Avalon, bishop of Lincoln 1186–1200.[13] The passage refers to Hugh's visits to hospitals (*matriculae*) where many lepers were maintained on certain of the episcopal estates of the bishops of Lincoln.[14] Attention to the distribution of leper-houses and the estates of the bishops of Lincoln indicates the passage refers to estates associated with towns rather than rural manors.[15]

In an indeterminate number of instances, the distribution of rural hospitals was influenced by feudal geography. Baronies, whose tenants held their estates from their crown by payment of baronial relief, represent the only sort of feudal tenure for which a reasonably comprehensive set of central places (*capita*) can be established in the twelfth and thirteenth centuries and included some of the wealthiest lords in the country.[16] Of 81 rural *capita*, those at Bolam, Embleton, Staveley, and Wormegay were near rural hospitals.[17] In the first three instances the role of baronial lords in the genesis of these institutions is suggested only by geographical proximity. Wormegay provides a clear illustration that some baronial lords did found hospitals at their rural capita. A confirmation charter of Henry II of 1174–5 concerning a leper-house in the vicinity of the island of Wormegay states that the leper-house was built by Reginald de Warrenne. A younger son of earl William II de Warenne, Reginald de Warenne, held the barony of Wormegay from 1166 until 1178–9.[18]

The distribution of rural hospitals was more strongly influenced by ideas associated with the general Christian duty to provide hospitality to wayfarers and guide them through dangerous places and across hazardous waters. Inextricably intertwined with these ideas was the material importance of the alms of such travellers to the slender economies of most rural hospitals. The situation for leper houses was different. While they received alms from passers-by, they consisted of permanent communities of the sick, and if they provided temporary accommodation for outsiders at all, it was only for mendicant lepers, as with the rural leper-house of *Gilduswad*.[19] This coupled with the greater concentration of alms-traffic to be found on the approach roads to towns may partly explain why the percentage of leper-houses which are urban rather than rural (92.3%) is significantly higher than other types of hospitals (74.3%). The importance of traffic is apparent from the hospitals associated with rural settlements with strong links to land or more rarely waterborne travel. The relationship is implicit in the numerous examples, where a rural hospital was associated with a settlement on a main road.

In a few instances the importance of travel by water is suggested by hospitals associated with tiny ports and landing places, such as Lode – a diminutive inland port on the fen-edge of east Cambridge-shire and Denhall – an outport of Chester located some nine miles (14.5 km) north-west at a small inlet on the estuary of the River Dee, Horning on the Bure, and Wyndham in Shermanbury, which was the head of navigation of the Adur *c.* 1700.[20] The leper-house of Wans-ford was associated with a place where road and water traffic intersected. Wansford was the head of navigation of the Nene, and an important crossing of the Great North Road.[21]

The reception of travellers from ships is apparent in the instance of Denhall. Geophysical and earthwork surveys of the site of the hospital and its environs revealed its location right on the edge of the cove adjacent to the remains of three probable medieval quays.[22] The maritime associations of the hospital are also explicit from its earliest charter of 1238. This refers to it as 'the hospital [...] by the shore of the sea', details its purpose as giving aid to the poor and the ship-wrecked (*pauperes et naufrages*), and records the dedication of the hospital to St Andrew, the patron saint of fishermen.[23]

In two instances it is tempting to associate hospitals on estuarine or coastal locations with religious ideas concerning the importance of guiding travellers across hazardous waters as exemplified in the *vitae* of saints, such as St Julian and St Christopher.[24] North Ferriby was the point of embarkation for one of the ferries that linked the Lincolnshire and Yorkshire banks of the lower Humber. North Ferriby had a ferry before 1086 and had apparently acquired a hospital-priory before 1183.[25] The probable location of the house, near what was the edge of the inter-tidal area, was well placed to serve the ferry. The position of the hospital of Cockersand on the Lune estuary 6 miles (9.6 km) south-west of Lancaster may reflect a role of the hospital in guiding wayfarers travelling along the sands at low tide, a role certainly played by the priory which succeeded it.[26]

In emphasising the importance of travel one important caveat must be made. Despite the importance of pilgrimage routes in the literature concerning hospitals, it is difficult to discern much of a relationship between pilgrimage and the distribution of English rural hospitals.[27] This in part reflects the nature of pilgrimage in England. Most English saints were only of regional or local importance and were unlikely to attract pilgrims in sufficient numbers to generate and sustain a hospital infrastructure along the routes beyond their cult centre. Only the shrines of international importance – Canterbury and perhaps Walsingham by the last quarter of the thirteenth century – are likely to have had this effect. Many hospitals lay along the London–Canterbury road, which was the most important overland route to the shrine of St Thomas Becket. All of the hospitals were associated with towns, an unsurprising relationship given the density of towns along this stretch of road. The Walsingham routes were far less urbanised, but are harder to characterise. Ickburgh and perhaps Great Massingham lay on routes to Walsingham and had rural hospitals.[28] The apparent failure of other cults to generate specific rural hospitals does not mean that rural hospitals did not on occasion dispense hospitality to pilgrims, but it cannot be said to be their primary purpose.

Insight concerning the relationship of the rural hospital to settlement is restricted to the twenty-five rural hospitals whose precise location is known. Perhaps most interesting is the relationship of rural leper-houses to settlement, though generalisation is difficult since only six sites can be located with precision. Some rural leper-houses did occupy sites which were distant from settlement. The leper-house of *Bradebusk*, for example, lay beside the Nottingham–Southwell road at the northern extremity of the vill over 0.6 of a mile (1 km) from the village of Gonalston and even further from the nearest neighbouring village Thurgarton (see Fig. 9.2A). The leper-house of Alkmonton lay beside what was probably the main road from Derby to Newcastle-under-Lyme (Staffordshire). The house was sited just in the township of Alkmonton at the boundary with the township of Hungry Bentley. The leper-house lay 0.4 miles (0.7 km) from the nearest settlement (see Fig. 9.2B).

Such isolated locations were not universal. The leper-house of Ickburgh (Norfolk) lay beside what was regarded as the Brandon–Swaffham section of the London to Wells road in 1675 and about 120m from the nearest settlement (see Fig. 9.2C).[29] The leper-house of West Somerton (Norfolk) lay beside the church of the township (see Fig. 9.2D). The hospital's location probably derives from its taking over the existing manorial complex, because in this part of England manorial halls were generally sited beside parish churches and the founders of the leper-house, the royal justiciar Ranulph de Glanville and his wife Berta, had granted the manor of Somerton to the hospital.[30] The sources concerning the foundation of the leper-house are too meagre to identify the agents who chose its site, but the location of the house at the heart of the community reflected power and status. The scenario that, as members of a richly endowed, high status com-

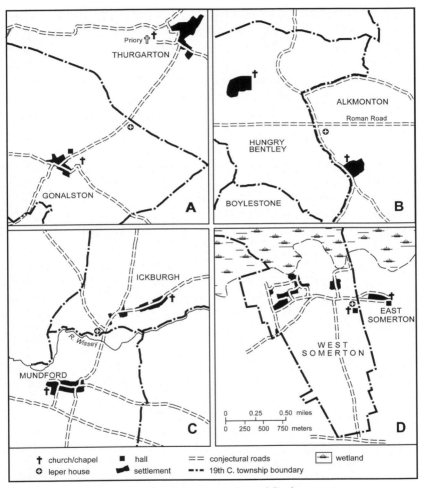

Figure 9.2 Rural Leper-Houses and Settlement:
    A: Gonalston   C. Ickburgh
    B: Alkmonton   D. West Somerton

unity, the lepers had the power to dictate where on their estate they would live, is speculative but plausible.

Non-leper hospitals also occupied a variety of locations in relation to settlement. Some were integrated within existing settlement and well away from the bounds of their township as at Mere or Greatham. The central siting of the hospital of Mere and the clear intention of its founder, Simon de Roppel, to give it such a location is apparent from his foundation charter. De Roppel referred to it as 'the hospital of St John the Baptist that I have built in my court'.[31] Mere Hall, the probable site of the manorial complex, lay in the centre of the township of Mere.

In three instances it is tempting to attribute the isolated locations of rural hospitals to eremitic ideas. The exposed location of the hospital of Cockersand, on a promontory extending into Morecambe Bay is wholly consistent with eremitic ideals, especially as the hospital site was largely cut-off from the mainland to the east and north by an extensive area of peat moss and west and south by the sea (see Fig. 9.3). This apparently limited access by land to periods of low tide.[32] The extreme location of the hospital reflects the circumstances of its foundation. A charter of William de Lancaster II (d.1184) confirms the original grant of the area to Hugh the Hermit (*heremita*) 'for the maintenance of a hospital'.[33] A later account names the hermit as Hugh Garth and states that he founded the hospital, collected alms for its building, and became its first master.[34] In the other instances explicit documentary evidence linking hospital location to eremiticism is absent, and we are reduced to speculation concerning why these rural hospitals occupied such striking locations. The leper-house of Bolton, for example, was sited far from main roads in a marsh on what is described in medieval documents as an island (*insula*). Were the connections of this leper-house with the Cistercian order important in its siting? The leper-house of Maiden Bradley was established on the margins of one of the heavily-wooded parts of the royal forest of Selwood.[35] Maiden Bradley was unusual in that it was originally conceived as a hospital for leprous women rather than a mixed community. Was its location influenced by the general appeal of eremetic ideas to religious women, as has been suggested for a number of rural English nunneries with similarly isolated locations?[36]

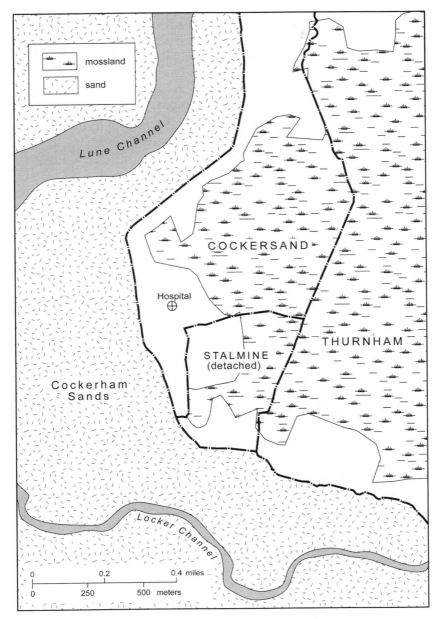

Figure 9.3 Cockersand Hospital

Isolation was of course relative. Something has already been said of the connection between Cockersand and travel, and the village of Maiden Bradley was bisected by what was regarded as the London–Barnstaple road in 1675.[37]

Locations isolated from settlement usually reflected more arbitrary reasons. For example, the isolation of the non-leper hospital of Whittlesford Bridge from the village of Duxford, and its proximity to the boundary of its township reflects the role of a main road as marking the boundary between the townships of Duxford and Whittlesford and the general attraction of roads for hospitals. Here topographical coincidence was important: it was not that the hospital owing its location to any concerns about 'liminality'. In some instances non-leper hospitals occupied locations some distance from settlements because they had been granted and lay within substantial estates, as with the hospitals of Anglesey and Clattercote.

In terms of terrain, rural hospitals appear to have avoided high ground (see Fig. 9.4). Only one rural hospital was sited higher than 200m Ordnance Datum. In addition to the obvious environmental difficulties, this may also reflect the nature of the road network. Wherever possible main roads in highland England appear to have followed circuitous lower routes along valleys ahead of more direct routes over high ground.[38] The influence of this characteristic of the road network on hospital distribution is well illustrated by one of the few clear exception to it – the trans-Pennine section of the Great North Road crossed Stainmoor between Swaledale and the Eden valley – and was also the focus for England's highest known hospital at Reycross sited at 420m. With more uncompromising terrain and greater traffic flows, highland England might have had hospitals in locations as spectacular as those of the great monastic hospitals on the pilgrimage routes over the Alps and Pyrenees, such as Mont-Joux on the route to Rome below the Col du Grand–Saint-Bernard (2469m), or the hospital of Santa Christina below the Col de Somport (1631m), on the Toulouse–Jaca leg of one of the routes through the Pyrenees to Santiago de Compostella.[39]

Rural hospitals unsurprisingly also seem to have preferred sites which combined good water supplies and access to passing alms

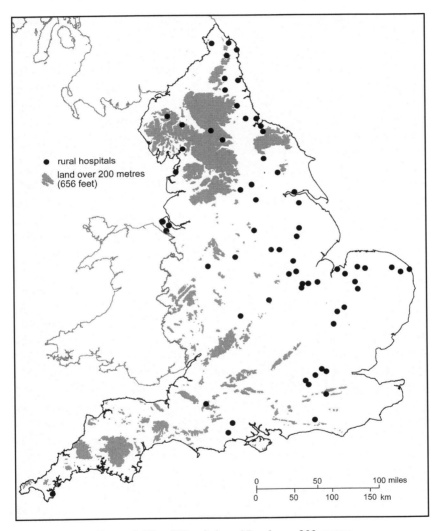

Figure 9.4 Rural Hospitals and Land over 200 metres

traffic. This is apparent from the many rural hospitals that took their names from crossings of watercourses, such as the hospitals of Aberford and Warenford (Northumberland), where the Doncaster–Knaresborough road crossed Cock Beck and the Berwick–Alnwick road crossed a minor watercourse, respectively. Similar locations of other rural hospitals are indicated by place-names which derive from the Old Norse *vath* (ford) and its Old English cognate *gewæd*, as at *Gilduswad*, a crossing of the Lowther near Bampton (Westmoreland); *Vadotavelli*, a crossing of the Avon in Charlecote (Warwickshire); Langwade in Cockley Cley (Norfolk), a crossing of a tributary of the Wissey; and *Boycodeswade* in East Rudham, a crossing of the Tat.[40]

Attention to the layout of the sites of rural hospitals is also revealing. It is probable that the boundaries which enclosed rural hospitals were made of modest materials and encompassed small amounts of land compared to monastic houses. No rural hospitals had layouts comparable to the large walled precincts of the principal hospitals of major urban centres, such as St Leonard's, York, and the four great London hospitals, or other major foundations, such as the hospital of Burton Lazars near Melton Mowbray, which was the main English house of the Order of the Knights of St Lazarus.[41] Even the rural hospital of Maiden Bradley, which was unusually wealthy, and may have required more room because it housed canons as well as leprous women, only occupied a site of *c.* 2.5 acres (1.0 ha).[42] It is probable that most rural hospitals had modest enclosures with boundaries defined by ditches and banks rather than stone walls, which were more expensive in most areas. A probable example is a small banked enclosure 22 x 13m that apparently marks the site of the hospital of Hartford Bridge.[43] The modest nature of most rural hospitals may explain the virtual absence of two other features: fishponds, an important indicator of high status diet, restricted to Alkmonton, Clattercote and perhaps Maiden Bradley; and moats, restricted to Clattercote.

The fertility and tractability of the soils within and beyond the boundaries of the hospital varied enormously from one hospital to another but is difficult to characterise. The leper-house of West Somerton provides an instructive example that a founder could grant prime agricultural land. Its rich estate, with a high value of £60 in 1292, reflected its location on the Isle of Flegg, an area which combined some of the finest arable in England with extensive wetlands for grazing livestock and cutting peat.[44] Most rural hospitals were probably far less well endowed. Many were probably limited in their capacity to feed the population of the hospital because of the inherent limitations in the fertility of their arable land, its small area, and problems in terms of cultivation, especially human and animal labour to work the land. Examples of rural hospitals associated with deserted medieval settlements, such as Alkmonton and Great Hautbois, underline how the fortunes of rural hospitals were bound up with those of their neighbours. A more detailed understanding of the rural communities associated with rural hospitals would cast light on the disappearance of many rural English hospitals in and after the fourteenth century and perhaps changes in the context and provision of rural poor relief in general.

On current research the rural hospitals of England in the twelfth and thirteenth centuries cannot yet be placed within a wider context. The most obvious point of comparison is the wave of English almshouse foundations that took place from the fifteenth century but they remain under-researched. Drawing meaningful comparisons between English rural hospitals and those of continental Europe is a major undertaking and beyond the scope of this paper. A few fragments of evidence illustrate profound regional differences in the numbers of rural hospitals. In the Mosane region, for example, over half the hospitals established before 1500 were in villages or the open countryside, while Rhineland leper-houses were exclusively associated with towns.[45] Normandy, which is of obvious contextual importance, had much larger numbers of leper-houses than England and preliminary mapping of their distribution in the diocese of Rouen indicates concentrations in more densely populated rural areas.[46] Mapping regional and national distributions of rural and urban hospitals is an obvious but important prerequisite for future comparative study, which could contribute to an understanding of wider themes, such as the relationship between demographic structures and rural and urban welfare practices.

Part of such an exercise must also involve greater attention to the depositional processes by which hospitals entered the historical record. The ease with which different sorts of hospital could disappear from the historical record needs careful consideration, especially give the importance of the survival of hospital charters for indicating the existence of short-lived rural hospitals and smaller urban hospitals. The conclusions of such an exercise may make uncomfortable reading, but if we do not estimate the extent of our ignorance, we cannot assess what knowledge we have.

Notes

1   Versions of this paper were read at the Verona Conference, 2000, and the 'Hôpitaux et maladreries au moyen âge: espace et environment', Laboratoire d'archéologie, Université de Picardie, Amiens, 22 November 2002.

2   See, for example, M. Bailey, 'Peasant Welfare in England, 1290–1348', *Economic History Review*, 51 (1998), pp.223–51; E. Clark, 'Some Aspects of Social Security in Medieval England', *Journal of Family History*, 7 (1982), pp.307–20; idem, 'Social Welfare and Mutual Aid in the Medieval Countryside', *Journal of British Studies*, 33 (1994), pp.381–407; C. Dyer, *Standards of Living in the Later Middle Ages* (Cambridge, 1998 edn), pp.234–57, 311–4; C. Dyer, 'Did the Peasants Really Starve in Medieval England?' in *Food and Eating in Medieval Europe*, ed. M. Carlin and J.T. Rosenthal (London and Rio Grande, 1998), pp.53–71; R.M. Smith, 'The Manorial Court and the Elderly Tenant in Late Medieval England', in M. Pelling and R.M. Smith (eds), *Life, Death and the Elderly* (London, 1991), pp.39–61; Z. Razi, 'The Myth of the Immutable English Family', *Past and Present*, 140 (1993), pp.3–44; P. Horden, 'Small Beer? The Parish and the Poor and Sick in Late Medieval England', in C. Burgess and E. Duffy (eds), *The Parish in Late Medieval England* (Donington, 2006), pp.339–64.

3   P. Horden, 'A Discipline of Relevance: The Historiography of the Later Medieval Hospital', *Social History of Medicine*, 1 (1988), pp.359–74; R. Gilchrist, 'Christian Bodies and Souls: the Archaeology of Life and Death in Later Medieval Hospitals', in S. Bassett (ed.), *Death in Towns: Urban Responses to the Dead and Dying 1000–1600* (Leicester, 1992), pp.101–18; C. Rawcliffe, 'The Earthly and Spiritual Topography of Suburban Hospitals', in K. Giles and C. Dyer (eds), *Town and Country in the Middles Ages*, Society for Medieval Archaeology Monograph, 22 (Leeds, 2005), pp.197–210.

4   For this study the following were classed as 'towns': Christopher Dyer's unpublished list of 882 large and small medieval towns, which where possible is based on occupational and population data; 115 early boroughs which either

did not retain or in some instances may never have acquired basic urban characteristics, and 91 settlements omitted by Dyer which Alan Everitt classified as
sixteenth-century market towns: A. Everitt, 'The Marketing of Agricultural Produce', in J. Thirsk (ed.), *Agrarian History of England and Wales*, 4 (Cambridge, 1967), pp.466–592 at 468–75. The Dyer list underpins C. Dyer, 'Small
Towns 1300–1600', in D. Palliser (ed.), *The Cambridge Urban History*, 1
(Cambridge, 2000), pp.505–37. My thanks to Chris Dyer for providing me with
a copy of his list. Data concerning hospitals comes from M. Satchell, 'Medieval
English Hospitals GIS Database', Department of Geography, University of
Cambridge (abbreviated hereafter as MEHGIS).

5   The greatest distance for a hospital associated with a town is the leper-house of
Stourbridge which lay 2,291 metres (1.42 miles) beyond the Cambridge town
ditch.

6   MEHGIS.

7   M. Rubin, *Charity and Community in Medieval Cambridge* (Cambridge, 1987),
pp.135, 136–7; D. M. Owen, *Church and Society in Medieval Lincolnshire*
(Lincoln, 1971), pp.55–6.

8   The author is grateful to the Wellcome Trust who funded the creation of the
MEHGIS database (Grant no. 066400). All maps were created by the author in
conjunction with Phil Stickler of the Cartographic Unit, Department of
Geography, University of Cambridge.

9   Dyer, 'Small Towns 1270–1540', pp.507–8, 509.

10   MEHGIS. See Fig. 9.1 nos 10, 11, 22, 34, 52, 57, 61.

11   The foundation of the hospital is apparently indicated by the charter of William
Turbe, bishop of Norwich, concerning the appropriation of the church of
Horning to the abbey for the support of the poor and the construction of 'out-
buildings' (*officinae*): C. Harper-Bill (ed.), *English Episcopal Acta VI, Norwich
1070–1214* (Oxford, 1990), no. 98, pp.83–4.

12   MEHGIS; T. Foulds (ed.), *The Thurgarton Cartulary*, Paul Watkins Medieval
Studies, 8 (Stamford, 1994), p.cxlvi.

13   N. Orme and M. Webster, *The English Hospital 1070–1570* (New Haven and
London, 1995), pp.41, 176.

14   Adam of Eynsham, *Magna Vita Sancti Hugonis. The Life of St Hugh of Lincoln*,
ed. and trans. D.L. Douie and H. Farmer, 1 (London, 1961), p.13.

15   MEHGIS; *The Registrum Antiquissum of the Cathedral Church of Lincoln*, ed.
C.W. Foster, 1, Lincoln Record Society, 27 (Hereford, 1930), no. 250, pp.193–
5.

16   This dataset derives from Sanders' listing but excludes *capita* which lack clear
evidence for baronial tenure, baronies in Wales, *capita* whose location is
unknown and those that either share the name of, or are within 500 metres of a
town: I. J. Sanders, *English Baronies: A Study of their Origin and Descent,
1086–1327* (London, 1960); MEHGIS.

17   MEHGIS. For the hospitals see Map 1 nos. 6, 7, 24, 52.

18   N. Vincent, 'The Foundation of Wormegay Priory', *Norfolk Archaeology*, 43 (1999), pp.307–12, esp. 309–11.

19   Cumbria Record Office (Carlisle), D/Lons/L medieval deeds AS6.

20   For the navigability of the rivers see J. Langdon, 'Inland Water Transport in Medieval England', *Journal of Historical Geography*, 19 (1993), pp.1–11; p.5, table 1, no. 34; B.M.S. Campbell, *English Seignorial Agriculture 1250–1450* (Cambridge, 2000), p.270 note 41; D. Hall, *The Fenland Project, 10: Cambridgeshire Survey. The Isle of Ely and Wisbech*, East Anglian Archaeological Report, 79 (Cambridge, 1996), pp.112–13; *Victoria County History, Sussex*, 6 (3), p.151.

21   Sea-going vessels are documented at Wansford in 1184: *Transcripts of Charters relating to Gilbertine Houses*, ed. F.M. Stenton, Lincolnshire Record Society, 18 (Horncastle, 1922), p.74, no. 2.

22   M. Jecock, 'St Andrew's Hospital, Denhall: Cheshire, An Archaeological Survey Report', unpublished report, RCHME, 1998.

23   Staffordshire and Stoke-on-Trent Archive Service, Lichfield Record Office, B/A/1/5ii, fol. 62r; calendared as *The Registers or Act Books of the Bishops of Coventry and Lichfield. Book V. Being the Second Register of Bishop Robert de Stretton A.D. 1360–1385*, ed. R.A. Wilson, Collections for a History of Staffordshire, new ser., 8 (London, 1905), p.132.

24   In the *vita* of St Julian, he and his wife 'departed [...] and went till they came to a great river over which much folk passed, where they edified an hospital much great for to harbour poor people, and there do their penance in bearing men over that would pass': F.S. Ellis (ed.), *The Golden Legend*, 3 (London, 1900), p.4.

25   The ferry was longstanding. The place-name, Ferriby, is first recorded in 1086 and derives from the Old Norse *ferja* 'ferry': M. Gelling and A. Cole, *The Landscape of Place-Names* (Stamford, 2000), p.71. The monastic community referred to in a charter of *c.*1164–83, is apparently the same as that referred to as a hospital in 1219: *Early Yorkshire Charters*, ed. C.T. Clay, Yorkshire Archaeological Society Record Series, Extra Series, 9 (Wakefield, 1953), no. 18, p.99; *Rolls of the Justices in Eyre being the the Rolls of Pleas and Assizes for Yorkshire in 3 Henry III, 1218–19*, ed. D.M. Stenton, Selden Society, 56 (London, 1937), no. 160, p.66. The journey was not without risk – the Humber is about 2 miles (3.2 km) wide between North and South Ferriby, the two embarkation points of the ferry.

26   M. Higham, 'Dark Age and Medieval Roads', in A. Crosby (ed.), *Leading the Way: A History of Lancashire's Roads* (Preston, 1998), pp.29–52: 51–2; *Collectanea Anglo-Premonstratensia*, ed. F.A. Gasquet, Camden Society, 3rd ser., 6 (London, 1904), no. 15, p.247.

27   R.M. Clay, *The Hospitals of Mediaeval England* (London, 1909), p.9.

28   *Ordnance Survey Map of XVII Century England* (Southampton, 1930), Ogilby route no. 52 (Ogilby routes hereafter are referenced by numbers alone). When Edward I visited Walsingham in 1296, 1299 and 1302 he travelled via Massing-

ham: E.W. Safford, *Itinerary of Edward I, II, 1291–1307*, List and Index Society, 103 (London, 1974), pp.84, 132, 188.

29   Ogilby, no. 52.

30   R. Mortimer, 'The Priory of Butley and the Lepers of West Somerton', *English Historical Review*, 43 (1980), pp.99–103, esp. 100.

31   'hospitali Sancti Johannis Baptiste quod construxi in curia mea de Mera': Cambridge University Library, MCD 959, fol. 77v.

32   R. Middleton et al., *The Wetlands of North Lancashire*, North West Wetlands Survey, 3 (Lancaster, 1995), pp.127–8.

33   *Chartulary of Cockersand Abbey*, 3 (I), Chetham Society, new series, 56 (Manchester, 1905), pp.758–9, no. 2.

34   *Heraldic Visitation of the Northern Counties in 1530 by Thomas Tonge*, ed. W. Hylton Dyer Longstaffe, Surtees Society, 41 (Durham, 1863), p.91.

35   M. Garvie, *The Bounds of Selwood*, Frome Historical Research Group, Occasional Papers 1 (1978).

36   R. Gilchrist, *Gender and Material Culture: The Archaeology of Religious Women* (London and New York, 1994), pp.65–7, 90–1.

37   Ogilby, no. 32.

38   Examples include the medieval routes around the Dartmoor massif and through the Pennines via the Tyne Gap and the Aire Gap.

39   A. Durán Gudiol, *El Hospital de Somport entre Aragón y Bearn* (siglos XII y XIII) (Zaragoza, 1986), p.13.

40   M. Gelling and A. Cole, *The Landscape of Place-Names* (Stamford, 2000), pp.94–5; Cumbria Record Office (Carlisle), D/Lons/L medieval deeds AS6; J. McN. Dodgson, *The Place-Names of Westmoreland*, II, English Place-Names Society, 48 (Cambridge, 1967), pp.199, 297; *MA*, 6 (I), 369, no. II; Norfolk Record Office (Norwich), Norwich Consistory Court Harsyk Register, fol. 17v. The place-name *Vadotavelli* (modern Thelsford) is from the legend of the hospital's seal: *Victoria County History, Warks.*, 2, plate 1 facing pp.74–5.

41   A.E. Brown, 'Burton Lazars, Leicestershire: A Planned Medieval Landscape', *Landscape History*, 18 (1996), pp.31–45, esp. 32.

42   Unpublished survey, South Wilshire Project, Royal Commission on the Historical Monuments of England, Salisbury.

43   Northumberland SMR (Morpeth), NAR No. NZ 27 NW2.

44   Mortimer, 'The Priory of Butley and the Lepers of West Somerton', p.100. For the fertility of the Isle of Flegg see Campbell, *English Seignorial Agriculture 1250–1450*, pp.335, 343–4; A. Young, *General View of the Agriculture of the County of Norfolk* (Newton Abbot, repr. 1969), p.12. About a third of the township of West Somerton including the site of the leper-house consists of deep loamy soils of the Wick 2 association (Soils Association no. 541 S) and is rated Grade 1 agricultural land.

45   J. Fray, 'Hospitäler, Leprosenhäuser und Mittelalterliches in Lotharingen (*c.* 1200–*c.* 1500), in F. Burgard and A. Haverkamp (eds), *Auf den Römerstrassen*

ins Mittelalter: Beiträge zur Verkehrsgeschichte zwischen Maas und Rhein von der Spätantike bis ins 19. Jahrhundert, Trierer Historische Forschungen, 30 (1997), pp.407–26, esp. 411; M. Uhrmacher, 'L'Implantation des léproseries en Rhénanie, réflexion à l'échelle d'un région', paper delivered to the Colloquium 'Hôpitaux et maladreries au Moyen Âge: espace et environnement', Université de Picardie, Amiens, 22 November 2002.

46   J. Fournée, 'Les maladreries et les vocables de leurs chappelles', *Cahiers Léopold Delisle*, 46 (1997), pp.49–142. Preliminary mapping was based on the gazetteer in A. Fouré, 'Lépreux et léproseries dans le diocese de Rouen', *Revue des sociétés savantes de Haute-Normandie*, 31 (1963), pp.7–16.

Sergio Onger

Chapter 10: The Formation of the Hospital Network in the Brescian Region between the Eighteenth and Twentieth Centuries

The formation of a network of hospitals in the Brescian region took place in the first decades of the nineteenth century, but not as the result of any precise planning. The country hospitals in particular, were set up piecemeal as works of private charity, although this concept had been updated in a new economic and social context.[1] For the first time, this health structure was no longer one that generally saw poor patients from the villages cared for at home while those in the city were admitted to the large city hospitals. Historically, this was the structure – with all the limitations and ties that this implies – on which the current hospital system has developed. And yet, at least initially, its spread was determined by local circumstances. Even the municipal authorities' contribution took place within a definitive framework of spontaneous generosity from private citizens.

It was not inevitable that this situation would develop in this way, above all in Lombardy, where under Joseph II, the government had undertaken definitive reforms that formally recognised the health of citizens as a state responsibility,[2] even if traditional charitable bodies still played their part. Even the province of Brescia, though it had not benefited from the influence of late-Enlightenment Austria, had experienced de-privatisation and rationalisation of public health during the Napoleonic period. It was with a new concept of sovereignty created at the end of the eighteenth century – i.e., the passage from the 'territorial state' to the 'population state' that really initiated reform. In addition to maintaining order and privileges and increasing the power of the state by territorial expansion, sovereignty was also expected to include looking after the well-being of its own citizens.[3] In the 'population state', health was a common asset of society and no longer a blessing allocated to individuals by virtue of Divine Providence; public charity, rationalised and controlled by the state, overlaid and replaced Christian charity. Thus hospitals began to be structured as organisations which were principally therapeutic, with their own rules, order and their own scientific–didactic role. Hand-in-hand with the profound transformation of the concept of care, went a change in the status of the inmates of a hospital. While these still continued to be mainly found among the local population, they also had to be ill to have the right of access to the structure; if not they were directed to other charitable institutions.

The object of this paper is to study the creation of the network of health institutions in the Brescian province which took on responsibility for its citizens' health, initially through the spontaneous impulse of private charities, but which later came increasingly under the control of public authorities. In contrast, the origins and consolidation of the hospital infrastructures will be looked at through a comparative analysis of different cases, and by identifying certain general trends. The history of individual institutions, although significant, will not be dealt with here.

In little more than a century the number of Brescian hospitals tripled, from eleven to thirty-seven, accompanying the growth of agricultural and manufacturing districts. Side by side with the quantitative imbalance went a qualitative one which, with few exceptions, penalised rural institutions. The urban hospitals were far ahead of the rural ones in terms of scientific and clinical specialisation, while the rural ones continued for a long time to offer a service that was closer to that of traditional beggars' hospices.

In demarcating the geographical area to be studied, we need to take into account the territorial variations the province experienced during the nineteenth century. The Camonica valley and Asolano area, integral parts of the province under Venetian rule, were respectively incorporated into the Department of Serio (later the Province of Bergamo) and into the Department of the Mincio (later the Province of Mantua) in 1801. With some minor modifications, these territorial changes remained until 23 October 1859 when the Camonica valley was returned to Brescian jurisdiction. In order to ease the problems posed by these geographical-administrative variations, we have limited our research to the area of the modern province adding only the Camonica valley. On the other hand, if we exclude the newly founded hospital at Malegno, this valley lacked hospitals for a long period (the first was created at Breno after 1848). This meant that in the first half of the nineteenth century, encouraged by a system of exchanges and contacts that traditionally gravitated around Brescia, 'many patients and women in labour, despite having different legal residence, preferred to go down to Brescia to invoke the city's charity'.[4]

I   The Napoleonic Period and the Restoration

The history of Brescian hospitals in the nineteenth century starts, at least on paper, in a revolutionary fashion. The decree of 5 September 1806 reformed the entire health system of the Italian Kingdom, creating medical commissions in all departments and proposing to strengthen the old hospital structures making these an ideal instrument for the policy of popular consensus.[5] The administration of public charity was entrusted to the Ministry of Religion where four inspector generals each governed one of the four administrative districts into which the Kingdom had been divided. The administration and funds of all welfare institutions of the principal regional cities were concentrated in the hands of the 'Charitable Congregations' composed of the Prefect, the Bishop, the President of the Court of Appeal or the Prefect of the Courts of Justice, by the 'Podestà' (or mayor) and by other members nominated by the Viceroy and proposed by the ministry.[6]

Despite these aims, there was no increase in the number of hospitals in the Italian Kingdom; the thirteen hospitals registered in the census of 1808 continued to exist, offering around 861 beds or one for every 354 inhabitants. The two city hospitals – the Ospedale Maggiore for male patients and the corresponding Women's Hospital – with 350 and 250 beds respectively – covered 70 per cent of the available places. The remaining beds were divided among the hospitals of

Bovegno, Carpenedolo, Castrezzato, Chiari, Desenzano, Lonato, Orzinuovi, Palazzolo, Rovato, Salò and Verolanuova. This imbalance between the city and its surrounding territory is even clearer if we compare the data of patients actually admitted: 474 out of a total of 584, that is 81 per cent of the whole, were admitted to the city hospital. In the hinterland, only Chiari with forty patients admitted and Salò with twenty could be considered welfare institutions of any importance.[7]

The city hospitals had a complex, highly developed operative structure. The Ospedale Maggiore had two clinics, one for medicine, the other for surgery, with a total number of 300 beds, it had rooms set aside for those suffering from venereal and other infective diseases and a pharmacy for the hospitals and the poor of the city.[8] Within the Ospedale Maggiore, there was also space for the newly founded hospital[9] and, from October 1797 a hospital for psychiatric patients with twenty beds and its 12-bed female counterpart[10]. On the other hand, in the provincial hospitals, only Bovegno, Chiari, Salò and Verolanuova accepted patients from outside their own districts.

Although the Napoleonic era passed without substantially altering the number of hospitals in the province, it did focus on the need to extend the right to be admitted to hospital to the surrounding populations and, consequently, to increase the capacity of the hospitals to accept further patients. An authorative exponent of the Brescian political class of the period, Antonio Sabatti, noted the importance of creating a hospital network in the Department, aimed at 'immediate relief for the suffering poor', without obliging patients to undertake strenuous journeys to reach the city hospital. To do this he believed it was necessary to re-capitalise the hospitals in order to 'make it possible for them to admit the sick from a specific administrative district'.[11] However the consequent project to channel all funds derived from legacies and donations into a few important and well placed institutions to guarantee an efficient, rationally distributed service came to nothing, hindered by local diffidence and by the financial difficulties of the Kingdom.

Furthermore, the hospital network did not change during the first two decades of the restoration of the Austrian monarchy, while the legislative situation did. The decree of 14 December 1821 redefined the organisation of small rural hospitals entrusting the management of their resources to a single administrator and medical direction to a general practioner employed by the town. In 1823 the plan for staffing the institutions was approved by the provincial delegation and three years later it was held that 'the reform was almost generally followed [...] in the administration of establishments'.[12]

In 1835 there was exactly the same number of hospitals as in 1808. In this period of apparent stagnation, some institutes had however started to function effectively and the service was better, ending disorder, economic difficulties and in some cases, inadequacies in the buildings and lack of personnel.[13]

The thirteen hospitals were divided into three classes. To the first category belonged those hospitals with more than 1,000 patients admitted per year: i.e., the Ospedale Maggiore and the Women's Hospital; in the second group were those with 200 patients, Chiari, Orzinuovi, Salò and Verolanuova, and in the third class were those with less than 200, Bovegno, Carpenedolo, Castrezzato, Desenzano, Lonato Palazzolo and Rovato. The city hospitals, designated as 'provincial', admitted patients from all over the region with the exception of the inhabitants of towns where there was already a hospital. The hospitals of Chiari and Salò aided the sick in their surrounding districts and the remaining hospitals, called 'municipal', limited their services to residents in their own specific area.[14] The greater efficiency of municipal hospital services can be seen in the average increase in daily patients rising by 84 per cent between 1808 and 1833. In addition, four new municipal hospitals were under construction. The hospital institution began in fact to consistently intercept the flow of funds coming from private charities.

Indeed, it was in the early nineteenth century that the hospital began to take on a primary position for acquiring merit and prestige in the eyes of the community. These new institutions could therefore be dedicated to the most generous benefactors by both participating in their planning or administration as well as contributing to their funding. Thus the local notables committed themselves to a complex form of aid that placed the idea of curing social ills together with traditional ideas of housing the needy in almshouses etc. Hospitals could therefore be understood as a response to the capitalist transformation of the countryside. This had eroded peasant property by forcing those who worked the land to stipulate work and rent contracts that undermined their consumer capacity. This is in fact the economic and social background in which the Lombardy hospital network developed: a society where four-fifths of the population was employed in agriculture, but in which the breakdown of consolidated production systems regulating the delicate balance that partially protected tenants and workers had worsened the nutritional, hygiene and health conditions of the lower classes.[15] It was in the Po valley where the process of impoverishment was most intense, that the growth of the hospital network was most marked. In particular, hospitals in the lower Brescian region increased from three to fourteen between 1797 and 1920.

In redefining the concept of charity that occurred with the process of capitalist transformation, rural hospitals became a place where the ruling classes sought to reconstruct the social contract broken by the lack of paternalistic ties uniting master and labourer under the *Ancien Régime*. Alongside a philanthropic spirit of solidarity by benefactors, there was the concrete interest in maintaining the workers' health, a concept completely different from previously inspired Christian precepts of charity. Philanthropy was no longer only a means to enter Heaven, but a sort of *humanisme nécessaire*, intended to maintain the workers' health to assure their contribution for production.[16] This idea was clearly expressed at that time by a doctor, Pietro Maggi, who effectively summarised the social scope of medicine:

> It [medicine] alone can say at what age of Man's life he is fit for work, that is ordered for production; what work is suitable for children, adults, old men; what can be done by women and what by men; so that work, instead of creating ordered production, is a means of building physical strength by exercising it, and does not become a means that exhausts the springs of life.[17]

It was therefore imperative to keep workers healthy as only increased output could ensure social progress.

Confirmation of the close link between worsening living conditions for country workers during rural transformation and the need to respond to this through the creation of rural hospitals comes from the role played in founding new hospitals caused by the spread of pellagra and epidemic crises: i.e. the epidemic of petechial typhus in 1816–1817 and those of cholera in 1836, 1849 and 1855. Each time an epidemic created a health emergency there was a spate of bequests to hospitals.[18] The examples of Manerbio, Montichiari, Travagliato and Leno (where the bureaucratic process to obtain government authorisation had been in progress since 1821), fit perfectly into this picture. These hospitals, which began working immediately after the 1836 outbreak of cholera were also all located in areas of the lower Brescian region where pellagra was most endemic. While the largest city hospitals were given increased importance by the clinic, those in the municipalities sprang from renewed charitable donations that for almost half a century took the helm of public health from the Austrian state, preoccupied at that time almost exclusively with balancing its finances while covering a role where its responsibilities were expanding as never before.

In contrast to what the 'medical policy' of Joseph II and the Napoleonic plans had forecast, the Austrian government after the Restoration did not believe it could plan the development of health structures nor indeed help charity orientated towards hospitals. Austrian policy towards pious works was much more concerned with inheritance (and what was due to the State) than in using assistance as a lever to enlarge and consolidate consensus. It was therefore slow and even reluctant to concede authorisation to create new hospitals. The Treasury's economic policy was expected only to fund new hospitals and maternity hospitals as well as lunatic asylums. Other welfare, charity or socially useful institutes (e.g. educational institutes which were pressurising the public authority for attention, funds and protection – see the emblematic case of nursery schools)[19] had to rely on their own efforts, on contributions from alms giving institutions, on municipal authorities and on private charity.[20] To overcome government resistance and obtain authorisation to set up a hospital, it was necessary to demonstrate that the new body would be entirely self-supporting; autonomy that could be achieved only through legacies and private donations. To add to their difficulties, in many cases local administrations were prevented from participating in founding hospitals due to restrictions on contributions.

In 1844 the hospitals in the province, excluding its principal city, had risen to seventeen out of seventy for the whole of Lombardy. Brescia was in second place after the province of Bergamo (that had twenty-one), and more than Mantua, in third place with nine. Statistics from a short time later showed that, out of eighty-eight public hospitals registered in the region's census, eighteen were in the Brescian province.[21] With the usual approximation, caused also by the 'fluid' concept of what constituted a hospital, administrative sources were not homogeneous in their tally of structures and, above all, in indicating how many beds they had; although these were estimated in 1843 as a total of 1,524. Of these 720 were in the city hospitals (including the principle, maternity and mental institutions), 90 in Chiari and 34 in Salò.[22]

The architectural aspect of hospitals in this period allow us to glimpse at the idea that the ruling classes had of the hospital as a modern form of assistance. They were no longer principally as ostentatious as a monument to the generosity of the benefactors, but a structure that aimed as far as possible at being functional, reducing costs to a minimum. Early nineteenth century hospital architecture simply modified the interiors of large exterior shells built in the preceding centuries through complex re-conversions of buildings that had once belonged to the religious orders abolished during the Napoleonic period. This answered the need to contain the costs of poor relief as much as possible.[23]

In the case of the Ospedale Maggiore it was transferred in 1847 to the monastery of San Domenico, thus creating a vast complex which communicated with the Women's hospital. So, in a single structure, afterwards known as the Ospedale Civile, there were both male and female hospitals, the two lunatic asylums, again for separate sexes, an institute for contagious diseases and a new hospital with a maternity annex. With its numerous wards, each with no more than thirty beds, the new hospital allowed clear separation between medical and surgical departments, while contagious diseases and the insane were housed in separate, isolated buildings. The fitting of operating theatres, that ended the practice of operating directly on the patient's bed, the creation of a consulting surgery, together with a series of lesser measures that improved hygiene conditions inside the hospital, were all indications of the increasing importance of implementing strictly therapeutic policies.

However, the buildings themselves did not lend themselves to the concept of a modern hospital and, indeed, were not redesigned simply along the needs of health care as expressed by the medical staff. The political class had another aim besides limiting expense; i.e. to banish the sight of the poor and suffering from Corso del Teatro, the city's most elegant and popular thoroughfare.[24] Indeed there was no lack of severe criticism from medical circles:

> the new hospital in Brescia is very badly built as far admission and care of the sick is concerned, and great sums have been spent on the healthy, that is for buildings destined for Executive offices, the Administration, the private dwellings of the Director, while a 'prison cell' has been set aside as a room for the medical assistants who must remain there continually [...] this indecency would have been avoided if the Administration, limiting itself to carrying out its duties, had left [...] the study of the construction and lay-out of the Hospital to the Director.[25]

The criteria on which the hospital in Montichiari was built were not dissimilar. Here, the seventeenth-century church of San Rocco that had become municipal property after the abolition of the lay brotherhood was re-adapted for use as a hospital, to the satisfaction of the Directory of Public Works in Milan.[26]

Only a few, very small hospitals were constructed *ex novo* in Lombardy at this time. The municipal hospitals in Travagliato, Manerbio and Pontevico, planned following the directives of doctors responsible for health in the province and the Directory of Public Works are examples of what was considered to be the functional requisites of a hospital. The location had to be on an elevated site, possibly outside the urban area, the building had to be well ventilated and in a sunny spot with abundant water supplies. Inside the building there had to be: a porters' lodge to oversee the patients who were kept in seclusion, two wards – one for each sex – a chapel, a contagious diseases department that was 'sufficiently' isolated, washing and toilet facilities, and some 'service' units that generally meant a kitchen and a store-room. The availability of a portico or arcade for the convalescent patients to walk in during the summer, a practice which the medical theory of the time held to be of high therapeutic value, was considered to be very important, even if not strictly indispensable.

The monumental character of the building continued to be an important element and was not neglected – financial means permitting. This was true of the pronaos on the Palladian villa in Travagliato designed by the architect Rodolfo Vantini and the façade with arches and columns in the ashlar work in Pontevico. But the form of these buildings was no longer conditioned, as previously, by religious but rather by secular ideas with the 'lay' architecture of the villa (around a central courtyard at Pontevico and on three sides of an open space at Travagliato and Manerbio) set in greenery and open to the air and light. The secularisation of architecture in fact mediated between the persistent but no longer predominant demand for monumentalism and the functional needs of the medical class.

II   After Unification

The annexation of Lombardy by Piedmont in 1859 did not substantially modify the hospital system, given that the new unified state was no less preoccupied with containing the increasing costs of public welfare. The administration of the health service and public health were regulated until 1888 by the Ratazzi law of 20 November 1859 and by the law of 20 March 1865, which, although repeating more or less the text of the preceding law, introduced mainly administrative changes.[27] The supervision of municipal hospitals was now entrusted to municipal commissions 'with a purely role of consultation delegated by the mayor and without precise ties to the panels of the Administrative and Provincial Councils'.[28] Only with the approval of the Crispi health law (22 December 1888), later completed with the approval of the law reforming pious works of 1890, would there begin to be a real distinction between hospitals and the other welfare institutions.

By the end of Austrian rule, the number of hospitals had risen to twenty-one. Besides the Rizzieri Infirmary in Breno, founded in 1848, that came under the Brescian hospital system with the inclusion of the Camonica valley, there were three other new institutions. First, the Vanzago hospital in Paratico, on Lake Iseo, opened in 1850 and was run by the religious order of the Fatebenefratelli. This was charged with accepting poor patients from the eight surrounding districts. There was then the hospital in Remedello Sopra, set up on the initiative of the parish priest Giovanni Battista Vertua, and the Monauni hospital in Coccaglio for the admission and care of its poor patients, created in 1858 but functioning only from 1862. The hospitals now had 880 beds available of which 371 (42%) were in the city and 509 (58%) throughout its territory.

The total number of places available had not substantially altered since 1808, and had indeed declined slightly in respect to the total population (a decline that can only be explained in part by the inclusion of the Camonica valley). The ratio of beds available between the city and the countryside had, however, seen a considerable shift. It was now the provincial territory that had most patients, increasing by 93 per cent. The city hospitals, transferred to San Domenico in the 1840s, had decreased by 37 per cent. Nonetheless, the city hospitals had increasingly abandoned the physiognomy of a hospice for the poor to take on that of a health care institute. Furthermore due to the chronic state of finances, more attention was paid to the type of patients accepted, and had allowed them to continue to help the same number of patients as in 1843, reducing hospital stay and therefore the need for beds. Furthermore, many of the sick from the hinterland were now accepted by rural hospitals and numerous patients, perhaps hastily classified as chronic, were doubtless sent back to their place of residence.[29]

In the 1861 statistics for good works, 109 hospitals in Lombardy appear in the census (twenty in the urban centres and eighty-nine in rural districts) with 8,125 beds or one for every 382 inhabitants. Of these hospitals forty-three or over 39 per cent had been set up after 1800. The Brescian province, which at that time also included the administrative district of Castiglione delle Stiviere, with its hospitals at Asola, Canneto sull'Oglio, Castelgoffredo, Castiglione and Ostiano, had most hospitals in Lombardy. However, where the regional average of beds per hospital was seventy-four, this number fell to thirty-six in Brescian territory with a bed for every 499 inhabitants.[30]

Between 1862 and 1920, sixteen new municipal hospitals including Bagolino were established. Once again the hospitals were set up without any coordinated planning for the territory and a tendency to favour building small rural hospitals with low specialisation and strong municipal links. As we have seen, this trend was the origin of the hospital network and indeed was reinforced in this period. However, the founders of the hospitals now had to deal with the growing costs of antiseptic procedures, which made the updating of surgical practice in many of the municipal hospitals impossible.[31] Thus a division of work evolved between the large city hospitals with their overcrowded surgical sections and the small territorial hospitals which often lacked surgical wards, acting as hospices for chronic cases.[32]

At the end of the 1870s, four new hospitals were created in Gardone Valtrompia, Gottolengo, Pisogne and Rudiano. Of these, two were established in ex-monastic buildings: Gottolengo, set up in 1863 thanks to the legacy left by the Rodella sisters, was located in the ex-Carmelite monastery in San Girolamo, while Pisogne was created in 1876 in the ex-Augustinian priory given by the municipal authorities to the Congregation of Charity. Again it was private legacies that allowed hospitals in Bagnolo, Darfo, Edolo, Ghedi, Gussago, Nave, Pezzaze, Quinzano and Verolavecchia to be founded. In 1901 the construction of the hospital at Adro had begun, but it did not start functioning until 1909 due to notable financial difficulties. It was followed by the hospital in Gargnano in 1903 thanks to the initiative of the Feltrinelli family and the institute in Ponte di Legno in 1905. The only hospital which closed in the whole period we have considered was the Cacciamatta in Paratico, after a decree dated 1873 withdrew it from the Fatebenefratelli's administration, creating a merger with the hospital in Iseo.

The most significant creation of a hospital in this period once more took place in Brescia itself, with the opening in 1902 of the 'Umberto I' children's hospital. The hospital filled the gap in medical assistance left by the Ospedale Civile which did not admit patients under the age of seven. It accepted poor children of both sexes from two to seven.[33] Set up provisionally within the Ospedale Civile, it consisted of two wards that initially had a total of fourteen beds, but only two years after its foundation these had risen to forty-four.[34] 'Umberto I' was then transferred to the building which had been the institution for rickets' patients, taking over this important function from the then abolished specialised departments. From 1912, following the Teresa Nava Contrini legacy, a convalescent home was added on the nearby hills for the rehabilitation of children.

At the end of the First World War, by 1920, the province's hospital network had 1,000 beds in the Ospedale Civile, eighty-four in the children's hospital and 670 in the Provincial mental asylum – all concentrated in the city itself. Outside the city, the hospitals totalled 1,147 beds (excluding Iseo and Ponte di Legno). Altogether, therefore, there were 2,231 beds or one for every 267 inhabitants leaving aside those in the mental asylum.[35] Compared to the data for 1861, the average beds per hospital had risen from forty to fifty-nine (an increase of 47.5%), although in the case of rural hospitals this was only thirty-two beds per institute, an increase of 28 per cent.

III Conclusion

The Brescian hospital network was formed with, on one hand, the capitalist development in the country and, on the other, according to the imitative logic of philanthropic creation. The results were in part unforeseeable, given that, for almost all the nineteenth century, public authorities were more interested in avoiding hospital services becoming a further burden on the Treasury. Nonetheless, a widespread infrastructure was formed throughout the territory and had a relevant role in modernising charity and maintaining cohesion among social classes after the *Ancien Régime* had been de-activated by the market economy.

The cure of typical rural and urban working-class diseases was not of primary importance due to the relative inefficiency of medical therapies until the last decades of the nineteenth century. This was underlined by the dispensary role of the new rural hospitals, despite the fact that these were set up just when the need to focus on the clinical and scientific aspect of the health structures was being encouraged by the medical profession and the more enlightened ruling class. Indeed, 'Hospitium humanitatis aegrotantis' ('Hospice for suffering humanity') is the ambiguous declaration on the elegant neoclassical pediment of the hospital in Travagliato, one of the few hospitals built *ex novo* during the nineteenth century.

However, following the spread of hospitals throughout the territory and their progressive specialisation, by the beginning of the twentieth century the hospital had already acquired a physiognomy which was much nearer the medical one than that desired by local notables and indeed perhaps by the local population. Furthermore towards the end of this period, hospitals admitted a new type of patient – the paying one; the fame of the consultant physician and the improved hospital environment became the new calling card for a hospital in search of new clients.

Notes

1   The Italian bibliography on this theme has grown particularly over the last few decades; see G. Albini, 'A proposito di studi recenti della storia della salute nel medioevo e nell'età moderna', *Nuova rivista storica*, 64 (1980), pp.143–64; M. Rosa, 'Chiesa, idee sui poveri e assistenza in Italia dal cinque al settecento', *Società e storia*, 10 (1980), pp.775–806; E. Bressan, *L''Hospitale' e i poveri: La storiografia sull'assistenza: l'Italia e il 'caso lombardo'* (Milan, 1981); G. Assereto, 'Pauperismo e assistenza: messa a punto di studi recenti', *Archivio storico italiano*, 141 (1983), pp.253–71; as well as the many regional studies published in P. Grisoli (ed.), *Atti del convegno 'Dalla Carità all'assistenza: Studi, metodi, fonti 1978–1988'. Torino, 21–22 ottobre*, in *Sanità scienza e storia*, 1 (1989), pp.57–226; A. Pastore, 'Gli ospedali in Italia fra Cinque e Settecento: evoluzione, caratteri, problemi', in M.L. Betri and E. Bressan (eds), *Gli ospedali in area padana fra Settecento e Novecento. Atti del III Congresso italiano di storia ospedaliera: Montecchio Emilia, 14–16 marzo 1990* (Milan, 1992), pp.71–88; E. Bressan, D. Montanari and S. Onger (eds), *Tra storia*

dell'assistenza e storia sociale: Brescia e il caso italiano (Brescia, 1996);
M. Cavallera, 'Per una lettura del sistema assistenziale periferico', in
M. Cavallera, A. Giorgio Ghezzi, and A. Lucioni (eds), *I luoghi della carità e
della cura: ottocento anni di storia dell'Ospedale di Varese* (Milan, 2002),
pp.17–28.

2   A. Malamani, 'La sanità pubblica tra Riforme e Rivoluzione', in M. Bona
Castellotti, E. Bressan, C. Fornasieri, and P. Vismara (eds), *Cultura, religione e
trasformazione sociale: Milano e la Lombardia dalle riforme all'Unità* (Milan,
2001), pp.139–48.

3   See M. Foucault, 'La politique de la santé au XVIII siècle', in *Les machines à
guèrire (aux origines de l'hôpital moderne)* (Paris, 1976), p.14.

4   See 'La riaggregazione della Valcamonica alla provincia di Brescia', an extract
from the *Gazzetta ufficiale di Milano*, 28 – 29 July 1858, p.13.

5   See C. Zaghi, 'L'Italia di Napoleone dalla Cisalpina al Regno', in *Storia
d'Italia* (Turin, 1986), vol. 18.I, p.436.

6   *Statistica del Regno d'Italia: le opere pie nel 1861* (Florence, 1868), pp.vi–vii.
See also: E. Bressan, *Povertà e assistenza in Lombardia nell'età napoleonica*
(Milan, 1985), pp.16–17; S. Onger, 'Il riassetto istituzionale della rete assistenziale nella Lombardia della Restaurazione', in V. Zamagni (ed.), *Povertà e
innovazioni istituzionali in Italia: dal Medioevo ad oggi* (Bologna, 2000),
pp.455–567.

7   See S. Onger, 'Gli ospedali "meschini": malattie e luoghi di cura nella pianura
bresciana occidentale (secoli XVIII–XIX)', in *Atlante della Bassa* (Brescia,
1984), vol. 1: *Uomini, vicende paesi dall'Oglio al Mella*, pp.243, 248.

8   A. Sabatti, *Quadro statistico del dipartimento del Mella* (Brescia, 1807),
pp.234–5.

9   S. Onger, *L'infanzia negata: storia dell'assistenza agli abbandonati e indigenti
a Brescia nell'Ottocento* (Brescia, 1985).

10   Sabatti, *Quadro statistico*, pp.235 and 239.

11   *Ibid.*, p.255.

12   Printed circular of the *Congregazione provinciale*, Brescia, 21 March 1826, in
the Archivio di Stato di Brescia (hereafter *ASB*), *Imperial Regia Delegazione
Provinciale* (hereafter *IRDP*), busta 3305.

13   Onger, *Gli ospedali "meschini"*, p.248.

14   W. Menis, *Saggio di topografia statistico-medica della provincia di Brescia
aggiuntevi le notizie storico-statistiche sul cholera epidemico che la desolò
nell'anno MDCCCXXXVI* (Brescia, 1837), 1, p.182.

15   F. Della Peruta, 'Le campagne lombarde nel Risorgimento', in F. Della Peruta,
Democrazia e socialismo nel Risorgimento, 2nd edn (Rome, 1973), pp.37–58;
idem, 'Per la storia della società lombarda nell'età della Restaurazione', *Studi
storici*, 2 (1975), pp.305–39; idem, 'Aspetti della società italiana nell'Italia
della Restaurazione', *Studi storici*, 2 (1976), pp.27–68.

272   Sergio Onger

16   A. Farge, 'Les artisans malades de leur travail', *Annales: Économies, Sociétés, Civilisations* (1977), p.999.

17   P. Maggi, *Alcune idee tendenti al miglioramento della medicina come fonte di produzione applicata giusta i veri principi morali all'individuo ed alla società, o Proposta d'associazione ad un giornale mensile 'La medicina politica' che verrà pubblicato in Brescia da una società di medici* (Brescia, 1850), p.24.

18   G. Cosmacini, *Medicina e sanità in Italia nel ventesimo secolo: dalla 'spagnola' alla II guerra mondiale* (Rome and Bari, 1989), p.293.

19   C. Sideri, *Ferrante Aporti sacerdote, italiano, educatore: biografia del fondatore delle scuole infantili in Italia sulla base di nuova documentazione inedita* (Milan, 1999). On the nursery schools in the Brescian area, see F. Bazzoli, *La carità educatrice: gli asili infantili a Brescia nell'Ottocento*, (Brescia, 1993).

20   B. Bertoli, 'Assistenza pubblica e riformismo austriaco a Venezia durante la Restaurazione: i "luoghi pii"', *Ricerche di storia sociale e religiosa*, 12 (1977), pp.28–31.

21   See G. Sacchi, 'Sulla pubblica beneficenza in Lombardia: memoria statistica', *Annali universali di statistica*, ser. II, 18 (1848), p.242. The data presented in this work are taken from G.L. Gianelli, *Dei miglioramenti sociali efficaci e possibili a vantaggio degli agricoltori e degli operaj* (Milan, 1847).

22   Provincial administrative report for 1843, in ASB, *IRDP*, busta 4198.

23   A. Scotti, 'Malati e strutture ospedaliere dall'età dei Lumi all'Unità', in F. Della Peruta (ed.), *Storia d'Italia, Annali 7. Malattia e medicina* (Turin, 1984), p.273.

24   S. Onger, *La città dolente: povertà e assistenza a Brescia durante la Restaurazione* (Milan, 1993), pp.84ff.

25   'Degli Spedali: Questione Sanitaria', in *La medicina politica*, 8–9 (1852), p.9 n. 10.

26   Sergio Onger, 'Poveri e malati a Montichiari (secoli XVIII–XIX)', in M. Pegrari (ed.), *La comunità di Montichiari: Territorio, vicende umane, sviluppo economico di un centro della pianura bresciana* (Brescia, 1996), pp.261–78.

27   F. Della Peruta, 'Sanità pubblica e legislazione sanitaria dall'Unità a Crispi', *Studi storici*, 4 (1980), p.740.

28   A. Appari, 'Cento anni della legge sanitaria', *Sanità, scienza e storia*, 1–2 (1988), p.12.

29   F. Soncini, 'Sul modo con cui si dichiarano e si licenziano i cronici negli Spedali provinciali, ed in ispecie negli Spedali di Brescia', *La medicina politica*, 3–5 (1852), p.370.

30   *Statistica del Regno d'Italia: le opere pie nel 1861*, pp.xv, 60–1, 194–5.

31   P. Frascani, *Ospedali e società in età liberale* (Bologna, 1986), p.136n.

32   *Ibid.*, pp.176–7.

33   Ospedale dei bambini 'Umberto I', *Statuto* (Brescia, 1903), p.6.

34   Ospedale dei bambini 'Umberto I', *Relazione del consiglio d'amministrazione sul Conto Finanziario e Consuntivo dell'Istituto a 31 dicembre 1904 (letta all'*

assemblea dei Benefattori nella tornata ordin. del 17 dicembre 1905) (Brescia, 1906), p.15.

35   The data are taken from the report of the Ispettore generale reggente, Brescia, 27 August 1920, in Archivio Centrale dello Stato di Roma, Ministero dell' interno, Gabinetto E, Direzione generale amministrazione civile, Serie diverse, div. III, busta 4.

STEVE CHERRY

Chapter 11: 'Keeping your hand in' and Holding On: General Practitioners and Rural Hospitals in Nineteenth- and Twentieth-Century East Anglia

Introduction

A century before the 1858 Medical Act defined the basis of qualified medical practice, traditional professional boundaries were already becoming blurred as surgeon-apothecaries established themselves in provincial centres.[1] They claimed 'regular' medicine for themselves, although a specific medical knowledge could not yet be demarcated from other forms of healing. Their model of general practice, initially based upon one-man and later one-woman family doctoring at commercial fees, was relatively expensive and subject to competition.[2] Wealthier patients were keenly sought after and sometimes 'poached' by other qualified practitioners, despite attempts to devise suitable medical etiquette. Friendly societies, works and sick clubs organised extensive rival forms of care, employing qualified practitioners at reduced remuneration. Various 'irregulars', notably druggists and herbalists, persisted into the twentieth century, not least because their remedies were accessible, relatively cheap and sometimes no less ineffective. As more qualified practitioners entered medical markets, the business of making a medical living remained precarious until the introduction of state national health insurance in 1911. This confirmed the GP as the provider of primary care and gatekeeper to the sickness benefit system for approximately 13 million insured workers, simultaneously offering most doctors a substantial guaranteed income.[3]

In other respects the position of the GP seemed less assured. The constituents of public health care varied historically, but GPs often felt threatened by state or local authority involvement, whether in sanitary reform or personalised services.[4] In the formulation of policy well into the era of the NHS GPs were frequently identified with sectional interest, exponents of individualised treatments rather than collaborative seekers of community health roles.[5] Insofar as 'scientific medicine' became increasingly influential, whether its progressive, technological or entrepreneurial aspects are emphasised, the teaching hospital, specialism and then laboratory medicine are identifiable at the leading edge.[6] Bedside medicine had its place but the specifics of disease-based approaches and identification of 'the case' paid little attention to the patient as a whole person reporting illness. Specialist medical examination, increasingly reliant upon scientific data from the patient's body, established his or her condition and became the hallmark of twentieth-century hospital medicine.[7] As the first point of contact for the lay public, GPs could personify medical orthodoxy and invasive measures, notably in regard to maternity and infant care, yet they were also depicted as isolated, outmoded and even dangerously over-extended in surgical practice.[8] More than a little self-interest featured in efforts by hospital specialists to exclude GPs, restricting them to a primary care role symbolically covered by the medical shorthand of 'Trivia'. This division of medical labour, largely completed by 1948 in Frank Honigsbaum's view, may have been operative in 1900, according to Rosemary Stevens' depiction of 'a referral system that gave all but the richest patients to the GP and all but the smallest hospitals to the specialist'.[9]

Medical innovation is associated with urbanisation, advanced hospital facilities and centres for dissemination via professional journals and research networks. Urban and rural medical markets were very different and specialist medicine rarely featured in the latter. There are no rural parallels with the teaching hospital and, with the possible exception of poorhouse or workhouse sick wards, there was so little continuity in rural England from the medieval alms house or hospice that rural hospitals were effectively re-invented.[10] Yet to regard rural medicine as a stagnant backwater or simply to assume weak emulation of urban practices subject to time lags seems an inadequate response to two centuries of development. Although this paper cannot address such a diverse subject, particularly its lay healing and herbal medicines, it focuses upon GP involvement in local and cottage hospitals, a neglected but now topical question.[11] For this purpose, 'the rural' is confined here to the three English agricultural counties of Norfolk, Suffolk and Cambridgeshire beyond their county towns and ports.[12]

Local Medical Markets

The main sources are hospital records and county directories, which used local lists and, from 1859, the medical register to indicate medical practitioners. These contain inaccuracies but were updated to cover deaths and retirements, thus allowing summaries and information on individuals over time. Indications of public medical office, for example under the post-1834 poor laws, improved after the 1858 Medical Act limited such posts to registered practitioners. Most rural appointments were part-time, but expanded with local authority provision under the 1866 Sanitary Act, the 1871 and 1888 Local Government Acts and the Public Health Act of 1875.[13] Sufficient information exists to suggest a 'proto-public' sector before 1900, albeit limited in rural areas before World War Two, with a rural GP hospital profile long before this was scrutinised by Ministry of Health *Hospital Surveys*.[14]

Population growth in the three counties was comparatively slow. It reached 960,000 in 1851, was virtually stable by 1900 and did not exceed 1,250,000 until 1951. Beyond the principal county towns and ports, natural increase was undermined by emigration. 'Rural Norfolk' had 45,000 fewer inhabitants in 1911 than in 1851 and little growth afterwards.[15] A west-east movement was the main feature in an otherwise static inter-war Suffolk population, with slow growth in Cambridgeshire inflated by boundary changes.[16] Thus any additional medical provision was not driven by population pressure. The combination of new cottage hospitals in the three counties and hospital expansion in their main towns tripled the number of voluntary hospital beds between 1861 and 1938 to two per 1,000 population, although this was no better than national levels and the poor law infirmary provision was grossly deficient.[17]

Calculations using lists of practising doctors in the three counties make no allowance for social class, geographic or gender determinants of patient access, but are hardly compatible with concepts of 'overstocked' late nineteenth-century medical markets.[18] A slight improvement to one doctor per 2,000 population in Norfolk in 1881 was followed by deterioration until 1911 and recovery barely below 1: 2,000 by 1939. Corresponding figures for Suffolk were 1:2,400 by 1881, improving by 1911 but less rapidly afterwards to 1:2,000 in the late 1930s. There were roughly 1,800 people per doctor before 1900 in Cambridgeshire, but slightly more between the wars. If such ratios were less than in the poorest urban centres, they considerably exceeded suggested national inter-war averages of 1:1,300–1,600.[19]

National poor law statistics suggested that late nineteenth-century Norfolk and Suffolk had the greatest incidence of pauperism and Board of Trade data confirmed the lowest of wage rates there in the early 1900s. Inability to pay for family doctoring was a vital issue and a detailed study of Norfolk GPs found no evidence of attendance on the poor at commercial fees, none recorded at reduced rates and few indications of charitable practice.[20] Yet poverty and the lack of poor law medical facilities were cited as a stimulus to sickness club membership in evidence to the 1905–9 Royal Commission on the Poor Laws.[21] Medical club practice developed from the early 1800s under local patronage or poor law tutelage in smaller Norfolk towns such as Wymondham or Coltishall. That established in Eye, Suffolk in 1876 had 'between two and three thousand members' by 1883.[22] National federations such as the Ancient Order of Foresters were prominent and the Ipswich-Suffolk County Medical Club, with nearly 10,000 members, retained fifty-five doctors by 1900.[23] This was one-third of the county's medical practitioners and one-quarter of Norfolk practitioners were similarly engaged by 1880. Some doctors simply accumulated clubs and income: Dr Hamill at Burnham Thorpe, Norfolk had fourteen club contracts in the 1890s.[24] Most also ran their own clubs with Dr Stork, describing general practice in the area surrounding Bury St. Edmunds, observing, 'there is only one doctor that I can think of who has not got a private medical club of his own'.[25]

Friendly societies and works clubs used qualified practitioners to provide lower cost care but there were alternatives. Examples of chemists and druggists, but also of 'herbalist and poet', 'surgeon-druggist', 'doctress', 'medical, botanical and veterinary surgeon' and 'medical botanist (practical)' persisted in twentieth-century directories. Rural herbalism was only part-replaced by the upsurge of patent medicines and such alternatives were under-recorded, particularly their frequency of usage. A notable group were 'medical men' not registered under the 1858 Act but included within the 1861 census occupation categories, as with general practitioner and 'subordinate' in 1871. County directory 'medical lists' in 1865 included thirteen unqualified practitioners in Norfolk villages, twelve in Cambridgeshire and eleven in Suffolk.[26] Excesses of occupied practitioners in census returns over the names on qualified medical lists, by forty-five in Norfolk in 1911, also suggest the continuation of irregular or fringe medicine in the three counties.[27]

The GP and Hospital Work

From the eighteenth century doctors saw in hospital work the advantages of prestige, a potential clientele among philanthropic supporters, opportunities to research and enhance skills and to take pupils. Hospital sizes and workloads increased and patients benefited additionally from rest, diet and rudimentary hygiene, but few hospitals changed dramatically before the use of anaesthesia. County hospitals, established in Cambridge in 1766 and Norwich in 1771, had honorary medical staffs who acted in a consulting capacity and acquired reputations as specialists. John Green Crosse, the premier hospital surgeon in Norfolk by the 1840s, felt that 'the assemblage of medical sciences is too vast for the mind to cope with even during a lifetime: the way to excellence is to work in a particular department'.[28] Yet he did not specialise until his fame and fortune were partly made and he combined hospital surgery with private work as an accoucheur. His hospital enjoyed a national reputation for lithotomy, but staff tended to be experienced practitioners with particular interests rather than young career-specialists. There were three consulting surgeons in 1900, while 'three physicians were sufficient for the wards and [...] as many as the district could provide a living for as consultants'.[29] Even at this major hospital economic practicalities overrode the claims of medical specialism.

Local GPs saw attractions and threats in hospital practice. From the middle of the nineteenth century hospitals were increasingly identified with more advanced forms of care. An outcry over 'hospital abuse' and over-provision of general and special hospitals in urban centres, even as club medicine assumed mass proportions, suggests that people sought the hospital combination of rest, nursing and 'on account of the greatly superior medical attention they receive'.[30] With Norwich and Cambridge hospital facilities inaccessible for most inhabitants of the three counties, dispensaries in six other towns were converted or replaced by hospitals between 1825 and 1838.[31] All, excepting in part the East Suffolk and Ipswich hospital, had GP medical staffs, whose restricted numbers suggest that posts were prized. Near the beginning of the period reviewed, the West Suffolk General hospital's GP staff of three was unchanged for at least eighteen years: at its close, the Yarmouth General hospital staff was castigated as a clique of local GPs, hostile to outside specialists.[32]

Voluntary special hospitals offered another route to a medical reputation but an eye hospital (1825) and a children's hospital (1854) in Norwich were the only such facilities in the three counties. Poor law medical work might supplement a doctor's income but infirmaries were confined to the county towns and rural facilities were limited to workhouse sick wards. No county council had taken former poor law or public assistance accommodation into municipal control before the establishment of the NHS and these facilities were condemned as 'practically non-existent [...] of a very low standard and no credit to the counties concerned' by the 1945 *Hospital Survey*.[33]

Cottage hospitals were more significant for rural areas and general practitioners than their limited historiography suggests.[34] More than 300 were established in the forty years after the 1858 Medical Act and over 600 existed by 1935.[35] They varied from six-bed 'village' hospitals to small but active institutions in market towns, ports and industrial centres and all were GP-staffed. Their development marked the geographic extension of voluntary hospitals but its timing and expansion in suburban areas and dormitory towns suggest medical efforts to extend qualified practice and maintain important patient clientele. Cottage hospitals addressed local needs and their convenience and therapeutic advantage to patients was rightly emphasised. If many of treatments provided were relatively simple, these were no less necessary, particularly in the contexts of inadequate poor law facilities and defective domestic environments. But unlike the earlier voluntary hospitals, many cottage hospitals admitted private patients and most required the payment of fees, with even their poorest patients usually assessed for some contribution. This may have been reasonable where hospitals lacked benefactors or wealthy patronage, but it echoed GP concerns over medical charity and hospital abuse.[36]

Arguably the prototype cottage hospital had been founded in Shotesham, Norfolk in the early 1730s.[37] Early Norfolk examples included Ditchingham (1865) and Cromer (1866), with Woodbridge (1861) and Sudbury (1867) the pioneers in Suffolk. Their variable development has been outlined elsewhere and one-half of the twenty-two known examples in Norfolk and Suffolk survive as district or community hospitals.[38] Others at Litcham and Harleston existed only briefly, that at Mildenhall closed in 1930, with Watton an early closure under the NHS. A different pattern emerged in Cambridgeshire, dominated by Addenbrooke's hospital and featuring the development of Wisbech cottage hospital into the sixty-bed North Cambridgeshire hospital, though Newmarket and Royston cottage hospitals were no longer included after county boundaries were re-drawn. Specialist services were concentrated at Addenbrookes (later the NHS regional hospital), at the Norfolk and Norwich (the largest hospital) and the East Suffolk and Ipswich hospital. Otherwise all general and cottage hospitals were GP-staffed.[39]

According to one GP historian, 'practices in places where there is a cottage hospital have always been more sought after than others and often they command a higher purchase price'.[40] General practice included surgical work – agricultural labour and mechanisation produced substantial numbers of casualties – and the opportunity practise in a hospital environment, perhaps with the benefit of consultation with colleagues or even following some division of work on 'neutral ground', was often appreciated. Operating theatre facilities were better than domestic environments and generally improved over time, whilst patients had the benefit of competent nursing and a recuperative period. More specialised surgical instruments could also be accessed, an important feature when GP surgeries and facilities were often poor.[41]

There were further advantages to regular practice in operative surgery. As 'FRCS', 'a cottage hospital surgeon of eminence' put it,

> besides the good to the hospital patients, the local surgeon is enabled 'to keep his hand in' at bad accidents and operations, and the rich resident often gets the benefit of this in an emergency. I tell my wealthy patients that, charity considerations aside, it is worth their while to keep up the cottage hospital for this reason alone.[42]

The traditional adage that 'the peasant's misfortune might aid the means of saving the life of the squire' could be re-worked at the cottage hospital and practitioners could 'hold on' to wealthier patients. This reduced the risk of a referred patient being 'poached' by a consultant also offering generalist services, or at least it gained the GP some recognition and economic advantage from a more defined referral process.

Cottage hospitals developed through a period in which the hospital was regarded as the apex of medical science, a site for the implementation of new techniques and discoveries. However, their GP staff practised family doctoring which, well into the twentieth century, involved a holistic approach to patients. Medicines, linctuses, expectorants and tonics often dealt with symptoms rather than underlying causes, but, in conjunction with professional advice, the securing of relief, placebo effects, faith in the doctor or knowledge that remedial action had been attempted may have benefited patients.[43] Yet even before the development of sulphonamide drugs and antibiotics from the late 1930s, scientific medicine could point to some successes. Effective treatments included quinine for malaria (still a feature in parts of west Norfolk, west Suffolk and north Cambridgeshire); Salvarsan for syphylis; antitoxins against diphtheria and tetanus; digitalis for some heart conditions and, in the 1920s, liver extract and iron preparations for anaemia and insulin in diabetes cases.[44]

As sites of treatment cottage hospitals presented the image of the 'modern' or 'hygienic' institution offering care rather than bacteriological research, blood counts or cystoscopy. New technology was often acquired but not always used effectively: X-ray equipment, for example, was prone to breakage and insufficient replacement stocks, incompatible electricity supplies, difficulties in developing plates or interpreting results.[45] Yet even limited success helped to establish a 'go-ahead' image for hospitals and medical officers. As with the status of science, this depended upon material improvements in the hospitals' physical fabric, systematised work and the results of treatment. It was also in part negotiated, relying upon public acceptance of technological benefits and successes claimed for 'new' developments familiar to the previous generation of teaching hospital staff. This is not to demean local achievements or reputations: the surgical excellence of Cromer cottage hospital GPs between the wars was readily acknowledged by consultants at the Norfolk and Norwich hospital. Arthur Burton, for example, performed 'one major operation almost weekly, with 100 per cent survival rate for the first fourteen years'.[46] Such results probably reflected his experience of military surgery and current skills and also the limited range of major operations at Cromer, but a perfect record meant endorsements, status and a plentiful supply of patients for Burton and enhanced local support for the hospital.

In Fig. 11.1 'medical lists' include all describing themselves as surgeon or physician before 1858. Their reduced numbers in 1865 give a better indication of qualified medical practitioners, who included full-time staff working in mental hospitals, medical officers of health and, later, in the schools medical service. Figures for 'all hospital posts' include consultants, but just sixteen of these were 'consulting only' or specialists in modern sense in 1900. Those in Norwich monopolised posts at the N&N, eye and children's hospitals. With one house physician and surgeon in the main hospitals, roughly one-half of Norfolk hospital posts before 1900 were held by GPs; slightly more in Suffolk and less in Cambridgeshire. Hospital GP numbers in the third column for each county are minimum figures, as all GPs were technically able to practise in local cottage hospitals, but particular associations developed and only named personnel are recorded. In Cromer, for example, it 'was agreed that the doctors should keep charge of the hospital three months in rotation', effectively as medical officer.[47]

Figure 11.1

Medical practitioners and voluntary hospital posts in East Anglia

Date	Norfolk			Suffolk			Cambridgeshire		
	on med lists	total hosp posts	GPs in hosps	on med lists	total hosp posts	GPs in hosps	on med lists	total hosp posts	GPs in hosps
1830	129	8		119				7	
1845	202	23	12	161	17	10			
1855	228	25	12	176	17	10	83	5	1
1865	162	34	13	148	20	12	76	8	1
1875	176	57	28	142	29	20	81	11	1
1888	217	57	28	158	25	20	93	21	9
1900	206	60	30	168	41	29	91	20	8
1912	202	65	35	185	44	32	112	35	15
1929	215	87	49	192	72	52	106	45	18
1938	253	111	63	193	85	65	111	51	29
				81*					78*

Notes: Cambridgeshire '1855' figure is actually 1858; after 1929 GP figures include GP anaesthetists in larger hospitals; 1938* includes GPs with posts in Public Assistance infirmaries, municipal or isolation hospitals.

Expansion of the three major hospitals produced more consultant and specialist positions after 1900, but the number of GP medical officers in cottage and district hospitals also continued to increase. Eighteen GPs assisted as anaesthetists at the N&N, Addenbrookes and ESI by 1938, for example, and five more also held house surgeon or physician posts at Addenbrookes.[48] An additional, unrecorded number practised as assistants or deputies to consultant specialists because, as one of the latter explained, 'by appointing as assistants men in general practice and therefore not dependent on their earnings as specialists, the evil of overloading the ranks of specialists is avoided'.[49] Others acted as 'GP-specialists', notably in ear, nose and throat or opthalmic surgery, in venereal diseases, obstetrics or pathology, particularly at county or district hospitals in Bury St Edmunds, Lowestoft, Great Yarmouth and Kings Lynn. Nine others were medical officers in convalescent annexes to the principal hospitals and nine more held posts in local TB sanatoria. Some indication of GP public assistance hospital numbers can be seen by 1938, but, excluding these, a minimum of 28 per cent of GPs in the three counties then had regular work in the voluntary hospitals.

This figure may be refined somewhat. Norwich was Norfolk's medical and population centre so 25 per cent of county doctors were based there before 1900 and 30 per cent during the inter-war years, including all consultants or specialists. Beyond the city there was a fluctuating but upward trend in 'other Norfolk' GPs with hospital posts, 20 to 25 per cent before 1912 and 30 to 35 per cent between the wars. In Suffolk a greater percentage of GPs had hospital work; in part because the county medical list grew more slowly and because there was a more restricted range of specialties at the ES&I hospital. There were fewer cottage hospitals in Cambridgeshire but Addenbrookes hospital had an unusual medical staff profile: two honorary physicians were still in general practice in 1938 and most routine or initial assessments were undertaken by GPs acting as house surgeons or physicians. A smaller county medical list also contributed to the higher proportion of GPs with hospital work than might have been expected, given the dissimilar network of hospital facilities. Contrary to national presentations, general practitioners in the three counties were 'keeping their hand in' at local hospitals.

Later Influences and GP Hospital Work

Were there 'rural' dimensions to the related issues of GP over-ambition, their continuing presence in hospital work and later exclusion from it? It is acknowledged that remuneration under state national health insurance enhanced the living standards of inter-war doctors, even compared with other professions. They could combine private practice with their NHI work to maximise income, accumulating panel patients in poor areas or concentrating upon private practice in more prosperous districts. Thus over 25 per cent of doctors obtained most of their earnings from the NHI scheme and 70 per cent of them derived at least 30 per cent of total incomes from this source.[50] Not all needed to do so. Herbert Cowley Dent, practising in Edwardian Cromer on a visiting clientele which included Princess Stephanie of Belgium, the Duke and Duchess of Devonshire, the Asquiths and Balfours, Sir Jesse Boot and Sir Henry Irving, refused to join the scheme.[51] But many rural GPs lacked dense blocs of panel patients and the dependants of agricultural labourers, excluded from the NHI scheme, provided no private business. Such doctors needed to keep up their 'club' and poor law work, which remained part of the rural medical scene. Local directories suggest that, between 1875 and 1938, the proportion of doctors with part-time poor law or 'proto-public' posts varied between 60 and 75 per cent in Norfolk, 56 and 63 per cent in Suffolk and 52 and 61 per cent in Cambridgeshire.[52]

Even though doctors referred more patients for treatments, voluntary hospitals received no meaningful funding under the state NHI scheme. Poor law hospital facilities in rural areas remained mediocre and voluntary hospitals introduced patient charges to bolster their own income as pressure on services increased. In response, people joined hospital contributory schemes, paying modest weekly contributions to secure exemption from charges for themselves and their dependants should they require hospital treatment. Such schemes became extensive in rural as in urban areas: versions dating from the 1870s in the three counties covered over 250,000 people in early 1920s and 435,000 by 1945, plus their dependants.[53] Cottage hospitals established contributory schemes but increasingly were forced into accommodations with larger hospital or independent schemes offering wider services and more advanced facilities for similar contributions.[54] Most opted for amalgamations, under which cottage hospitals received financial allocations based upon collections in 'their' area and payments according patient numbers. Hospital doctors, GPs as well as consultants, began to receive a percentage of these allocations, generally about 20 per cent by the late 1930s, making such posts still more attractive.

These arrangements stimulated the referral of patients between hospitals, usually on a reciprocal basis, with complex or specialist treatments provided in larger hospitals and post-operative cases or patients requiring simpler procedures transferred to smaller institutions, again with compensatory cash flows. Thus, of the 90 scheme members in the small town of North Walsham, Norfolk who were hospitalised in 1927, 71 went to the local cottage hospital, 9 were referred to the Norfolk and Norwich, 3 to the eye infirmary and 2 to the children's hospital in Norwich, and 5 were sent to convalescent homes.[55] Similarly the cottage hospital in Beccles, Suffolk had 290 inpatients in 1938, with 191 members of the hospital's own contributory scheme and 31 from others.[56] Beccles and other cottage hospitals also received direct grants from local authorities for other treatments provided, from which GP-staffs were paid. They often provided sole provision for midwifery cases with complications, for example at Wisbech, Cambridgeshire or Aldeburgh, Suffolk, and for children referred under the schools medical service for dental, ear, nose or throat surgery. No less than thirty-five of the eighty-four inpatients at North Walsham in the autumn of 1928 were 'Education Committee' child patients sent in for tonsillectomy.[57]

It has been estimated that GPs nationally performed 2.5 million surgical operations in 1938–9, an average of three per week, and that 20 per cent had access to hospital beds.[58] A greater proportion were likely to be involved in the three counties in surgery, which ranged from tonsillectomy and cleaning up of wounds following accidents through to complex skin grafting, mastectomy and hysterectomy procedures. Over-ambition in some GPs remained a serious concern but the growth of contributory schemes, by providing hospitals and specialists with additional income, encouraged special departments and patient transfers between hospitals. This enabled more suitable workloads to be undertaken by medical officers, although such rationalisation remained underdeveloped before the instigation of wartime emergency hospital services and the National Health Service.

Noticeably the 1945 *Hospital Survey* for eastern England focused upon the need for specialist services, identifying gaps in provision and suggesting their resolution via additional appointments or use of existing staff at the principal hospitals. Hospitals were implicitly judged on these criteria, with the N&N occupying foremost position, ahead of the ES&I, 'a first class hospital' and Addenbrookes, a teaching hospital 'owing to the fact that it is in a university town'.[59] Deficient facilities at some cottage hospitals were noted, although Yarmouth General Hospital was singled out as particularly outmoded and with a restrictive GP staff.[60] If these remarks were justified, subsequent discussion concerning a proposed replacement hospital and its medical staffing confirmed the tough stance adopted by Norfolk and Norwich hospital staff. With their economic position more assured, they reversed their earlier attitude to GP hospital work. A.J. Cleveland, acting chairman at the N&N, informed his opposite number that consultant specialists must prevail in Yarmouth: 'his colleagues were strongly opposed to nominal appointments [...] in future they would only be accepted on condition that a physician or surgeon was invited to take an active part in the work'. If deputies for consultants were required, their appointment was no longer a matter for local GPs but 'should be left to the Joint Medical Staff of the N&N and the new Hospital'.[61]

The lack of specialist and consulting services featured prominently in other regional surveys undertaken by senior medical figures, although questions such as the role of the hospital in relation to wider services or community health were barely mentioned.[62] Hardly a progressive force in health policy formulation, the British Medical Association nevertheless raised GP concerns over the need for continuity in treatments and local access, the persistence of inadequate domestic environments and the retention of 'a type of hospital or accommodation in which a general practitioner can treat cases falling within his sphere of competence'.[63] However, the Royal Colleges of

Physicians and Surgeons now made no secret of their desire to exclude GPs from hospital work.[64] Labour's Minister of Health and Housing, Aneurin Bevan, saw no friends and many political opponents among BMA leaders, but was already strongly inclined to equate hospital technology and consultant services with optimum standards of care.[65]

Postscript

The NHS had a tripartite structure based upon hospital, general and community services. Cottage hospitals, marginalised among more important institutions, were largely separated from GPs, themselves allegedly demoralised by 'trivia' and their role in referring patients to hospital or sickness benefits.[66] Revisions occurred not so much through the formation of a Royal College of General Practitioners in 1952 but in response to the alleged failings of large expensive hospitals and belated recognition in the 1970s of the need to develop community health services, which could also be provided comparatively cheaply. At this point there were still 350 'community hospitals' in England and Wales, with which 16 per cent of GPs were associated.[67] The latter still performed 25 per cent of surgery in the sixty-four Scottish 'GP hospitals' and those in England and Wales still undertook a great deal of minor surgery, easing pressures on larger hospitals.[68]

    This suggests revised but useful forms of 'holding on' by GPs, since

> dealing with minor trauma locally results in considerable savings in time and transport costs and is highly valued by the community; by contrast the requirements in terms of space and equipment are relatively small.[69]

Similar arguments may apply with post-operative, recuperative or continuing care and it remains a moot point, if not a legal argument, whether all hospital operations really require the appropriate specialists when resources are stretched and waiting lists increase.

Few GPs have worked outside grouped practices or community health teams but the greater role for Primary Care Groups or Trusts within a reformed NHS is beginning to address such issues. Features such as clinical interest; full usage of skills; greater professional contacts; and the focus upon community/patient relationships, are being associated with improvements in the role, morale and job satisfaction of contemporary medical practitioners. These might not be wholly unfamiliar to the GP 'keeping his hand in' at the cottage hospital of the 1860s.[70]

Notes

1   Nearly 84 per cent of the 3,120 practitioners listed in Samuel Foart Simmons, *The Medical Register for the Year 1783*, were described as 'surgeons and apothecaries'.
2   I. Loudon, 'The Concept of the Family Doctor', *Bulletin of the History of Medicine*, 58 (1983), pp 347–62.
3   A. Digby, *The Evolution of British General Practice 1850–1948* (Oxford, 1999).
4   C. Hamlin, 'State Medicine in Great Britain', in D. Porter (ed.), *The History of Public Health and the Modern State* (Amsterdam, 1994), pp.132–64.
5   See J.T. Hart, 'The *British Medical Journal*, General Practitioners and the State 1840–1990', in W.F. Bynum, S. Lock and R. Porter (eds), *Medical Journals and Medical Knowledge* (London 1992), pp.228–47; J. Lewis, *What Price Community Medicine?* (Brighton, 1986).
6   See respectively M.J. Peterson, *The Medical Profession in Mid-Victorian London* (California, 1978); L. Granshaw, 'Fame and Fortune by Means of Bricks and Mortar', in L. Granshaw and R. Porter (eds), *The Hospital in History* (London, 1989), pp.199–220.
7   J. Howell, *Technology in the Hospital* (Baltimore, 1995), pp.3–6.
8   Political and Economic Planning, *Report on British Health Services* (London, 1937), pp.243, 262; F.B. Smith, *The People's Health 1830–1910* (London, 1979); J. Lewis, 'Providers, Consumers, the State and the Delivery of Health Care Services in Twentieth-Century Britain', in A. Wear (ed.), *Medicine in Society* (Cambridge, 1992), pp.317–45.
9   F. Honigsbaum, *The Division in British Medicine* (London, 1979); R. Stevens, *Medical Practice in Modern England* (New Haven, 1966), p.34.

10   Rural hospitals, whether cottage, poor law or isolation, have received little attention; see M. Emrys Roberts, *The Cottage Hospitals 1859–1990* (Motcombe, 1991); M.A. Crowther, *The Workhouse System 1834–1929* (London, 1981), though county town hospitals and asylums took significant proportions of rural patients.

11   Current NHS reforms include a reorientation upon primary care groups and community hospitals.

12   For further discussion see S. Cherry, 'Medicine and Rural Health Care in Nineteenth Century Europe', in J. Barona and S. Cherry (eds), *Health and Medicine in Rural Europe 1850–1945* (Valencia, 2005), pp 19–62.

13   The 1866 Act required the appointment of sanitary officers and allowed local authorities to establish isolation facilities; the 1871 Act combined Poor Law and public health measures under the Local Government Board; the 1875 Act defined and codified appropriate aspects of public health and the 1888 Act established County Councils (with urban and rural district councils) as the responsible unit of local government.

14   E.g. Sir W. Savage, Sir C. Frankham and Sir B. Gibson, *Hospital Survey: The Hospital Services of the Eastern Area*, HMSO (London, 1945).

15   A. Armstrong, *The Population of Victorian and Edwardian Norfolk* (Norwich, 2001), p.11.

16   Population actually fell in West Suffolk 1891–1931. The Isle of Ely was added to Cambridgeshire in 1891.

17   Based on hospital annual reports; H. Burdett, *Hospitals and Charities* (London, 1914); R. Pinker, *English Hospital Statistics, 1861–1938* (London, 1966), p.69.

18   Cf. A. Digby, *Making a Medical Living* (Cambridge, 1994), p.13.

19   S. Cherry, *Medical Services and the Hospitals 1860–1939* (Cambridge, 1996), p.69. These ratios exceed Digby's earlier figures, generally within a band of 1,500–2,000.

20   M. Muncaster, 'Medical Services and the Medical Profession in Norfolk, 1815–1911' (unpublished PhD thesis, University of East Anglia, 1976).

21   *Report to the Royal Commission on the Poor Laws* (1909), Appendix XV, Part 2: A.C. McKay and H.V. Toynbee, p.109.

22   Kelly, *Directory for Norfolk and Suffolk* (London, 1883), p.872.

23   H. Burdett, *Hospitals and Charities* (London, 1900), p.511.

24   Muncaster, 'Medical Services', p.147.

25   *Royal Commission on the Poor Laws* (1909), vol. 1: Stork, p.332.

26   *Whites Suffolk Directory* (1865), pp.944–5; *Post Office Directory for Norfolk and Suffolk* (1875), p.754.

27   Muncaster, 'Medical Services', p.206.

28   V.M. Crosse, *A Surgeon in the Early Nineteenth Century: John Green Crosse* (London, 1968), p.138.

29   A. Cleveland, *The Norfolk and Norwich Hospital 1900–46* (Norwich, 1948), p.78.

30   *The Hospital*, 18 January 1890, p.243.
31   In Bury St Edmunds, Ipswich, Yarmouth, Lowestoft, Kings Lynn and Beccles.
32   *Suffolk Directories* (1865), p.944; (1883), p.834; *Hospital Survey* (1945), p.3.
33   Viz. Ipswich, 1938, Norwich, 1941. *Hospital Survey*, p.6; Crowther, *Workhouse System*, p.186.
34   E. Roberts, *Cottage Hospitals*; idem, 'Where was the First Cottage Hospital?', in R. Rolls, J. Guy, and R. Guy (eds), *A Pox on the Provinces* (Bath, 1990), pp.29–37; R.M.S. McGonaghey, 'The Evolution of the Cottage Hospital', *Medical History*, 11 (1967), pp.128–40; S. Cherry, 'Change and Continuity in Cottage Hospitals 1859–1948', *Medical History*, 36 (1992), pp.271–89.
35   Burdett, *Hospitals*, p.32; B. Abel Smith, *The Hospitals* (London, 1964), p.408.
36   Cf. Emrys Roberts, *Cottage Hospitals*, pp.149–50.
37   A. Batty Shaw, 'Benjamin Gooch, Eighteenth Century Norfolk Surgeon', *Medical History*, 16 (1972), pp 40–50.
38   Cherry, 'Cottage Hospitals', pp.275–7. Others included Sudbury (Suffolk), 1867; Mildenhall (S) 1868; Litcham (Norfolk) 1868; Royston (Cambs), 1870; East Rudham (N), Harleston (N), 1872; Beccles (S), 1874; Wisbech (C), 1875; Coltishall (N), Newmarket (C), 1881; Halesworth (S), 1882; Swaffham (N), Gorleston (S), 1888; Southwold (S), 1897; Thetford (N), 1898; Watton (N), 1899; Diss (N), 1900; Aldburgh (S), Wells (N), 1910 and North Walsham (N), 1924.
39   *Hospital Survey* considered the N&N 'by far the best hospital in every way in the Region', p.17.
40   McGonaghey, 'Evolution of the Cottage Hospital', p.138.
41   Digby, *General Practice*, pp.188–9, 194.
42   H.C. Burdett, *Cottage Hospitals, General, Fever and Convalescent* (London, 1896), p.127.
43   J. Riley, *Sick not Dead* (Baltimore, 1997), makes a similar point concerning the effectiveness of club medicine.
44   I. Loudon and M. Drury, 'Some Aspects of Clinical Care in General Practice', in I. Loudon, C. Webster and J. Horder (eds), *General Practice under the National Health Service 1948–97* (Oxford, 1997), pp.92–127.
45   L. Ramsay, 'The Diagnostic Use of X-rays in the UK 1896–1920s: A Regional Study' (unpublished MPhil thesis, University of East Anglia, 1999).
46   K. Hindle, 'Medical Provision in Cromer' (unpublished MA thesis, University of East Anglia, 1998), ch. 5.
47   Cromer Hospital Minute Book, 1903–25 October 1907.
48   *Hospital Survey*, pp.33, 35, 37, 39, 41.
49   Cleveland, *N&N*, p.81.
50   A. Digby and N. Bosanquet, 'Doctors and Patients in an Era of National Health Insurance and Private Practice 1913–38', *Economic History Review*, 41 (1988), pp.74–94.

51   H.C. Dent, 'Early Days of the Old Cromer Hospital', *Norfolk Chronicle*, 22 July 1932; Hindle, 'Medical Provision', ch. 4.

52   Includes part-time sanitary officer, factory certification, TB officers, county medical officer and full-time twentieth-century infant welfare and schools appointments. Excludes prison, police surgeons and asylums.

53   S. Cherry, 'Hospital Saturday: Workplace Collections in Late Nineteenth Century Hospital Funding', *Medical History*, 44 (2000), pp.461–88; 'Beyond National Health Insurance: The Voluntary Hospitals and Hospital Contributory Schemes', *Social History of Medicine*, 7 (1992), pp.455–82.

54   Cherry, 'National Insurance', p.482; 'Cottage Hospitals', pp.282–5.

55   North Walsham and District War Memorial Cottage Hospital, Minute Book 1927–31, 11 December 1927.

56   Beccles and District War Memorial Hospital, Admissions and Discharge Book, 1938–48, 1938–9.

57   North Walsham, Minute Book, 1927–31, 11 December 1928. The hospital received £1.65 for each tonsillectomy performed, so GPs also serving as schools' medical officers might organise their medical living!

58   J. Brotherston, 'Evolution of Medical Practice', in Nuffield Provincial Hospitals Trust, *Medical History and Medical Care* (London, 1971), pp.85–126, 100.

59   *Hospital Survey*, pp.3–4.

60   *Ibid.*, p.18.

61   N&N Medical Committee Memorandum, 19 July 1945, Norfolk County Record Office, NNH 65/27.

62   G. Godber, 'The Domesday Book of British Hospitals', *Bulletin of the Society for the History of Medicine*, 32 (1983), pp.4–13.

63   BMA Report, *A General Medical Service for the Nation* (1938).

64   F. Honigsbaum, *Health, Happiness and Security* (London 1989), pp.113–14, 127.

65   J. Campbell, *Nye Bevan* (London, 1994), pp.167–9.

66   D. Morrell, 'Introduction', in Loudon, Horder and Webster, *General Practice*, p.6.

67   Including one in Aylsham, Norfolk, developed from former poor law accommodation and opened in 1954.

68   A.J.M. Cavanagh, 'Contribution of General Practitioner Hospitals in England and Wales', *British Medical Journal* (1978), 2, pp.34–6.

69   RCGP Report, 'General Practitioner Hospitals', *RCGP Occasional Paper*, 23 (Exeter, 1983), p.3.

70   *Ibid.*, p.3. This is not to minimise current GP concerns over inadequate funding, excessive bureaucracy and threats of litigation.

Part Four: The Impact on the Patient

LOUISE GRAY

Chapter 12: Hospitals and the Lives of the Chronically Sick: Coping with Illness in the Narratives of the Rural Poor in Early Modern Germany

This study examines the experiences of the labouring poor who were suffering from chronic physical illnesses in the early modern period.[1] Despite the popularity of institutional history among medical historians, the perceptions of the sick poor themselves have hitherto been sorely neglected. Overwhelmingly, early modern hospital histories to date have either focused upon the organisation of a specific institution, or have considered such foundations within a wider historical agenda, particularly with regards to debates concerning Foucault and the medicalisation process.[2] While a few previous works have considered daily life within a hospital setting (*Alltagsgeschichte*), prior research into the motivation of the sick poor to petition for a place in a hospital has stemmed from a reliance upon statistical sources, such as patient lists, or upon the foundation ordinances which stipulated for whom the hospital was intended to cater.[3] It is the contention of this paper that an over-reliance upon such documentation omits an understanding of the experiences of those persons among the 'silent masses' who were living with a chronic ailment. Where studies to date have considered patient experience, it has predominantly been through bureaucratic records concerning complaints and punishments, and has frequently relied on second-hand comments written by an official or administrator. Research focusing upon the early modern period has been largely silent with regards to both the specific ways in which a prospective patient viewed a hospital, and the point in a sick person's life in which they would apply for admission into such an institution. Such a dearth of interest can be compared to the growing number of studies which relate to applications for poor relief and which concentrate upon the role of this aid within life-cycle strategies. A common theme of such investigations concerns the power that the poor applicants potentially revealed through these documents.[4] Questions focus on issues such as whether and how these individuals were able to manipulate the poor relief process to most benefit themselves. This study will offer a different perspective of the process of hospitalisation by studying the lives of the poor through a series of surviving petitions from applicants wishing to gain entry into hospitals in rural Hesse, Germany.[5]

The institutions at the centre of this study are the *Landesspitäler* (territorial hospitals), established by the Protestant Landgrave of Hesse, Philip the Magnanimous, on the eve of the Hessian Reformation. Four such establishments were founded – named Haina, Merxhausen, Hofheim and Gronau. All were former religious institutions that had been dissolved and transformed into hospitals as a direct result of the Reformation. Allowed to retain a proportion of their former monastic wealth (including many farm lands and forests from which the hospitals could draw resources), these establishments were, in theory at least, to be self-financing.

Two of these territorial hospitals (or *Landesspitäler*) were intended to cater for women and two for men. The examples mentioned in this paper will predominantly stem from one of the men's hospitals called Haina. Reference will also be made to Merxhausen, a women's hospital. These institutions were founded in 1533. The conception behind the *Landesspitäler* was that the sick poor from the surrounding countryside would find free shelter and care within these establishments. Given their rural location, a study of Haina and Merxhausen offers a different perspective of poverty, sickness and medical care in the early modern period than is usually provided by historians. Whereas most historical studies have focused primarily upon urban medical care in this era, the *Landesspitäler* specifically offered care to the sick poor in the Hesse countryside.[6] For the most part, this credential was adhered to, although it is clear that upon occasion mental patients were also taken from the towns, upon payment, usually if they were considered a threat to the community, and if the town in question was without the means to care for the patient.

In order to apply for a place in one of these institutions, one had to write a formal request to the Landgrave or, later on, the relevant hospital authorities. These petitions were written for, or on behalf of, patients requesting admission to these state hospitals. The requests were initiated either by the invalid themselves, or by their families or local communities. It is through these sources that I aim to gain a more nuanced perspective of the experience of the chronic incapacity among the poor petitioners of rural Hesse.

These documents offer a glimpse into the experiences of the 'silent masses', although the 'voice' of the applicants is frequently made known to us through the hand of a scribe. Moreover, the petitions had to reflect the fulfilment of the admissions criteria. At its most basic, entry into a *Landesspital* was dependent upon a person being poor, resident in the Hessian countryside (i.e. non-urban), and unable to obtain sufficient care, either from oneself, one's relatives or friends, or within the community in which one lived. One also had to be suffering from an incurable illness or ailment. Both mentally and physically ill patients were admitted – this chapter will focus predominantly on the latter cases. The afflictions suffered were usually of a chronic nature but were not life threatening.

The authorities were as aware as the historian of the problems of assessing the truths of the claims.[7] As a result, all testimonies had to be corroborated by many other witnesses – including at least local officials, priests, and, from the eighteenth century, a doctor. Such rigorous checking would have made lying futile.

Petitions were not pure 'ego-documents'. They were written with a clear goal in mind and had to contain elements of formulaic language and structure in order to fulfil the requirements of the hospital ordinances. Nevertheless, as this study will show, the petitions were personalised.[8] Briefly charting the applicants' life histories, these documents reveal a different perspective of the capabilities of the sick poor than is perhaps expected. Through these sources, I will analyse the self-perception of the sick poor in terms of their physical infirmities, and link this self-image to their view of the hospitalisation process. This issue will be considered from two key vantage points: the pre- and post petition situation. What did it mean to suffer from a chronic physical condition if one was a pauper who relied on one's labour to support oneself?[9] How did this identity carry on into an individual's role as a hospital patient?

This chapter will focus upon two aspects of capacity and incapacity as experienced by the hospital inmates. The first instance will concern the pre-petition situation, namely the ability of an individual to cope with a chronic illness (frequently for a not inconsiderable time) prior to requesting hospitalisation. Far from the onset of a chronic illness or a chronic condition (such as blindness, lameness, and a variety of disabilities that affected one's mobility) signalling the immediate need for institutionalisation, this study will illustrate the (frequently) gradual nature of this process. In spite of their infirmities, many of the applicants reveal a striking resilience in the face of their afflictions, having coped with their situation for many years before seeking admittance into a hospital. An invalid would adapt his or her lifestyle (most notably their occupation) in order to accommodate their affliction. Depending upon the age and personal situation of the invalid, the role of the carer and their ability to provide continued assistance could have been of crucial importance in determining a chronic invalid's capacity to survive in a domestic setting. Applications only arose as a last resort, when all other options had failed – the invalids could no longer provide for themselves, and they had exhausted all other sources of familial and communal assistance.[10]

The second section of the chapter will detail notions of work, capability and self-identity within the hospitals themselves. It will be argued that such issues should not solely be regarded as an indication (in a Foucauldian sense) of the state imposition of its authority over the poor. As will be shown, a person's ability (and willingness) to be productive also influenced their social identity within the hospital.

I Coping with a Physical Illness – Work, Capacity and Lifestyle

In 1577, Adam Bingel described himself as 'a poor, old, lame man without means' who had always supported himself and his children through hard (manual) work. When however his 'age and inability (*unvermögen*)' meant that he was no longer able to undertake such activities, he turned instead to herding cattle, and had been employed in this way by his neighbour for quite a number of years. His age (and the physical changes that this brought with it) did not prevent him from working, but merely ensured that he altered his career to fit in with his physical capabilities. Bingel's application arose when he was unable to unable to undertake even this employment.[11] The reason for his petition was not however specifically, connected to his age, but rather to misfortune. As a result of a 'darned fall' he was now 'completely lame in one arm', and could no longer work.

Similar circumstances preclude the 1709 application of seventy-year-old Johannes Bretzen. Johannes had been involved in some accidents, 'some [unspecified] years previously'. A dung-cart had run over his right leg and, whilst working as a shepherd, he had broken his left leg in two. He had also lost his hearing, and had no-one to care for him – his three sons had been killed in military service. While not the primary cause of his misfortune, it would appear that Bretzen's advancing years placed an added strain upon an already tenuous situation – the cumulative effect of these physical conditions meant that Bretzen was no longer able to make any sort of living.[12] In common with the majority of the applicants to the *Landesspitäler*, Bretzen and Bingel were dependent upon their ability to labour to support themselves. Low-paid, low-skilled, manual work was a common theme in the petitions. Such occupations also lacked the support of guilds or other social networks that other forms of employment enjoyed.[13] Emphasis was also placed upon the availability of work – all too often these individuals relied on others to employ them – and upon the individual's physical capabilities.

These cases (and many others like them) offer many perspectives regarding the experience of chronic physical ailments among the labouring poor in early modern rural Hessen. The petitioners' attitudes with respect to their physical condition is particularly noteworthy. Many of the reports stress as the overwhelming reason for appealing for entry into the hospital, not one's physical frailties, but one's current inability to feed oneself. Evidently, the former had contributed to the latter, but it is of great significance that the applicants had coped for so many years under physical conditions that most of us would assume to be grounds for hospitalisation. These documents serve to remind us that if one merely looks at hospital lists of patients which offer details such as name and affliction, one arrives at a wholly different conclusion as to which illnesses would render people incapable of fending for themselves; or, more to the point, at which stage the medical condition would lead a person to seek hospitalisation. It is undoubtedly true that physical conditions such as lameness and blindness would frequently prevent people from working in a traditional sense, but the evidence in the petitions reveal that most of the applicants laboured with these afflictions for many years before seeking help. Many of the applicants had managed their conditions and the various ailments that they suffered by changing their occupations and lifestyles as far as possible to fit their physical capabilities at any given time.

The labouring poor of the Hessian petitions revealed a remarkable ability to have coped with their chronic condition for long periods of time prior to their application for a place in a hospital. An additional, and perhaps surprising, stage is added to the process of adapting one's employment to one's capabilities: begging. Having been forced through infirmity to give up 'work' in the conventional sense, the applicants had frequently supported themselves by begging. It would seem that begging was an accepted strategy of self-help among the chronically sick. The epileptic, Anna Maria Westermännin, detailed how she had previously supported herself by travelling 'from district to district' in search of alms. As her condition deteriorated, she was no longer able to undertake these journeys. Her admission of begging did not however prevent the hospital superintendent from agreeing to her request to enter Merxhausen.[14]

The search for alms was regarded a form of work – although theoretically forbidden in Protestant Hesse, it is repeatedly referred to in the petitions and seems to have been largely accepted by the ruling authorities. This tolerance appears to have largely stemmed from the fact that these persons were the 'worthy poor' – their medical conditions (rather than some moral failing) were responsible for their inability to continue working. They were thus 'worthy of alms'. This state of begging would last until immobility set in and they were unable to go out and search for alms. The experience of Anna Schultzin, 'a very poor, old, decrepit and infirm widow who can only move with the use of crutches', echoed that of Westmänin. Schultzin had been a widow for just over thirty years, and had hitherto managed to support herself. Lameness eventually both forced her to give up her previous occupation of weaving and rendered impossible any other form of work. Initially she had survived upon the alms given to her by 'kind-hearted Christians'. Her application to Merxhausen arose as a result of her advanced old age and increasingly deteriorating health meaning that she was physically incapable of seeking this form of assistance.[15]

Immobility was a key factor in determining an individual's application to the *Landesspitäler*; particularly among those persons who had previously relied solely or predominantly upon their own earnings to support themselves. Wendel Rauch, a blind man, explained that he had previously sustained himself as a musician – a violinist – until his mobility was compromised.[16]

II Caring for the Chronically Ill: Work, Capability, and Lifestyle

Emphasis upon an ability to work also features in documentation relating to individuals who had suffered from chronic illness from childhood, and had always been dependent upon the care of others for their survival. Overwhelmingly, this support had hitherto been supplied by relatives. Applications arose when the family member was no longer able to sustain this level of care; usually due either to old age and the increased incapacitation of the carer, or due to a change in the carer's personal circumstances. The latter cause most commonly relates to widowhood (in the case of parents as carers) or to a change in the family structure (either through remarriage or through the birth of children). In all of these situations, the underlying theme is poverty. The carers are themselves impoverished, and they have reached a juncture in their lives in which they are no longer able to shoulder the burden of an extra mouth to feed; especially when the incapacitated individual could only ever constitute a drain upon the household resources. The epilepsy of Conrad Meister's seventeen-year-old son exacerbated an already precarious economic situation for the family. Conrad was a day labourer. The family owned an extremely small property (*gar kleine Häußgen*), but were otherwise wholly without means. Conrad had previously worked as a cowherd, but had been forced to become a day labourer. He had been badly injured while serving in the Landgrave's artillery in Mainz, and has since been unable to undertake any other form of employment. Conrad's son had suffered severely from epilepsy for ten years, and was unable to support himself; in addition, Conrad also had a ten-year-old daughter to provide for. [17]

Inherited poverty was a common problem for those individuals who were unable to support themselves and who had recently been orphaned or widowed. Annen Gertraudt, for instance, was the epileptic daughter of the late Henrich Daniell Drolzich, a cowherd. Unable 'to earn her bread by working for others', she was also without any form of accommodation. As the district official stated, her parents were wholly without means and had to work hard to feed themselves through cowherding. As the family lived from hand-to-mouth, Annen received no inheritance and was not capable of earning her own living; hence the petition. [18]

Insight into the effects that chronic illness had on the wider family are apparent in the petition of the pastor, George Alberti. In 1702, Alberti applied for his eldest (twenty-two-year-old) son, Moritz, to be taken into Haina. Moritz had suffered from epilepsy for many years, and it was believed that this condition was responsible for his mental illness. Moritz's illness had clearly been a strain on the family; George recounts that, having lost his reason through a severe attack of epilepsy, Moritz had lain for over a year in a '*paroxismo*, [...] neither able to live nor to die'. He had broken both ankles and also had suffered various other injuries. Clearly all of these conditions required treatment and this was a huge burden on the pastor's limited means.

In cases of epilepsy and mental illness in particular, a further motivation for requesting hospitalisation is evident: danger. George describes his son's angry and violent outbursts, lamenting that, at such times, everyone feared both for their lives, and also that Moritz would damage either a person or property with fire – a common concern in the petitions. Previously the family had hoped that Moritz would recover. His behaviour has now become so erratic that it is believed that it would be safer for all if he were taken into Haina.[19] Similar concerns are evident in the petition of Anna Catherina Sprangs. Anna recounted that, the previous year, her husband, Diedreich, had been 'struck with frenzied madness (*raserey*)'. Since this date he had been incarcerated, under guard, within his community (Ehringen, in the district of Wolfhagen) on several occasions. As a result of his dangerous behaviour, she and her children had been forced to leave home and return to live with her parents. The reports of the pastor and local officials clearly show that Diedreich was considered to be a great danger, not just to himself, but (more importantly, perhaps) to the wider community.[20] Acceptance of a petition did not reflect an immediate resolution however. Delays were commonplace; not infrequently individuals died before their theoretical place became a reality. In spite of the desperate plight of his family and community, records show that Alberti Mortiz did not enter the hospital until July 1704.[21]

III   Incapable Inmates?

Perhaps the most important lesson of which these petitions remind us is that we should not automatically equate chronic physical illness with a total inability to perform any form of work. Even if the application stemmed from the inability of a principal carer to provide assistance, the key point was often that the invalid was unable to earn enough to support themselves. Johann Auel, for instance, explained that his daughter's physical and mental state meant that her earnings were insufficient to allow her to be self-supporting. Should she be awarded a place in Merxhausen, she would be able to use her sewing skills to contribute to the hospital economy.[22]

The petitions also reveal that we should not blithely equate chronic medical conditions with an immediate desire to seek some form of institutionalisation. The poor in these documents clearly tried all other means first. This might be partially explained by the fact that, once accepted, an individual was entitled to spend their remaining days within the hospital (provided that they did not sufficiently recover nor were expelled through bad behaviour). The vast majority of petitions offer no indication that an applicant had previously entered any other form of hospital or poor relief institution. The key issue at work in the applications was that an individual was no longer sufficiently able to support him- or herself, either off his/her own bat, or through the care of others. This state of affairs was mirrored in the hospital ordinances. Any inmate who sufficiently recovered their health to be able to earn their living independently was to leave the hospital. Such 'success stories' did exist, although they are relatively few in number. This is unsurprising, given that applicants had to be suffering from a seemingly incurable condition to be deemed eligible for consideration in the first place.[23]

In spite of their physical afflictions, some of the petitions reveal a specific desire on behalf of some of the patients to continue working within the confines of the hospital. In his application, Georg from Scholley stressed that, 'as his community could testify', he was 'still able to assist others with wood carrying and other menial tasks.'[24] The crucial point however is that he was unable to earn enough through the small amount of work that he could perform to support himself.

Some persons clearly believed that they were able to work in spite of physical incapacity, but applied to the hospital as their earning capabilities were insufficient to sustain them. Hubert Vitterer, a former, injured (*blesirter*) soldier explained that the frailty of both himself and his wife meant that they were unable to work. As 'they [still] wished to earn their bread', he requested that he be considered for the next vacancy as a porter at Haina.[25] This case differs from the other petitions above as Vitterer was requesting to become a hospital employee rather than a patient – his wife would be able to accompany him to the hospital. The monetary pay for this position however was however meagre. The job's attraction was that the individual (and his immediate family) would receive shelter and protection from the hospital network, including food and clothing. Nevertheless, Vitterer offered similar arguments in requesting this post that the other (inmate) petitioners used; namely that his physical condition was sufficiently weakened to mean that he was unable to support himself (and his wife) through his earnings alone.[26] Acceptance into the hospital would ensure the sustenance of Vitterer and his wife and would mean that he was perform a socially useful function by working within the wider care network of the hospital.

The belief in the potential for invalids to become productive members of both the hospital, and wider, community was not restricted to adults. All children resident within these institutions were to undertake some form of apprenticeship that would then enable them to function in the outside world when they reached maturity. Even the parents of sick children did not rule out the possibility that their offspring could learn a trade, as illustrated by Anna Elisabetha Simonin, a 'poor inmate (*Mit Hospitaliten*)' in Merxhausen. At the time of her petition, Anna had resided in the hospital for thirteen years. Approximately seven years previously, she had been allowed to have her 'two minor children, namely two twins [...] one son and one daughter' join her in the hospital. She cared for them there, and they were allowed to remain in the institution until they were confirmed. Her daughter had been confirmed the previous year and had duly left the establishment. Her son was due to be confirmed later that year (at

Whitsun). She requested that her son be allowed to remain within the
territorial hospitals' care (moving to Haina) so that he could be trained
to be a tailor – this would take two years. Further reports indicated
that due to the boy's 'weak nature', he would be unable to perform
any 'heavy or hard work' (*schwerer arbeit*). Unable to support himself
in the outside world, the boy was taken into Haina and contributed to
their economy through his apprenticeship.[27] It is highly unlikely that
he would have been offered this opportunity in the wider world.

IV Work, Identity and the Self-Perception of the Hospital Patient

If capable, a hospital inmate was expected to perform daily light work
within the institution. This was not a profit-making exercise, but was
instead intended (according to the foundation ordinance) to prevent
idleness and temptation by the Devil. The work was to be of a light
nature and was supposed to fit in within the individual inmate's capabilities. Only the bedridden and the incarcerated insane were exempt
from duties. Failure to abide by these rules resulted in punishment
(frequently in the form of a reduction of food), and could, theoretically, lead to an individual's expulsion from the hospital.

Research to date which has looked at issues of work within
hospitals (or indeed within poor relief) has largely considered it as an
expression of the imposition of elite authority over the masses. It
primarily concerns issues such as the idleness of the poor and the
foundation of workhouses. This focus gives an overwhelmingly negative view of the poor from an elite or middling perspective. Comparatively work on poor relief has revealed ways in which the poor were
able to obtain relief in return for working for the parish in some form.
Perhaps the best known of such studies are those which concern
England, notably Margaret Pelling's work on Norwich, and Andrew
Wear's article on the parish of St Bartholomew, London[28] While this
viewpoint is not so negative, it still finds its basis in forms of work

which are effectively imposed upon the poor by authorities – at its most basic, a failure to accept any of these job offers would result in a reduction of poor relief for the individuals concerned. This paper is not denying the enforced nature of the work ethic within the Hessian institutions. A close analysis of sources suggests however that this interpretation does not reflect the whole reality of the situation.

Documentation from 1717 and 1719 relating to one of the hospital brethren, Johan Diedrich Simmersbach is indicative of the tensions that could occur when an individual's perception of his role as a hospital patient differed from that of the institution and indeed also from the ideas of fellow patients. Simmersbach complained to the hospital visitation committee that his food allowance had been cut and that he had been imprisoned for his inability to work. He stressed that his action was due to a physical weakness and incapability rather than a shirking of responsibilities. He also mentioned that he had requested clothing but had received neither of these items to date.

Correspondence from the hospital superintendent confirmed the situation, but stated that the punishments were implemented because the patient (*Hospithalit*) refused to go to work like other individuals. These restrictions were to be kept in place until he '[conformed and] worked'.[29]

At present, I have been unable to discover the ultimate outcome of this case. Nevertheless the accompanying inquest offers some interesting insights regarding a person's identity and their capacity to labour. When questioned, the fifty-two year old Simmersbach described himself as 'old and weak'. He stated that the injuries that he had received through his many years of military service had rendered him incapable of any form of strenuous work (*starcker arbeit*).

A report from hospital officials detailed the types of work that capable patients were expected to undertake. Winter activities included chopping the required wood for the kitchen and for their accommodation. Summer work included haymaking and fruit picking. For this work, inmates would receive certain perks such as extra bread and cheese. The authorities believed Simmersbach to be capable of such menial tasks. Indeed, he was believed to be one of the 'healthiest' (in comparative terms) patients within Haina at the time. It was specifically stated that his age (he was fifty-two years old) did not exempt him from these duties.

When further questioned, Simmersbach stated that his military wounds rendered him incapable of undertaking the forms of work of which other impotent inmates were capable. Due to the nature of his injuries – he had been stabbed – he became short of breath when he worked. Contrary to Simmersbach's assertions however, was the claim that he had told a hospital attendant that 'he could work as well as the best [workers] but he did not wish to do this'. Moreover Simmersbach had allegedly stated that the Landgraves had ordained that he be exempt from all work. Simmersbach dismissed such reports, asserting that 'the attendant [Peter Schneider] sometimes spoke many untruths'.

Schneider stood by his claims however and swore that 'his wife [and] also other competent (*verständigen*) brothers' had also heard Simmersbach make these statements. Under interrogation, Schneider was further asked if, during the time that Simmersbach had been under his care, he (the patient) had been confined to bed and had been weak (*bett lägerig und schwach*). He answered that 'he had not seen or heard anything to even slightly' suggest this condition. In fact, quite the opposite was true. One of the barber surgeons ('quite which one he could not remember'), had reported to the attendant that 'he had seen no brother who was healthier or livelier (*frisch*) than' Simmersbach. Attacking Simmersbach's moral character still further, Schnieder stated that he had appeared drunk on several occasions, and that he had also hit his [seemingly Schneider's] wife on one occasion. He was punished by the governor for the latter offence.

Johann Friederich Halbach, the hospital surgeon, was also questioned. His report claimed that he had been requested to visit Simmersbach and had found a 'severe' (*schlechter*) bodily/flesh (*haupt*) wound on his right side; he had been stabbed approximately twelve years previously whilst in military service. The wound in his chest was two fingers wide, and the sword had gone straight through his body, under his ribs and out through his back. Halbach concluded however that this wound had been 'cured', meaning that Simmersbach was able to undertake the 'minimal work' in the hospital as required of other inmates who were of a similar physical condition to the plaintiff. [30]

This paper is not denying that the interconnection of a comprehension of illness as being directly linked to an inability to work was widespread in the early modern period. Numerous historical studies have already shown this to be the case. Neither am I wishing to suggest that the authorities did not impose their power in forcing those inmates that they felt capable of work to work – punishments included having their food taken away and imprisonment. The Simmersbach case, and others like it, suggest however that there was also another force at work here that was linked to the notion of identity and a division between the stages of chronic incapacity experienced by hospital inmates. It would seem that the inmates – just as the authorities – distinguished between those of the brethren who worked and those who did not. In spite of the physical afflictions of all of the hospital population, it would appear that the inmates considered those who were unable to perform any duties to be 'ill' in a different manner to those who were able – in a sense it was as if the former group were deemed to be more ill or at a more advanced stage of their illness than the latter. The reality of this might have been wholly different, for some patients were described as bedridden and yet spent many years in this state within the hospital. Nevertheless, one's standing within the patient community depended, in part at least, upon one's (legitimate) ability or inability to perform the socially useful action of 'work'.

As the Simmersbach case reveals, an individual's notion of their capabilities did not always tie in with that of the authorities – nor indeed with the rest of the patient population. Simmersbach was a problematic patient for many reasons. A key theme of his case however was that he did not behave like a person who was unable to work – he had not proved himself to be bedridden and suitably weak. This failure also meant that his behaviour did not match that expected of an inmate (*Hospithalit*). Such issues are echoed in other documents in which patients complained about the actions of their fellow inmates. Thus in both 1683 and 1742 a group of sisters in Merxhausen petitioned about the behaviour of their fellow female patients. One cause of complaint related to work. These women were (in comparison to the plaintiffs) relatively young, yet they deemed themselves incapable of work. The correspondence from 1742 stated that the types of 'light work' that the sisters were asked to perform were considered to be of a nature that 'even the smallest child' would be able to perform them – this included involvement in cloth manufacture, assistance in the kitchens and bakery, work in the garden and the carrying of fruit. Their inability to perform these tasks was deemed by the authorities and the other inmates to be a charade and a further sign of their insubordination. The other patients, however, seemed to regard it as a sign that the younger, marginally more mobile patients were not behaving in a manner that suited their position (and by implication their medical condition) at this point in time.[31]

V   Conclusion

This chapter has considered aspects of capability and incapacity among the patient population, arguing for the extended ability of the chronically ill to both cope with their illness and to adapt their lifestyles accordingly. An ability to labour was also of fundamental importance in cases in which an individual relied upon the care of others for their survival. I have also suggested that one should not equate suffering from a serious medical condition with the automatic inability of a person to perform any sorts of task. Irrespective of the provision of the hospital that those who could work should do so, it would appear that many persons found it important that they be allowed to continue to work once within the hospital. An ability to do so was important to their identity and self-perception – the application for hospitalisation only arose as their decreased work capabilities (including no doubt, the speed at which these individuals were able to perform tasks) meant that they were no longer able to earn sufficient monies to provide for themselves. This work-based identity carried on into the hospital itself. One can see patients distinguishing between those persons who were capable of performing some menial tasks, and those who were immobilised by weakness or who were bedridden.

The latter stage was deemed by many to be the only time at which one was 'honourably' able to claim to be incapable of working. The patients themselves seem to have made distinctions in these matters and classified those persons within the hospital who failed to work as 'unworthy' of a place therein – they questioned their infirmity and suggested that they were in fact healthy and workshy, using much the same language that the authorities used against the unworthy beggars and vagabonds.

Far from merely equating illness and poverty with a request for hospitalisation, the petitions of the Hessian poor suggest that the whole process of the experience of chronic illnesses is one which needs a more subtle and in-depth analysis than it has hitherto been afforded.

Notes

1   Research for this paper was funded by the Wellcome Trust, and this work forms part of an ongoing project focusing upon welfare provision in early modern Hesse, Germany. I wish to thank the Trust for their continuing support.

2   M. Foucault, *The Birth of the Clinic: An Archaeology of Medical Perception*, trans. A.M. Sheridan Smith (London, 1973); idem, *Madness and Civilisation: A History of Insanity in the Age of Reason*, trans. R. Howard (London, 1967). For a critique of Foucault's ideas, see M. Dinges, 'Michel Foucault's Impact on the German Historiography of Criminal Justice', in N. Finzsch and R. Jütte (eds), *Institutions of Confinement: Hospitals, Asylums, and Prisons in Western Europe and North America, 1500–1950* (Cambridge, 1996), pp.155–74; R. Porter, 'Foucault's Confinement', *History of the Human Sciences*, 3.1 (1990), pp.47–54. See also the collection of essays, C. Jones and R. Porter (eds), *Reassessing Foucault: Power, Medicine and the Body* (London and New York, 1994).

3   Regarding Alltagsgeschichte, see U. Knefelkamp, *Das Heilig-Geist-Spital in Nürnberg vom 14–17 Jahrhundert: Geschichte, Struktur, Alltag* (Nuremberg, 1989); M. Mayer, *Hilfsbedürftige und Delinquenten: Die Anstaltsinsassen der Stadt St Gallen 1750–1789*, St Galler Kultur und Geschichte, 17 (St Gallen, 1987); A. Mischlewski, 'Alltag im Spital zu Beginn des 16. Jahrhunderts', in A. Kohler (ed.), *Alltag im 16. Jahrhundert: Studien zu Lebensformen in spätmittelalterlichen Städten* (Vienna, 1987), pp.152–73. See also the com-

ments of A. Goldberg, 'Institutionalizing Female Sexual Deviancy: Women, Rural Society, and the Insane Asylum in Nassau, 1815–1849', in R. Blänker and B. Jussen (eds), *Institutionen und Ereignis: über historische Praktiken und Vorstellungen gesellschaftlichen Ordnens* (Göttingen, 1998), pp.275–94, esp. p.276. Regarding the problems of an over-reliance upon censuses as a source-base, see M. Chaytor, 'Household and Kinship: Ryton in the Late Sixteenth and Early Seventeenth Centuries, Sources and Problems', *History Workshop Journal* (1980), pp.25–60, esp. 26–7.

4   T. Sokoll, 'The Position of Elderly Widows in Poverty: Evidence from Two English Communities in the Late Eighteenth and early Nineteenth Centuries', in J. Henderson and R. Wall (eds), *Poor Women and Children in the European Past* (London and New York, 1994), pp.207–24. See also other essays in this volume, and in the following collection: T. Hitchcock, P. King and P. Sharpe (eds), *Chronicling Poverty: The Voices and Strategies of the English Poor, 1640–1840* (London and New York, 1997), pp.1–18; K. Snell, *Annals of the Labouring Poor: Social Change and Agrarian England, 1660–1900* (Cambridge, 1985).

5   Obviously, the findings in this study relate to a specific group of the poor – those persons who (for the most part, successfully) applied for a place in one of the Hessian *Landesspitäler* – rather than offering sweeping statements regarding the experience of chronic illness among all of the Hessian paupers.

6   The best general history to date of Haina and Merxhausen is W. Heinemeyer and T. Pünder (eds), *450 Jahre Psychiatrie in Hessen*, Veröffentlichungen der Historischen Kommission für Hessen, 47 (Marburg, 1983).

7   Compare to D.G. Troyansky, 'Balancing Social and Cultural Approaches to the History of Old Age and Ageing in Europe: A Review and an Example from Post-Revolutionary France', in P. Johnson and P. Thane (eds), *Old Age from Antiquity to Post-Modernity* (London, 1998), pp.96–109, esp. 106.

8   For wider discussions on the use of petitions in historical inquiry see, among others, S. Hindle, *On the Parish? The Micro-Politics of Poor Relief in Rural England, c. 1550–1750* (Oxford, 2001), pp.155–64; A. Würgler, 'Voices From Among the "Silent Masses": Humble Petitions and Social Conflicts in Early Modern Central Europe', *International Review of Social History*, 46 (2001) (Supplement 11), p.34.

9   While the ordinances stipulated that poverty was a necessary prerequisite, this condition was not always adhered to. This paper will primarily focus upon pauper petitions. For admissions policies from the sixteenth to early eighteenth centuries, see L. Gray, 'The Self-Perception of Chronic Physical Incapacity among the Labouring Poor: Pauper Narratives and Territorial Hospitals in Early Modern Rural Germany' (unpublished PhD thesis, University of London, 2001). For the situation in the eighteenth century: C. Vanja, 'Leben und Arbeiten im Hohen Hospital Haina um 1750', in J.H.W. Tischbein, *Das Werk*

des Goethe-Malers zwischen Kunst, Wissenschaft und Alltagskultur, ed. A. Friedrich, F. Heinrich, and C. Holm (Petersberg, 2001), pp.33–45.

10   There is a vast literature concerning care networks. See especially, S. Cavallo, 'Family Obligations and Inequalities in Access to Care (Northern Italy Seventeenth–Eighteenth Centuries)', in P. Horden and R.M. Smith (eds), *The Locus of Care: Families, Communities, Institutions and the Provision of Welfare since Antiquity* (London, 1998); Gray, 'Self-Perception', ch. 5; Gray, 'Family, Institutions and Care in Sixteenth-Century Rural Germany', European Social Science History Conference (Amsterdam, 2000), unpublished paper (published version forthcoming).

11   Archiv des Landeswohlfahrtsverbandes Hessen (henceforth LWV), *Bestand 13*, Reskripte, 1577. Regarding the issue of old age in these petitions, see Gray, 'Self-Perception', ch. 4; eadem, 'The Experiences of Old Age in the Narratives of the Rural Poor in Early Modern Germany', in S.R. Ottoway, L. Botelho, and K. Kittredge (eds), *Power and Poverty: Old Age in the Pre-Industrial Past* (Westport, Conn. and London, 2002), pp.107–24.

12   LWV, *Bestand 13*, Reskripte, 1709.

13   Regarding the role of guilds in medical history, see A.-M. Kinzelbach, *Gesundblieben, Krankwerden, Armsein in der frühneuzeitlichen Gesellschaft: Gesunde und Kranke in den Reichstädten Überlingen und Ulm, 1500–1700* (Stuttgart, 1995), pp.172–80.

14   LWV, *Bestand 13*, Reskripte, 1700.

15   *Ibid.*, 1698.

16   *Ibid.*, 1702.

17   *Ibid.*, 1713.

18   LWV, *Bestand 17*, Reskripte, 1711.

19   LWV, *Bestand 13*, Reskripte, 1704.

20   *Ibid.*, 1722.

21   *Ibid.*, 1704.

22   LWV, *Bestand 17*, Reskripte, 1605–25.

23   Regarding 'work', see Gray, 'Self-Perception', ch. 6.

24   LWV, *Bestand 13*, Reskripte, 1576.

25   *Ibid.*, 1712.

26   Similar arguments have also been noted in studies of applications for poor relief. See Hindle, *On the Parish?*

27   LWV, *Bestand 13*, Reskripte, 1717.

28   M. Pelling, 'Illness among the Poor in an Early Modern English Town: the Norwich Census of 1570', *Continuity and Change*, 3.2 (1988), pp.273–90; A. Wear, 'Caring for the Sick Poor in St Bartholomew's Exchange, 1580–1676', *Medical History*, Supplement No. 11 (1991), pp.41–60.

29   LWV, *Bestand 13*, Reskripte, 1717, 1719.

30   *Ibid.*

31   LWV, *Bestand 17*, Reskripte, 1683, 1742.

ERIC GRUBER VON ARNI

Chapter 13: 'Tempora mutantur et nos mutamur in illis': The Experience of Sick and Wounded Soldiers during the English Civil Wars and Interregnum, 1642–60

The title of this paper has been taken from an inscription written on the inside cover of a small leather-bound account book compiled by John Holhead, the Overseer of a Parliamentary military hospital that functioned in Parson's Green, West London, between March 1645 and September 1646, which translates roughly as 'the times they are changing and we are being changed with them'.[1] Coming as they do from someone who was closely involved in coping with the effects of a brutal war these words may appear reasonable but can his sentiments be equally applied to the nature of contemporary military hospital care?

The earliest recorded attempt by any army at forming a regular camp field hospital occurred during the War of Granada, 1492, when Queen Isabella of Castille provided a number of large tents, known as the 'Queen's hospitals', permanently reserved for the sick and wounded, and furnished them with appropriate attendants and medicine at her own charge and, during the long history of conflict that involved Spain, France and the Dutch in the Low Countries, the Spanish Army of Flanders devised a sophisticated medical support network for its troops.[2] From 1585, a major military hospital was sited at Malines equipped with 330 beds, augmented during prolonged sieges or active fighting by temporary field hospitals at strategic locations or by the requisitioning of civil hospitals.[3]

During Elizabeth I's Irish campaign of 1598–1603, English troops experienced notoriously high sickness rates, particularly as a result of dysentery. Poor communal hygiene, bad and inadequate food, the climate, a hostile local population and poor lodgings all combined to seal the fate of many raw recruits within a very short time of landing on the island.[4] Many soldiers died in the streets for want of assistance and it was obvious that a more satisfactory solution to the care and disposal of casualties was needed. Eventually, on 10 January 1600, after two agents of the Secretary of State, Lord Robert Cecil, had proposed the establishment of military hospitals within Ireland itself, the Privy Council decreed that hospitals for sick and injured soldiers were to be provided in every province, funded by allowing each regiment to draw a fictitious soldier's daily rate of pay to cover property rental and bedding.[5]

Four hospitals were planned for Cork, Drogheda, Dublin and at Derry where a wooden building, erected within the walls of an old church, was opened in September 1600 containing just twenty-eight beds and a kitchen, besides some other small rooms.[6] Each hospital was to be supervised by two unpaid civilian overseers appointed from 'honest householders in the towns'. Salaried staff were allocated to each hospital including a Master, a physician or surgeon, his servant, who probably also acted as the hospital clerk, and four female nurses.[7]

The lessons of Ireland were not, however, fully appreciated and, in the hard school of the Thirty Years' War, they had to be re-learned by bitter experience. Despite England's official policy of noninvolvement in that conflict, large numbers of Britons offered their services, particularly to the Protestant participant countries. In 1620, Sir Horace de Vere raised a large body of English volunteers in support of James I's son-in-law, the Elector Palatine, taking a number of surgeons with him.[8] Their presence set the pattern for medical establishments during subsequent expeditions for the next forty years. Nevertheless, although planning was undertaken by the most experienced military officers of the day, there was no mention of medical or hospital stores amongst the minutely detailed stores inventories.

Other countries relied upon local militia forces to form the basis of their military structure in times of war, but, when each crisis was over, such formations dissolved as rapidly as they were raised. The Swedish army's organisation was innovatory in providing the first conscripted, permanent national force financed by a national budget.[9] Gustavus Adolphus, conscious of the need to husband his forces as a national asset, introduced a standardisation programme throughout his army which included a thorough reform of its medical support. Whereas other armies passed responsibility for the provision of soldiers' health care to individual captains, who frequently neglected this aspect of their duty, the Swedish king regarded the provision of adequate medical facilities as an enhancement of morale and a recruiting incentive.[10] France's record in this regard was nowhere near so impressive albeit, during the Franco-Italian wars of Louis XIII, the need for military hospitals was clearly recognised. Cardinal Richelieu created a military hospital at Pinerolo, near Turin in Northern Italy, and attempted to institute a complete military medical service including a 'train of army hospitals' but a lack of financial support limited their development.[11]

In England during the 1630s there were fewer than 1,000 men in military service, but, when the Bishops' Wars, the Irish Rebellion and the Civil Wars erupted, up to 20,000 English and Scottish adventurers serving on the Continent returned home bringing with them considerable experience of the ways of war. Despite the destructive effects on health care provision wrought by Henry VIII's Dissolution of the Monasteries that destroyed the medieval facilities where, formerly, hospital-based health care was provided to all-comers, the outbreak of civil war in 1642 found large numbers of citizens ready to regard the task of caring for the needy as a patriotic duty. The surviving documentary evidence indicates that, regardless of the ever-present evils of wanton destruction and pillaging common to all wars, large numbers of men and women across the country strove to provide care and comfort to the victims of the fighting in a manner that would do credit to a similar section of society today.

Surviving documentary evidence for the provision of care to Royalist forces is relatively scarce. The King's attitude towards his army's casualties was ambivalent at best. In addition, lackadaisical administrative paperwork and the wholesale destruction of documents following the surrender of Oxford combine to cloud our appreciation of their facilities. Nevertheless, even contemporary Royalist sources conceded that their enemy's medical services were far superior to their own.[12]

By comparison, Parliament appears to have been genuinely committed to establishing and maintaining high standards of care for wounded soldiers by adopting a strongly positive approach towards them and it is possible to compile a comparatively comprehensive dossier on these achievements. This chapter will therefore concentrate on the medical facilities afforded Parliamentary troops in hospitals.

Control of the City of London and the Exchequer was an ace up Parliament's sleeve. Along with possession of the nation's financial centre came access to the City's five ancient poor hospitals. Throughout the war St Thomas' and St Bartholomew's hospitals in particular – received a steady flow of wounded soldiers, but, significant as their contribution was in caring for military casualties, they were only able to handle a small proportion of those needing assistance. Their duty of care towards the capital's civilian population meant they could not be relied upon to provide all the hospital requirements of the army. Specific arrangements were required.

On 25 October 1642, within forty-eight hours of the opening battle at Edgehill, Parliament passed an Act that, for the first time, acknowledged the State's responsibility to provide for the welfare of its wounded soldiers and also for the widows and orphans of those killed.[13] On 14 November, with the pressure for hospital beds rising, Parliament formed 'The Committee for Sick and Maimed Souldiers' to take full control of the organisation and implementation of its casualty care arrangements (Fig. 13.1).[14]

An extensive series of accounts, which provide a broad insight into the work of this committee, survives in the Exchequer papers. Five distinct audit periods can be identified. The first, managed by Robert Jenner and Cornelius Holland, both Members of Parliament, with assistance from William Foster, an accountant, lasted from the Committee's foundation in November 1642 until 31 May 1643. The second, in the hands of four new treasurers, ran from 1 June 1643 until 31 March 1645 and the third, the most lengthy and extensive, was uninterrupted between 1 April 1645 and March 1653. In 1653 the Committee for Sick and Maimed Soldiers was abolished and authority was transferred to a new body known as the Hospitals Committee with a single Treasurer. The fourth accounting period, May 1653 to 1657, was followed by a fifth and final series covering the remainder of the

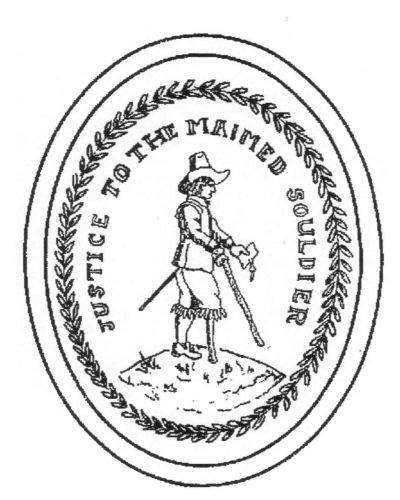

Figure 13.1 The Seal of the Committee for Sick and Maimed Souldiers.
(Drawing by A.Turton and E. Gruber von Arni from an original seal at Wiltshire and
Swindon County Record Office)

Protectorate and Commonwealth years to 1660. The two sets of account papers for 1653–60 have not been discovered, but their contents are indicated by associated letters and documents. While all of these accounts are unreliable, both in respect to their arithmetical accuracy and their failure to record every transaction, by noting payments for everyday items such as utensils, sheets and blankets, clothing and laundry, wages and a variety of minutiae, it is possible to gain an unparalleled insight into the lives of the patients and staff.[15]

It was decided to establish a hospital specifically reserved for the care and treatment of sick and wounded soldiers and the Savoy Hospital in the Strand, an ancient poor hospital originally founded by King Henry VII, was chosen (Fig. 13.2). Admission to the Savoy was restricted to army casualties and the College of Physicians and the Barber Surgeons' Company were given a direct order to provide physicians and surgeons to work at the hospital.[16] On 3 December a daily clinic was instigated for non-resident wounded, who, in addition, received 8d a day for food and lodging whilst under care.[17] Four nursing sisters of the original staff remained in the hospital. These were further augmented until eventually at least twelve nurses were employed to work under the directions of an overseer.[18]

The Savoy remained the sole military hospital for over two years until March 1645 when a second was opened in the western suburbs of London.[19] Apart from identification as 'the hospital at Parson's Green', this hospital's exact location is not clearly described in extant documents, but the premises used must have been reasonably substantial as they were capable of holding over seventy patients. In the mid-seventeenth century there were only three buildings in the Parson's Green and Fulham area large enough and, of these, the most likely site for the military hospital was the house of Sir Nicholas Crispe. This building sat alongside the Thames between Fulham and Hammersmith and was described in a contemporary report as a 'great brick house lately built by Sir Nicholas Crispe, knight, situate and being near the town of Hammersmith'. The Churchwardens' accounts for St Paul's, Hammersmith record several entries relating to disbursements for maimed soldiers and also a payment of 2s 4d to the sexton for digging seven graves for soldiers that had died at Sir Nicholas Crispe's house.[20] More recently at least two other historians have claimed that

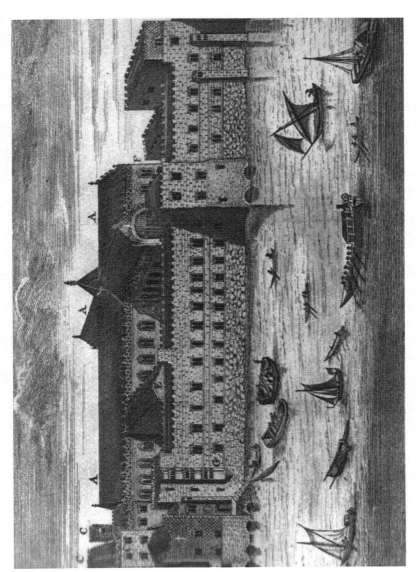

Figure 13.2 The Savoy Hospital from an eighteenth-century print. (Author's collection)

Crispe's house was used as a military hospital during the Civil War and reported that human bones were often found buried in the Crabtree area and were believed to have been the remains of parliamentarian soldiers who had died at Sir Nicholas Crispe's house when it was in use as such.[21]

The Overseer's account book for the hospital in Parson's Green, from which the title of this paper is taken, confirms both the payment of weekly pensions to the in-patients as well as routine weekly housekeeping expenditure. Like the Savoy, Parson's Green was ideally suited for river access and several account entries recorded payments for the carriage of patients to and from the hospital by water. Soldiers were admitted from the armies of the Earl of Essex, Sir William Waller, the Earl of Manchester, the Earl of Denbigh as well as the various London Trained Bands and some captured soldiers from the Royalist Army. Admissions peaked when casualties arrived from the siege and fall of Basing House on 14 October 1645.[22]

Each nurse at Parson's Green received 5s a week in wages and, although there was an occasional reduction to three as the work-load varied, for the majority of the time the staff consisted of four ladies. This figure temporarily rose to five during November and December 1645 to cope with an influx of wounded following the storming of Basing House, but, towards the final closure in August 1646, only two remained in employment. The hospital staff formed a small community and on one occasion even held a lottery to raise money for sick and wounded soldiers. There were regular payments for labourers and to someone called 'Roger', possibly a child who helped with general tasks such as errand running and, on one occasion, a child was paid 1s 9d for mending bedding. Other entries included regular weekly expenditure on sundries such as candles, brooms, spoons, malt for beer making and earthen pitchers, soap and ashes, the latter being used for making lye for use in the laundry.[23]

When Parson's Green hospital was closed at the end of the First Civil War, the overall demand for hospital beds did not, however, decline and, although the accounts record that the last patients remaining at Parson's Green were transferred to the Savoy Hospital, a desperate shortage of beds for military patients persisted. Two years later, in 1648, with the outbreak of the Second Civil War, the Savoy was again placed under pressure and an urgent need for more beds arose. Ely House, which lay at the end of High Holborn, was the former London palace of the Bishops of Ely and had been used as a prison for Royalist prisoners of war for the past six years. In September 1648, after considerable and expensive refurbishment, its doors were reopened as a military hospital (Fig. 13.3).[24] The main buildings of the extensive property consisted of a large hall, a chapel and a cloistered quadrangle where patients could walk in the fresh air with protection from the elements in inclement weather. On the south side large gardens, including a herb garden with medicinal plants, provided a pleasant amenity. It was there, throughout 1654, that a man named Walker was officially paid to feed a pet fox that was presumably kept for the amusement of patients.[25]

So, what do we know of the experiences of the wounded soldier on admission to one of these hospitals? On entering one of the London military hospitals the new patient would find himself comfortably housed in clean surroundings, albeit aware of an all-pervading aroma from the burning pitch used to fumigate the wards (Fig. 13.4). He would have been allocated one of the heavy wooden beds that were set around the walls of the wards and supplied with a clean pair of sheets and pillowcases each week. He would also have been provided with any clothing that he needed and two or three weekly changes of underwear. The beds as well as the windows were curtained and screens were made available if necessary. Warming pans heated the beds in winter and, with rugs on the floor, chairs and settles available for mobile patients and benches around the dining tables, the patients were made reasonably comfortable.[26] The bed-ridden were provided with pewter chamber pots stored in bedside 'close stools' (commodes) and supplied with tow for hygiene purposes. A woman known as Goody Swayne was paid 2s weekly to empty the close stools every morning and evening and a man was employed to bring coals from the cellar to the wards for general heating and cooking purposes.

The number of patients for whom each nurse was responsible naturally varied according to circumstances, but, as the following table demonstrates, with an average nurse to patient ratio of 1:10, the military hospitals experienced better staffing arrangements than their civilian counterparts.

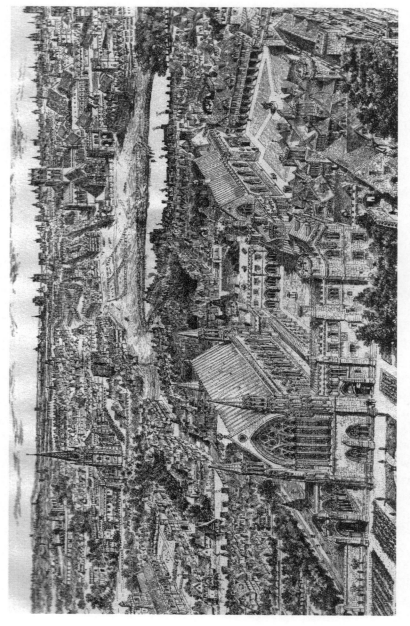

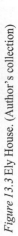

Figure 13.3 Ely House. (Author's collection)

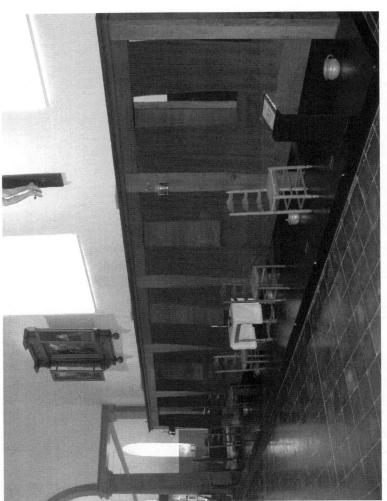

Figure 13.4 Reconstructed ward scene showing layout similar to that at the Savoy Hospital and Ely House. (Author's photograph, Hospice de Notre Dame de la Rose, Tournai)

Figure 13.5
Comparative Patient to Nursing Staff Ratio

Hospital	No. Nurses	No. Beds	Ratio
a) Military			
The Savoy	Up to 15	Approx 150	Approx 1:10
Ely House	Up to 15	Approx 150	Approx 1:10
Parson's Green	Up to 5	Average 50	Approx 1:10
b) Civilian			
St Thomas'	15	200	Approx 1:13
St Bartholomew's	15	249	Approx 1:16

Sources: The National Archives, SP28/141B; St Bartholomew's Hospital Archives, Ha 1/4 and 1/5, Hospital Journal and Committee Book, IV and V, *passim*; F.G. Parsons, *The History of St Thomas' Hospital*, 2 vols (London, 1934), pp.51–91

Just as in contemporary civilian hospital practice, care of the patients at night in the military hospitals does not appear to have been a normal part of the nurses' regular responsibilities. Although one nurse, Nurse Gunston, received at least three payments for 'watching a man at night' during April and May 1654, the most common arrangement was to employ men and, less often, women from outside specifically to watch over particular patients at an average rate of 8d for each night-duty shift.[27] Occasionally ex-patients were employed for these duties, as in the case of 'one Hunt a poor man [...] lately a patient, [for] watching that night and his labour that night in the same ward' who was paid 1s on 20 March 1653. Other payments were made to members of staff for escorting patients to other hospitals for appointments or treatments, and to coachmen for transportation, such as the 6d paid for someone to go with a patient to St Thomas' Hospital, 2s for a coach for a soldier and, on 15 April 1654, the hire of a coach to convey two lame men to the Savoy cost 1s 6d. A few children or young persons, possibly the children of soldiers' widows, may have found employment in and around the hospitals as errand boys and general labourers.[28]

The head nurse of each ward was responsible for food preparation for the patients in her charge, but little evidence remains of the diet provided for patients in the Savoy or Ely House. Nevertheless, we are fortunate that comparable alternative information has survived relating to the period of Parliament's military administration in Scotland, between 1653 and 1659, when an army facility was opened in Heriot's Hospital, Edinburgh. There, instead of the nurses preparing the patients' food, a staff Cook and an assistant toiled over two fires, one for roasting and the other for boiling.[29] In 1655 Heriot's was only equipped for thirty in-patients and, of these, twenty-two were each provided with a pint of gruel or milk for breakfast and, on four days each week, a pint of beer, five ounces of butter, five ounces of cheese and two pounds of bread. On the other three days one and a quarter pounds of meat were substituted for the cheese. The eight soldiers not included in the stated allowance were too weak for this diet and were granted 3s 6d weekly from which suitable food was purchased. The following table provides a comparison of relative food values between this Heriot's Hospital diet and modern recommendations:

Figure 13.6
Food and calorific values in the Heriot's Hospital diet

Element	Heriot Diet	Recommended daily intake for males 19–50 years: 1992	Surplus/ Deficit
Calcium	1,217.6 mgm	700.0 mgm	517.6 mgm+
Vit C	3.7 mgm	40.0 mgm	36.3 mgm–
Iron	27.0 mgm	8.7 mgm	18.3 mgm+
Protein	152.1 g	55.5 g	96.6 g +
Kcal	4,189.4 kcal	2,250.0 kcal	1,839.4 kcal +

Source: Dietary calculations kindly provided by Mrs F. Bowen, Senior Dietician, Frimley Park Hospital

By way of further comparison, the official target calorific value for the military diet provided to British troops during World War One, was 4,300 calories per day.[30] It will be noted that for calories, protein, calcium and iron, the Heriot's diet contained much higher quantities than modern recommendations for the average male aged between

nineteen and fifty years, albeit these are for white-collar workers.
Even after an appropriate adjustment for arduous physical activity or
convalescence from injury, a considerable imbalance remains between
the two sets of figures. The Heriot's diet certainly compared favourably with that provided to troops on garrison duties or in the field as
shown in the following table.

Figure 13.7
*Comparative daily values for Heriot's Hospital, garrison and
marching soldiers' diets*

Item	Heriot's Hospital	Chalfield Garrison	On the March
Bread & biscuit	2 lb	8 ozs	10½ ozs
Peas & beans	Unrecorded	4 ozs dried or ¼ pint Fresh Peas	3 ozs dried or 6 ozs cooked
Meat & dairy produce (on 3 days a week)	1¼ lb	1 lb	5 ozs
Salt	Unrecorded	Unrestricted	1 oz
Beer	1 pint	2½ pints	½ pint
Oatmeal (Gruel ± milk)	1 pint	¾ lb	Nil
Cheese	5 ozs (on 4 days a week)	2 ozs	Nil
Butter	5 ozs	Unrecorded	Nil
Fish	Unrecorded	Unrecorded	Nil

Source: The National Archives, S.P. 28/128, Part 28, fol. 26; S. Peachey, *Civil War
and Salt Fish* (Leigh on Sea, 1988), p.7; J.H.P. Pafford, *Accounts of the
Parliamentary Garrison of Great Chalfield and Malmesbury, 1645–6*, Wiltshire
Natural History and Archaeological Society (Devizes, 1966)

Although, as shown, military hospital food was better than standard
military rations, both remained short on fresh fruit and vegetables and
lacked essential vitamins, particularly C, minerals and other dietary
elements. The soldiers' potential for recovery was therefore prejudiced
even before their moment of injury. Even so, the Civil War soldier's
diet still managed to compare favourably with the average diet available in the United Kingdom during the food rationing of World War

Two, when, for example, the weekly cheese ration varied between only 1 and 8 ounces depending on availability.

Care for the mundane, temporal needs of the patients was augmented by an equal consideration for their spiritual welfare. Religious worship figured largely in the patients' daily lives. Two ministers were attached to the hospitals and religious books were distributed throughout the wards.[31] The first two paragraphs of the hospital rules stipulated that every soldier (who was able) was to attend church twice every Sunday and a Bible reading twice a day. Failure to attend either incurred financial penalties.

In addition to the patients' physical and spiritual needs, the hospital appointments and surroundings also received care. Account entries indicate that the expression 'cleanliness is next to godliness' was a reality in these hospitals as it was a highly important factor in hospital routine. Bed frames were regularly painted with lime-based whitewash, which has mild disinfectant properties, but, when a ward was to be thoroughly cleaned, all the beds and fittings were removed to another area and replaced afterwards at considerable expense.

The high incidence of amputations carried out in the surgical treatment of battle casualties was reflected in both the resources and relatively sophisticated equipment provided for the comfort and care of patients who had suffered the loss of limbs. Amputation cases were nursed under bed cradles supplied by the hospital carpenter. Crutches were supplied in various lengths. The carpenter was frequently required to provide prosthetic limbs and the associated attachments for them. For example, one soldier was provided with a wooden hand whilst another, who had suffered an above-knee amputation, was supplied with a prosthetic limb described as 'a new artificial leg with a leather box, plated all over with iron, complete with swivels and pins'.[32] These resources remained available to patients following their discharge from hospital providing on-going maintenance.

Although the services of a 'bone setter' were sometimes employed, the Savoy was provided with an eminent surgical staff headed by Thomas Trapham, Cromwell's personal military surgeon and Surgeon-General.[33] Fortunately, the writings of Richard Wiseman, a Royalist surgeon, later appointed Serjeant-Surgeon to Charles II, survive as evidence of contemporary military surgical practice describing every stage of treatment. In the main his methods follow closely the sixteenth-century teachings of Ambroise Paré and there is no reason to doubt that the methods of Trapham and his colleagues differed in any marked way.

Whilst surgeons held sway at the Savoy, physicians were pre-eminent at Ely House, where they treated a wide variety of conditions, including infective, systemic and psychiatric disorders. The only, somewhat limited, sources of identification for the various ailments suffered by patients admitted to Ely House are the Order Books of the English Commanders-in-Chief in Scotland which record transfers of patients from Heriot's Hospital to London. These documents restrict themselves to such terms as 'lameness', 'diseased' or 'sickness', but a few are more specific. For instance, Arthur Coleman, a Corporal, was referred to Ely House having contracted 'consumption and a cough of the lungs'.

The prevalence of psychiatric disorders is unclear, as such conditions were often misunderstood, poorly recognised and diagnosed, and seldom documented. Two cases of 'fitting' were recorded at Ely House as requiring 'watching' at night and we learn that two soldiers with psychiatric conditions were identified at Heriot's Hospital prior to transfer to London. One, Edward Hodgson, was described as 'a very sad object deprived of his understanding and totally helpless' and another, Thomas King, suffered from 'a lameness wherewith he is troubled in his head'.

Also at Ely House, the opening of a ward known as the hot-house was a novel experience for the soldier patients. Inspired by the work of Peter Chamberlen, a physician of some influence, these rooms were used to provide the 'sweating treatment', primarily for those suffering from venereal infections and involved placing the patient in a heated room and administering a small quantity of mercury morning and evening, either orally or in the form of an ointment. This treatment, which was recommended by such influential practitioners as Harvey, Wiseman and Sydenham, was continued for three to eight weeks until the patient began to suffer excessive salivation and other signs of mercurial poisoning. Meanwhile, he was kept warm, either in bed or seated by the fire and fed a liquid or soft diet.[34] Interestingly, there appears to have been a refreshingly non-judgmental approach to the needs of these patients.

No expense was spared in running the hot-house facility. Two male nurses supervised the soldiers who sat or reclined in cubicles whilst smoking from issued clay pipes, and wearing special caps and heavy baize coats in the atmosphere of a Turkish bath created by a copper bath stove from which heat was channelled to each cubicle. Their regular provisions included an ample supply of claret wine and sugar. In St Thomas' hospital, where the need for increased fluid intake by the patients undergoing this treatment was equally appreciated, the 'sweat wards' were issued with a healthier three barrels of beer or ale weekly and no wine or spirits. I have no doubt that the soldiers at Ely House felt theirs was the superior arrangement. Sadly, the effects of such a high consumption of alcohol in a heated environment are not recorded.[35]

The most expensive single item recorded was the provision of spa water treatment. As early as August 1645 the Committee for Sick and Maimed Soldiers paid £4 5s for military patients to travel to Bath in Somerset for treatment. Significant groups of sick soldiers again visited the city in 1647 and 1648. After Dr John French, a proponent of spa water treatment, was appointed senior physician at Ely House in 1649, large sums of money were allocated to this annual event until, in 1653, the largest allocation, up to £1,600, was authorised.[36]

Why was Parliament prepared to commit such a huge sum of money to such an undertaking? Altruism and the desire to provide the most up-to-date treatment available are considerations, but, in terms of hard cash, a reduction in overall expenditure would, inevitably, have resulted from a rapid cure in Bath compared with expensive on-going in-patient care at the Savoy or Ely House.[37] This would certainly have been a major factor in the later years of the Protectorate. As the country's financial base became increasingly unsteady, shortage of ready cash became a significant factor in the lead up to the Restoration of the Monarchy in 1660 and the subsequent final demise of Parliament's military hospitals in 1661.

So, is it possible to assess the quality, availability and effectiveness of care provided in the military hospitals of the Civil War and Interregnum in the light of surviving evidence? It may seem anachronistic for an observer, viewing the situation from a distance of 350 years, to attempt to define acceptable standards of care and make comparisons with those of the twenty-first century. However, there are many aspects that have remained constant over the centuries.

Despite the mainstream changes in political thought and attitudes that emerged during the Reformation, many traditional work-practices and values survived. Mid-seventeenth-century nursing inherited many attitudes, traditions and regulations from earlier, medieval practice. These included the 'Comfortable or Corporal Works of Mercy' listed in St Matthew's Gospel which Protestants could accept without difficulty:[38]

> For I was an hungred, and ye gave me meat:
> I was thirsty, and ye gave me drink:
> I was a stranger, and ye took me in:
> Naked, and ye clothed me:
> I was sick, and ye visited me:
> I was in prison and ye came unto me.
> Matthew, 25, vv.35–6.

The *regimen santitatis*, medieval regulations written to govern the day-to-day existence of staff and patients in hospitals, were compiled to define the practical application of the 'Comfortable Works' in the belief that the role of physicians and nurses was to support and enhance the six non-naturals deemed necessary for life. These included the provision of a congenial environment and an equable state of mind, adequate rest and exercise, sufficient, restful sleep, the management of excretion, and repletion with appropriate food, drink and medication. The original 1515 statutes for the Savoy Hospital had incorporated these elements and it is not unreasonable to suggest that the same standards were inherited by the nurses of 1642.[39]

Using a modern 'nursing model', developed to offer guidelines when determining appropriate nursing practice, it is possible to determine how closely these factors are in tune with our perceptions of care today.[40] The 'Activities of Daily Living', developed by Roper, Tierney and Logan, have been selected as an appropriate tool:

Maintenance of a safe environment
Mobilisation
Communication
Breathing
Eating and drinking
Elimination
Personal cleaning and dressing
Controlling body temperature
Working and playing
Expressing sexuality
Sleeping
Dying[41]

These twelve components bear an uncanny similarity to both the 'Corporate Works of Mercy' and the *regimen sanitatis* and, if we address each of them in turn, we may arrive at some interesting conclusions.

The patients' environment was certainly safe. They were comfortably housed in well-appointed rooms and close attention was paid to security by a porter who manned the gates which he locked at night. The safety of individual patients who were in danger of injury by virtue of their illness, such as epileptic and 'disturbed' patients, was supervised by 'watchers' hired for the purpose. Requisite treatments, both medical and surgical, were provided and wounds were appropriately dressed.

During a patient's recovery, his mobilisation was assisted in a variety of ways, even including the provision of a rope hoist to assist in re-positioning himself in bed.[42] Many of the patients were confined to bed for prolonged periods and for them the essential nursing task of preventing the occurrence of 'bed sores' was well appreciated. In the words of Brugis, a contemporary surgeon and author, it was essential to enable the patient to 'air his back and hips lest they excoriate with too much lying'.[43] Assistance with mobilisation was particularly relevant for those who had lost limbs, for whom prostheses and crutches were available. It has been noted earlier that Ely House became a centre for the supply of these items to both in-patients and out-pensioners, including maintenance and after-care services.

Communication was clearly facilitated, especially the voicing of patients' grievances. On admission to a hospital the individual surrendered many of his personal freedoms in exchange for his treatment, bed and board. Any complaints he might have had were forwarded through the military chain of command and, indeed, patients' petitions often arrived on the desk of Sir Thomas Fairfax, Commander-in-Chief of the New Model Army. Fairfax was an active supporter of soldiers' rights and he expended considerable effort in bringing these petitions to the attention of Parliament.

As regards breathing, the frequent fumigation of wards with burning pitch resulted in a thick, heavily laden atmosphere exacerbated by tobacco smoke and the odour of infected wounds, compounded at night by closed windows and the common contemporary belief that nocturnal air was unhealthy. It is therefore most unlikely that ventilation was adequate. It is not surprising that expectorants and bronchial medications, including inhalations, were amongst the frequently prescribed treatments.

In assessing diet I have presented an analysis of the average patient's diet which, when compared with that of contemporary civilians could be described as adequate. It was even superior to that supplied to their healthier colleagues in the regiments, despite a probable deficiency in fruit, vegetables and vitamins.

Elimination of bodily waste was assisted by various laxatives and diuretics prescribed when necessary and a variety of contemporary medical texts show that the importance of maintaining normal bodily functions during periods of bed rest was well appreciated.

Personal hygiene was promoted and it was the nurses' specific responsibility to ensure that their patients were kept 'clean and sweet smelling'. No doubt, they assisted mobile patients in dressing themselves in the specially made clothing provided.

The maintenance of an appropriate body temperature was a prominent feature in most treatment regimes. The need to keep patients warm was recognised with each ward being allocated its own coal allowance which varied according to the season.

It is a much more complex task to assess the support for enabling patients to express their sexuality. As this function includes the provision of help in shaving and personal grooming it is possible to confirm a positive approach to the task. However, the wider aspects of sexuality were actively repressed throughout contemporary society during this period. Compared with the high degree of prominence afforded this topic in the twenty-first century, the subject was then taboo. During the early years of the seventeenth century the Church had pursued an active programme of repressing sexual immorality and, assisted by Puritan influence, all classes of society experienced an unprecedented fall in the level of sexual permissiveness.

Sleeping was assisted by the comfortable beds provided and, when necessary, sleeping draughts were prescribed. If undue noise was created during the hours of darkness, the offender was liable to punishment.

Death was much more a familiar part of everyday life and was viewed as a natural and expected event and ample evidence survives to demonstrate that, except in the immediate aftermath of battle, soldiers expected and normally received a formal religious burial service.[44] Ministers provided spiritual support for the dying, and the dead were treated with reverence and respect. The presence of representatives from dead soldiers' regiments at military funerals was a legal requirement.

At the conclusion of this analysis it appears that, overall, the balance sheet shows that the soldier patient was remarkably well cared for in the military hospitals of Parliament throughout the period under discussion. Can the inscription written by Overseer Holhead at Parson's Green, used as the title for this paper, be said to be an accurate comment on his experience? It may be argued, on the one hand, that the work of his hospital staff was conducted along the same lines that had been employed for centuries past. On the other hand, this was very much a time of innovation and change. Parliament had accepted for the first time that it had a duty of care towards those killed and injured in its service as well as to the relatives of those who suffered.

All of Parliament's achievements were swept away at the Restoration of the Monarchy in 1660 when the hospitals were closed. Although the Royal Hospitals at Chelsea and Kilmainham were opened some twenty years later as shelters for soldiers worn out by service, it was more than 100 years before a permanent, acute receiving hospital dedicated to military patients was again established in London. It is in this light that Parliament's achievements have to be reviewed.

We do not know at what point in his hospital's eighteen months' existence Holhead wrote his inscription but, if we read his words in the context of the unsettled events of his time, with political and other changes seemingly turning his personal world upside down, perhaps we can understand why he wrote what he did.

Notes

1   The National Archives (hereafter TNA), SP 28/141B, part 4.

2   W.H. Prescott, *History of the Reign of Ferdinand and Isabella*, 2 vols (London, 1841), 2, p.345; *Journal of the Society for Army Historical Research* (hereafter *JSAHR*), 4 (1925), p.219, Reply No. 179.

3   G. Parker, *The Army of Flanders and the Spanish Road, 1567–1659* (Cambridge, 1972), p.169.

4   TNA, SP 63/44, fol. 49; J.J.N. McGurk, 'Casualties and Welfare Measures for the Sick and Wounded of the Nine Year War in Ireland, 1593–1602', *JSAHR*, 68 (1990), pp.22–35, 188–204.

5   *JSAHR*, 68 (1990), pp.331–4, 396.

6   *Calendar of State Papers (Domestic)* (hereafter *Cal. SP. Dom*) 1589–1600, p.209; McGurk, 'Casualties', p.34.

7   *Cal. SP. Dom, 1589–1600*, pp.375 and 448; *Calendar of the Carew Manuscripts*, ed. J.S. Brewer et al., 6 vols (London, 1867–73), vol. 3: *1589–1600*, p.275.

8   C.R. Markham, *The Fighting Veres* (Boston and Cambridge, 1888), pp.456–7; J. Adair, *Roundhead General: A Military Biography of Sir William Waller* (London, 1969, republished Stroud, 1997), pp.7–8.

9   M. Roberts, *Gustavus Adolphus*, 2 vols (London, 1953–8), 2, p.676; idem, *Gustavus Adolphus*, rev. edn (London, 1973), pp.96–101; idem, *Essays in Swedish History* (London, 1967), pp.56–81 and 195–225; M.S. Anderson, *War and Society in Europe of the Old Regime, 1618–1789* (London, 1988), pp.33–76; J.F.C. Fuller, 'The Thirty Years War: The Military Operations', in J.A. Hammerton (ed.), *Universal History of the World*, 8 vols (London, 1927–9), 6, pp.3645–6; A.F. Steuart, 'Scottish Officers in Sweden', *The Scottish Historical Review*, 1 (1904), pp.191–6.

10   Wellcome Library for the History of Medicine, Royal Army Medical Corps Muniments Collection, RAMC 562, box 123.

11   In his 'Code Michau' of 1629, Richelieu had stipulated that every regiment and fortress was to be equipped with an infirmary and a surgeon and evidence

survives to demonstrate that this was put into effect: C. Jones, 'The Welfare of the French Foot Soldier', *History*, 65 (1980), pp.193–213; J.A. Lynn, *Giant of the Grand Siècle* (Cambridge, 1997), pp.421–2.

12   G. Bernard (ed.), 'Life of Sir John Digby', in *Camden Miscellany*, 18, Royal Historical Society (London, 1910), pp.67–119; C. Hill and E. Del, *The Good Old Cause* (London, 1969), p.243.

13   E. Husband, *An Exact Collection of all Remonstrances, Declarations, Votes, Proclamations, Messages, Answers and other Remarkable Passages between the Kings' Most Excellent Majesty, and his High Court of Parliament, December 1641 to March 1643* (1645), pp.672–3.

14   TNA, SP 28/141B, fols 1–4; *Cal. S.P. Dom, 1660*, p.107; *Journal of the House of Commons, 1643–1644* (hereafter *JHC*), iii, 3, p.685; W. Steven, *History of Heriot's Hospital* (Edinburgh, 1859), pp.49–50 and 66–70.

15   TNA, SP 28/141B, fols 1 and 5.

16   E. Prescott, *The English Medieval Hospital, 1050–1640* (London, 1992), p.141; *JHC*, ii, pp.832–5.

17   *Ibid.*, 874.

18   TNA, SP Dom 28, Piece 104A; R. Somerville, *The Savoy: Manor, Hospital, Chapel* (London, 1960), pp.71–6; J. Henderson and K. Park '"The First Hospital Among Christians": The Ospedale di Santa Maria Nuova in Early Sixteenth-Century Florence', *Medical History*, 35 (1991), pp.164–88.

19   *JHC*, iii, 691.

20   Archive and Local History Centre, Hammersmith, Ref PAF/1/22, St Paul's, Hammersmith Parish Register, p.41v.

21   A. Sproule, *Lost Houses of Britain* (Newton Abbot, 1982), p.63; L. Hasker, *The Place which is called Fulanham*, Fulham & Hammersmith Historical Society (London, 1981), p.32. Unfortunately, both Sproule and Hasker fail to quote their sources.

22   TNA, SP 28/141B, fol. 4.

23   The process of making an alkaline liquid for washing clothes was commonplace before the introduction of caustic soda. Lye was made by allowing water to pass through wood ash and would loosen grease and dirt in the laundered clothing. It could be used by itself in the 'buck-wash' or added to fat to make soap: J. Seymour, *Forgotten Household Crafts* (London, 1987), p.88.

24   *JHC*, ii, 912 and v, 530.

25   British Library (hereafter BL) Map, *Faithorn and Newcourt's Map of London, 1658*; H.G. Nussey, *London Gardens of the Past* (London, 1939), pp.31–3; *JHC*, ii, 912; TNA, SP 28/141A, Part 4, fol. 141 *et seq.*

26   TNA, SP 28/140A, n.f., and 140B, fols 1–5; SP 28/141A, n.f.; J.J. Keevil, *Medicine and The Navy, 1200–1900*, 4 vols (Edinburgh and London, 1957–63), 2, pp. 24–5.

27   TNA, SP 28/141B, fol. 5.

28   SP 24/141B. The weekly payments of 1*s*. recorded to 'Roger' at Parson's Green, as mentioned in the text, typify such arrangements.

29   J. Thurloe, *Collection of State Papers*, 7 vols (London, 1742), 4, p.525.

30   P.E. Dewey, 'Food Production and Policy in the United Kingdom, 1914–18', *Transactions of the Royal Historical Society*, 5th series, 30 (1980), pp.71–89.

31   TNA, SP 24, n. f; SP 28/141B, fols 1–5.

32   SP 28/141B, Part 4, fol. 103.

33   London Metropolitan Archives (hereafter LMA), H1/ST/A6/2, St Thomas's Hospital, Grand Committee Minute Book, p.98.

34   J. Cam, *A Practical Treatise or Second Thoughts on the Consequences of the Venereal Disease with a Vindication of the Practice of Salivating* (1729); D. Turner, *A Practical Dissertation on the Venereal Disease* (1717).

35   LMA, Grand Committee Minute Book, p.61.

36   J. French, *The Yorkshire Spaw* (1652); TNA, SP 28/141A, fols 2 and 5 after 410; 28/141B, Part 3; TNA, AO 503/119; *Cal. S.P. Dom. 1652–3*, fols 320, 332, 341, 355.

37   Bath Record Office, unreferenced document, *The Survey of Bath 1641*, passim; J. Wroughton, *A Community at War* (Bath, 1992), p.36.

38   C. Rawcliffe, *Medicine and Society in Later Medieval England* (Stroud, 1995), pp.194–215; C. Rawcliffe, 'Hospital Nurses and their Work', in R. Britnell (ed.), *Daily Life in the Late Middle Ages* (Stroud, 1998), pp.43–64.

39   BL, MS Cotton Cleopatra C V, Statutes of the Savoy Hospital, 1524, fols 30–4.

40   D. Orem, *Nursing: Concepts of Practice* (New York, 1985); C. Roy, *Introduction to Nursing: An Adaptation Model* (Englewood Cliffs, 1984); M. Walsh, *Models in Clinical Nursing* (London, 1991); N. Roper, W.W. Tierney, and A.J. Logan, *The Elements of Nursing*, 2nd edn (Edinburgh, 1985).

41   Roper, Tierney, and Logan, *Elements of Nursing*, pp.5 *et seq.*; Walsh, *Models*, pp.53–89.

42   T. Brugis, *Vade Mecum, or a Companion for a Chyrurgion*, (1651), p.176.

43   *Ibid.*

44   L. Stone, *The Family, Sex and Marriage in England, 1500–1800* (London, 1977), pp.55–65.

FLURIN CONDRAU

Chapter 14: The Institutional Career of Tuberculosis: Social Policy, Medical Institutions and Patients before World War II

Introduction

The campaign against tuberculosis began in Britain and Germany during the late nineteenth century with the setting up of sustained efforts to treat patients in sanatoriums. By help of large schemes of social security and also influenced by ideas of national competition, both Britain and Germany started to provide sanatorium treatment for the working classes on a very large scale.[1] The provision for pulmonary tuberculosis was indeed larger than for any other disease, and only fairly recently have specialist cancer hospitals come close to matching the number of beds available to tuberculosis patients in the interwar period. Institutional treatment for tuberculosis patients was of course not limited to Britain and Germany, indeed virtually every country with a remotely developed Western medical system, provided for tuberculosis institutions of one form or another.[2] What makes Britain and Germany particularly important is the fact that sanatoriums were part of wider frameworks of tuberculosis control, which in one way or another embraced communities, medical elites as well as governments and official politics. In both countries, treatment was intended for the early cases of tuberculosis. Those patients, it was hoped, had a reasonably good chance for recovery from the deadly disease even though the efficacy of an unspecific treatment was questionable.[3] In fact, contrary to popular belief, the sanatorium was always challenged as inefficient by those not directly benefiting from its existence. Alfred Grotjahn, health spokesman for the Social Democratic Party (SPD) in the German parliament after 1918, denounced the sanatorium as an inefficient and ill-informed way to counter tuberculosis.[4]

Criticism notwithstanding, the sanatorium for tuberculosis involved impressive capital expenditure for all the buildings; in both Germany and Britain the number of sanatoriums built reached over 100 and despite a possibly dubious medical record, they represented the only location for medical treatment for the most important cause of death of adults until the interwar period. The German sanatoriums tended to concentrate on open-air treatment in rest halls whilst supplying a rich diet.[5] Provided the architecture was in place and the finance available, this scheme was relatively easy to follow for the various institutions. What critics called the 'Kadaverruhe' (carcasses' rest) was thus a relatively standardised and proven way of treatment until the introduction of modernised forms of treatment such as chest surgery.[6] The popularity of this institution stemmed from the agenda of social integration that has been very much part of the modern German welfare state since the 1880s. The sanatoriums, it was argued, had to cater for the working classes as iconic examples of the benefits of modern social policy. With the social policy aiming to create one nation in a context of a highly fragmentised imperial society, it was clear that the sanatorium had to play its role in the quest for social integration. The British institutions, however, followed the example of the Brompton Hospital Sanatorium at Frimley where Marcus Paterson started to treat patients with graduated labour therapy.[7] What he called auto-inoculation of tuberculosis was based on making labour an integral part of working-class treatment in the sanatorium. Even if not all the British sanatoriums followed this strict treatment regime to the full, they all provided a class-based treatment that was part of a systematic effort to single out the disease and its victims.[8] Indeed, tuberculosis was given special consideration in the National Insurance Act when the sanatorium benefit not only specified the disease for special support, but also virtually prescribed the only legitimate way to treat its sufferers. Given the opposition against the sanatorium, which in Britain came rather more from practitioners than from academic circles, this can only be seen as a remarkable feature of early British health policy.

Historiography has almost universally treated the sanatorium as a specialist development within hospital history. It has emphasised the sanatorium as one specific type of medical institution, a logical consequence of a specific form of medical treatment. More orthodox medical historians have drawn the attention to the architecture of the sanatorium and the elements of treatment provided.[9] This line of enquiry is based on the elementary assumption that there is indeed a link between design and purpose of medical institutions. Several studies of sanatorium design in international contexts confirm the *modern* roots of sanatorium design, which indicates that sanatorium design and medical theories are not one and the same thing.[10] This leads to an interesting hypothesis that suggests distinct motivations for design of medical institutions and medical change.[11]

However, the study of sanatorium architecture has remained a somewhat peripheral undertaking in modern history of medicine. Social history of medicine has, from the mid-1980s, started to map campaigns against tuberculosis.[12] Scholars have quickly negated any success of institutional treatment and instead focused on the 'true' intentions behind this puzzling institution. Looking at the sanatorium *from the outside* provided historians with a paradigmatic case of an institution that could never quite fulfil the high expectations of the time. But the prevailing perspective has been to study the sanatorium as an isolated institution both geographically and institutionally. Downplaying differences between those institutions within a national context and in an international perspective has led the term sanatorium to be universally used; the long shadow of Thomas Mann's *Magic Mountain* has kept historians from understanding it as part of an institutional framework that involves many other types of medical institutions. The genre of the sanatorium novel has created such a powerful image that historians find it difficult to establish a new interpretation.[13] Also, albeit noting that some patients may have returned for a second round of treatment, most scholars have tended to see sanatorium treatment as a one-off, often describing it as an ineffective way to cope with a chronic disease such as tuberculosis.[14]

This chapter offers a partial reinterpretation of the sanatorium by studying its *institutional career*. The fundamental hypothesis is that the sanatorium was very much part of a whole framework, where visits to more than one institution were the rule rather than the exception. It seems appropriate to study patients suffering from a chronic disease on an equally 'chronic' quest through medical institutions. This implies a longitudinal perspective on treatment that considers the long-term fate of tuberculosis patients *and* the historical change occurring within a considerable number of institutions involved in treating and caring for those patients. For not only are patients to be studied using a longer timeframe, the same logic applies to the institutions as these have seen quite considerable change themselves. Typically, studies of medical institutions look for extension, growth and specialisation, whilst non-medical change, standardisation, decline and crisis have rarely been studied. It is stating the obvious to consider that medical institutions change over time. But in what sense do they get older? Buildings simply age through everyday wear and tear, but treatment ideas become more widely known, develop a certain routine and patients may well be asking for something 'new'. Such a dialectic understanding of the institutional career of tuberculosis can help to tackle both the patients' and the institutions' change over time. This chapter will start out looking at various types of institutions available for treatment and the structural relationship between them. The analysis will then shift its focus to the patients and follow their careers in and with institutions.

The Career of Institutions

A growing interest in anti-tuberculosis campaigns starting at the end of the nineteenth century highlighted the range of institutions for the treatment and care of tuberculosis in Britain and Germany. Tuberculosis medicine has always been a fairly competitive field, which is not surprising given the fact that there was no causally successful treatment available until after World War II.[15] While limited therapeutic success led to conflicting ideas on how to explain the results, there was also an element of national prestige involved German and

British institutional schemes and treatment regimes.[16] In Britain, medical institutions were forced to cope with tuberculosis long before the arrival of the modern sanatorium. There were British sanatorium pioneers such as George Bodington, but in reality tuberculosis was a problem that was being dealt with in the realms of the poor law long before specialist institutions started to be promoted.[17] Looking at the German system of poor relief can help to understand better the specifics of the British case. The debates in Germany centred around the 'Elberfelder System', a modernised and economical system of non-institutional poor relief that was first introduced in the city of Elberfeld in 1853.[18] The purpose of this system was to cut back on poor relief expenditure through individually approved, strictly need-based benefits aimed at reintegrating the poor into the labour market.[19] While the system started out as an all-inclusive form of poor relief, the latter half of the nineteenth century and in particular the early twentieth century saw an increased specialisation and differentiation of benefits and providers.[20] However, the impact of disease on poverty, and the complex relation between poor relief being aimed at the labour-market and the consequences of long-term diseases such as tuberculosis is still in need of further research.[21]

The British story is different. Starting with the Commissioners Workhouse Rules Order in 1842, the introduction of more or less separated sick wards in workhouses brought the problem of institutional treatment of chronic diseases into the spotlight.[22] The scientific paradigm shift towards a new contagionism, ultimately leading to a bacteriological interpretation of the infectious nature of tuberculosis, contributed to the two-fold problem of how to achieve isolation and treatment at the same time. But with compulsory isolation being virtually impossible to achieve, the prevention of infection was being sought by a combination of isolation and treatment for advanced cases. Hence, the first steps in providing organised treatment for tuberculosis outside of private sanatoriums were not only taken in a poor law environment, they also were also closely linked to the prevention of infection by isolation.[23] While some specialist sanatoriums were founded under the auspices of the Metropolitan Asylums Board (MAB), the bulk of the burden in relation to tuberculosis was being carried by poor law infirmaries. The quality of treatment provided in these houses is extremely difficult to assess and has not, so far, been the subject of much historical attention.[24] There certainly was an extreme regional disparity, with London infrastructure generally being superior to the provinces. Yet even within London the standards differed enormously between richer areas such as Westminster and poorer locations such as Whitechapel.[25] It will be a fair over-all assessment to assume that most workhouse infirmaries initially did not offer much beyond basic care and were often stricken by high institutional mortality. Indeed, tuberculosis must have been the most important non-age-related cause of death as it accounted for at least 20 per cent if not more of all deaths occurring in these institutions. Around the turn of the century poor law infirmaries were essentially the only institutions available for terminally ill cases of tuberculosis throughout Britain as the few existing voluntary sanatoriums clearly stayed away from hopeless cases. An observer noted in the *British Medical Journal* of 1898:

> In the twenty-five large infirmaries now existing within the area [of London] a very considerable and distressing aggregation of such cases [TB] is to be found. [They] find their way to the infirmaries as a last resource, and the high mortality swells the death roll of the infirmaries. Indeed, it would not be overstepping the mark to say that tuberculosis in one form or another supplies almost a fourth of the mortality in these institutions.[26]

The problem of tuberculosis in poor law institutions soon received specific medical and political attention involving the MAB and other charitable bodies. A study commissioned by the British Medical Journal in 1902 confirmed that among all the institutions for the treatment of tuberculosis, only the Poor Law Infirmaries accepted patients in all stages of the disease including the terminally ill.[27] The drive to develop an effective sanatorium movement had a strong base within the Poor Law, aiming at both complementing the available institutions and improving them for the provision of sanatorium treatment.[28]

> The success which is said to have attended the open-air treatment of tuberculosis could not fail to arrest the attention of the metropolitan boards of guardians, in whose infirmaries a large number of phthisical patients are constantly in residence. On the suggestion of the Local Government Board, a conference of the metropolitan boards of guardians was convened in July to

consider the advisability of special accommodation and treatment being provided, under the management and control of a metropolitan authority, for the treatment by open-air methods of phthisical patients chargeable to the Metropolis.[29]

However, administrative problems, such as funding issues between the Local Government Board and the various Poor Law Unions, resulted in surprisingly little development in the sanatorium movement until the National Insurance Act of 1911, and only a handful of prestigious voluntary institutions were built before that. But the 1911 act did benefit the sanatorium; the interdepartmental committee led by Lord Astor decided to support local authorities in building sanatoriums, which in turn led to an increase in the number of beds available.[30] This happened within the context of the growing importance of hospitals and the problems modern hospitals had with infectious diseases. Throughout the nineteenth century, large and prestigious teaching hospitals saw an increase in importance as they developed in to centres of medical innovation (and intervention).[31] However, with tuberculosis largely being considered not only an infectious, but also an incurable and untreatable disease, hospitals were not keen on taking patients with tuberculosis.

For Germany, it has been shown that while hospitals regularly accepted tuberculosis patients for residential treatment, the relative number of such patients was only about 3.5 per cent of all adult patients during the early 1890s, which is low considering the fact that tuberculosis was the single most important cause of death for adults. But there can be no doubt that German general hospitals went out of their way to keep as many cases of tuberculosis as possible away from the hospital. In fact, part of the move to the modern hospital has implied a concentration on curable diseases, which tuberculosis certainly was not at this time.[32] One way to remedy the situation was to open specialist institutions; not surprisingly, therefore, the German sanatorium was statistically counted as a *general* hospital, which of course it was not.[33]

British voluntary specialist hospitals such as the Royal Brompton Hospital for the Diseases of the Chest in London, were founded during the first half of the nineteenth century to offer treatment for diseases that were unpopular or even overlooked in general hospitals.[34] Similarly to the German case, tuberculosis was a problem for these new hospitals, which they mostly relegated to their outpatient departments. Hence, while specialist hospitals were indeed most important in providing out-patient treatment, their provision of stationary treatment has probably been overestimated.[35] Apart from screening and diagnosis, there was little to be done for tuberculous patients, who ultimately had to be discharged to the very same living-conditions and to the same jobs that were partly responsible for their disease in the first place.[36] While often claiming to be the prime location for residential treatment of tuberculosis, hospital statistics on the duration of stay suggest that specialist hospitals never really lived up to their reputation and were quite reluctant to actually treat tuberculosis beyond the acute stages of the disease.[37] Economic considerations played a role for these institutions too as there was an apparent trade-off between the treatment of chronically ill patients suffering from incurable tuberculosis and the implied effects on hospital success statistics, which ultimately affected the hospital's donors.[38] One historian has even argued that the hospital economy was responsible for the Brompton Hospital *not* using its full capacity to accommodate tuberculosis patients, but rather leaving beds unoccupied.[39] On the one hand, specialist hospitals *did* provide a form of specialist institutional treatment that was not available before; as such they became centres of the modern research-led and later also surgery-based treatment of tuberculosis, whilst being used for clinical trials of medication such as tuberculin.[40] On the other hand, they were effective only for a very limited number of patients. Before the arrival of specialist treatment in the form of chest surgery, they most importantly served as feeder-hospitals for attached sanatoriums. Later-on, this hierarchy was reversed as the hospitals became the treatment centres, while relegating the sanatoriums to the role of rehabilitation clinics where patients could recover from more invasive treatments provided in hospitals.[41]

It is worth noting, though, that the sanatorium was neither the first nor the only medical institution to provide treatment for tuberculosis. Its historical importance came from the fact that sanatorium doctors were the first medical specialists to claim ability to heal the sick rather than just to care for them.[42] Hermann Brehmer, one of the early pioneers of the German sanatorium movement, said: 'Tuberculosis is in its early stages always curable'.[43] The sanatorium has received considerable scholarly interest, but transnational studies on treatment regimes, social political decisions on funding and implications of the wider issues of health policy are relatively scarce.[44] The British way of doing sanatoriums for working-class patients was geared around labour therapy. Marcus Paterson's 'Auto-Inoculation' of Tuberculosis was an ingenious attempt to sell an unspecific treatment to a bacteriologically informed audience.[45] But as a voluntary sanatorium, it owed as much to its funding structures as it did to the medical treatment.

> First, it would do much to meet the objection that members of the working classes are liable to have their energy sapped, and to acquire lazy habits by such treatment; secondly, it would make them more resistant to the disease, by improving their physical condition; and thirdly, would enable them by its effect upon their muscles to return to their work immediately after their discharge.[46]

In this most revealing passage, Paterson actually made these issues very clear because his points mainly address the charitable donors and the employers. Labour therapy, it seems, was first and foremost the logical extension of the workhouse in as much as it may have provided treatment without ever doubting the merits of solid, hard work for working-class patients. This led the British working-class sanatoriums to being relatively low-prestige institutions, even though Paterson won a prize at the 1908 international tuberculosis in Washington. But patients had to expect a fairly rough sojourn, an impression that probably got even worse after World War I, when Paterson's quasi-bacteriological approach became redundant.

The German sanatorium followed a different agenda, which was more openly linked to the aims of German social policy. Bismarck, the big political figurehead behind Germany's first instalment of social insurance during the 1880s, left no doubt about his intention to create a system of social integration by providing insurance to the working classes. Through individualisation of rights, contributions and benefits, but also by making the socially coded medical treatment accessible to most, the German system was largely successful in its efforts both to contribute to social integration and to the medicalisation of the German society.[47] One sanatorium doctor commented: 'After many years of experience as a sanatorium doctor, I cannot but say that the sanatorium treatment is more important for the balance of the society than old age pensions'.[48]

This was the strongest of all arguments in favour of the social value of the treatment as old age pensions were the core ingredient of producing social balance in society. Professor Ernst von Leyden, a well-known clinician in Berlin and a strong voice in the sanatorium movement, conceded that: 'We never claimed to offer miracles in our sanatoriums. Instead, we have always stressed the need to give the same help to the poorest which the rich and the well-off can easily afford'.[49]

The welfare system, however, aimed at producing more than mere loyalty to the state. Ever since its foundation, the German Central Committee against Tuberculosis (DZK) put special emphasis on the educational component of sanatorium treatment. The working classes should be taught how to establish a middle-class life-style, whilst also preventing the spread of infection. This educational programme gradually replaced the therapeutic agenda of the sanatorium. Even the local tuberculosis dispensaries, structurally opposed to the sanatorium, recognised that a prolonged stay in the sanatorium had an effect similar to a medical boarding school. Food and daily hygiene were the core ingredients of this education. Some German sanatorium doctors went as far as to call their patients 'hygienic apostles' who upon discharge were supposed to act as messengers of the 'sanatorium gospel' in their families and peer groups.[50] The treatment itself was no longer intended to be a cure for the sick, but, rather, should teach them a healthy lifestyle in order to prolong what was left of their life. The patients should become accustomed to a specific way of life and particularly to a specific diet, but this alleged medical treatment was clearly based on social values. Professor von Leyden stated: 'I never said that every worker should be given champagne, partridge or oysters, he will be happy enough with a roast, potatoes and a good beer'.[51]

Naturally, sanatorium treatment did not help much to resolve the social tensions in German society. For one thing, their 'success statistics' showed that sanatorium treatment had only limited therapeutic value. Even though the sanatorium was usually the only institution in Germany providing medical treatment for tuberculosis, whilst offering the opportunity for research to its doctors, it came under heavy criticism for not up-holding its claims. Alfred Grotjahn, an outspoken opponent of sanatorium treatment, commented on the statistical results of success control: 'How anyone could ever enjoy these figures is beyond me.'[52] And in fact, the shift towards an educational rather than a medical agenda reflects an acknowledgement that the sanatorium idea was a failure in terms of helping to cure people suffering from tuberculosis. While commentators regularly observed that the sanatorium was a viable business idea, there were serious doubts as to whether they represented a legitimate way of using the scarce resources of insurance contributions coming from the workers themselves. Brehmer himself was even discredited as a 'business minded hotelier'.[53] But to make matters worse, the German sanatorium system was particularly inept to survive times of crisis. In this respect, it differed substantially from the British institutions which were quite resistant to external shocks. The First World War, and in particular the period of hyperinflation brought most German sanatoriums close to bankruptcy and fundamentally wrecked the idea that social integration in medical institutions was such a good idea. This crisis in confidence led most sanatoriums to look elsewhere for survival, and they found what they needed in the arrival of new medical therapies such as chest surgery which led medical science to have a stronger influence in the German sanatorium.[54]

The institutional career of the sanatorium itself can thus be described in three stages. First, it was of peripheral public health importance and served mainly as an institution for the upper classes. Private sanatoriums and their chief medical officers were often part of the medical periphery in terms of academic standing. The second stage of the sanatorium movement was the euphoric stage of large-scale sanatorium movements, which were made possible by large state funded social security schemes. The sanatorium idea was convincing at that time not because it was particularly successful, but because it provided a treatment where other treatments had failed. In fact, understanding the career of institutions for the treatment of tuberculosis requires a general understanding of the terms 'treatment' and 'medical success' during the late nineteenth and early twentieth century. Medical success, however, is a tricky field for the historian as the term 'success' or rather the frequently used words 'healed' or 'cured' have meant different things at different times.[55] The sanatorium was successful in the sense that it established a new line of thought about medical success by way of mass empirical studies.[56] The third stage of the sanatorium career is the gradual change into a specialist institution. This coincided with a gradual decline of the sanatorium and its popularity. It became more important for doctors to show that most patients would survive chest surgery rather than to study the long-term survival rates. The decline of the sanatorium was therefore probably not so much due to the existence of new antibiotic treatment after the Second World War, even though this clearly accelerated the crisis of institutional treatment. But the career of the sanatorium had already entered a terminal decline when doctors, patients and the health authorities began to shift away from thinking in average ratios of survival towards more individualised forms of treatment and expected to see immediate results for more active and invasive new treatments.

The Career of Patients

The second part of this chapter deals with the perspective of the patients suffering from tuberculosis as they went through a series of medical institutions.[57] The luckier of the patients kept (or regained) their health and did not require any more treatment after a singular round of sanatorium treatment. The ultimate outcome probably depended as much on the sanatorium as it did on finding suitable work after discharge and other adjustments in daily life of the patients. Also this touches on the difficult question of historical diagnosis and, to a larger extent, on the question of the admissions policy.[58] Often German public sanatoriums, such as the 600-bed sanatorium Beelitz near Berlin, used their capacity for tuberculosis patients for those in danger of contracting disease. In this context, the Imperial Health

Office spoke of preventive treatment of tuberculosis.[59] Clearly, this term could be taken to describe the initial function of the sanatorium, as it was hoped that treatment would delay disability and subsequent insurance claims.[60] However, it could also mean to accept people who had not yet developed clear signs of the disease, ignoring whether they were even suffering from it in the first place. Indeed it was a regular practice in German sanatoriums to have patients with unconfirmed symptoms or in danger of developing the symptoms.[61] This was made possible by the interests of sanatorium doctors, who were keen on diagnosing 'potential for tuberculosis', but it was also supported by the idea that the earliest cases offered the best chances for treatment. Logic dictates that the earliest possible case is one where the disease has not yet really been ascertained, but where circumstances suggest that it might not be long before such onset begins.[62] According to the official publications, a ratio of around 50 per cent of all sanatorium patients survived for a minimum of five years after discharge. But this could imply including those who did not suffer from tuberculosis in the first place.[63] Amongst the most famous cases of such patients being treated in a sanatorium for preventative rather than curative reasons was Katja Mann, Thomas Mann's wife whom he visited in Davos to gain the inspiration to write the *Magic Mountain*. Attempts in practical historical diagnoses suggest that she might never have suffered from tuberculosis in the first place regardless of her prolonged stay in the sanatorium.[64]

The notion of an institutional career of tuberculosis patients leads us in another direction, to address the question of repeated treatment in a range of institutions over time. This is ultimately connected to the aetiology of tuberculosis as a chronic disease. Infection normally took place during childhood and it was by no means certain that a much more dangerous outbreak would strike in the early adult years. In fact, studies performed at the beginning of the twentieth century showed that virtually the whole population at risk was infected sooner or later during their lifetime, with only a proportion subsequently developing the disease.[65] Those who became ill in their adult years, however, were looking at a prolonged period of suffering potentially lasting for years if not decades. Typical for tuberculosis, this was characterised by a largely unpredictable cycle of ups and downs of the individual's health status. In fact, it has been suggested that tuberculosis changed its character in the Western world from a deadly killer to a long-term chronic disease, a transition that reached its peak shortly after the introduction of effective antibiotic treatment during the 1950s.[66] The start of this transition into a chronic disease might well have to be backdated to the beginning of the century; sources record prolonged suffering more often than quick death.

A typical example of an early institutional career is Moritz Bromme, a young German worker who wrote most impressive auto-biographic material at the beginning of the twentieth century.[67] Married and a father of four (later five) children, he was found to be suffering from tuberculosis in his early twenties, and was sent to a sanatorium for treatment after getting his application approved by the invalid insurance. His experience during treatment can be seen as paradigmatic for those German sanatoriums that were well funded by insurances before World War I. Reasonably recovered after a three-month sojourn, he was sent home and advised to stay away from factory work. Yet after several weeks of job hunting, he decided that he could not afford to stay out of work any longer and was thus forced to go back to his old factory job. Once back in the factory, his health started to deteriorate right away and after a few months he was sent back to the sanatorium. His diary reflects the change in his confidence in medical success. While at first he was clearly hoping for a perman-ent cure, he became much more realistic once he started the second and third round of treatment. After returning from the second round, his factory foreman quite simply asked: 'How long will it be this time before you end up again in the cougher's castle?' His repeated stays in the sanatorium changed Bromme's opinion of such institutions. Not only did he become critical of therapeutic success, he also started to feel torn between the hygienic advice in the sanatorium and the reality of his problems to bring up his family.

This case is representative of unspecific sanatorium treatment for early cases of tuberculosis. It is very likely that the treatment helped to improve the health of a malnourished, overworked and stressed out factory worker. Paired with changing living conditions and a different job, the treatment might have had a fairly lasting outcome. However, as in Bromme's case, a better job was usually not available and the need for looking after a family seriously hindered any longer lasting effects of the treatment. It is revealing that the sanatorium doctor routinely discharged Bromme as cured. Cured in the sense that he was ready to resume working. It was not in the doctor's interest to specify for how long the patient was likely to be able to work. This contrasted clearly with the survival rates which were measured by the funding bodies.

This institutional cycle was directly influenced by the prevailing economic principle of the German invalid insurance and its tuber-culosis treatment. The insurance covered the treatment as long as it could reasonably expect that the patient could go back to work long enough to recover the cost through insurance contributions.[68] Calcula-tions of the Imperial Health Office showed that twelve to fourteen months of working was enough to support a three months' stay in a sanatorium.[69] But what happened to those whose health did not allow a full working year after discharge from a sanatorium? The tubercu-losis asylums movement was a complete failure in Germany, while sanatoriums were extremely careful to discharge hopeless patients in time as institutional deaths were perceived to be a serious threat to their prestige.[70] Hence no specialist type of institution was available for advanced cases. Either the invalid insurance office (LVA) was well-meaning. In this case it could try to find a place in a cheaper sanatorium as there was quite a considerable price spread between in-stitutions. Or, it was not so well-meaning or could not provide a place in any therapeutic institution at all. Most of the advanced tuberculosis cases stayed at home and received occasional help from the tubercu-losis dispensary. Care for terminal cases was therefore often provided by families, only occasionally supported by stays in general hospitals. German general hospitals saw a growing number of terminally ill cases after the turn of the century as they gradually changed into institutions where people also came to die.[71]

More evidence to support the idea of an institutional career on the part of the patients comes from British poor law infirmaries, and more precisely, from two reports that were being commissioned by the London County Council in 1922 and 1923.[72] This chapter has argued above that while sanatoriums were being built in Britain at a fairly frantic pace, the poor law infirmaries remained the backbone of much of the institutional care for tuberculosis patients. The LCC reports cover twenty-five London infirmaries offering on average around 615 beds, between 9 per cent and 10 per cent of which were usually devoted to tuberculosis patients. This report confirms the importance of infirmaries for the provision of tuberculosis care. Against an estimated total number of beds in non-poor law sanatoriums and specialist hospitals in England and Wales of 13,300, the London poor law infirmaries alone made 1,430 beds available for tuberculosis care.[73] However, it must be noted that the overall contribution of poor law infirmaries was in relative decline; this mainly stemmed from the drive of local authorities to build up tuberculosis accommodation. The big advantage of the poor law infirmaries in relation to sanatoriums from the point of view of the patient was the very short time required to become a patient. Typically, the district's medical officer could send the patients more or less directly to an infirmary. The tuberculosis officers of the various tuberculosis dispensaries, since 1911 responsible for applications for sanatorium treatment on behalf of their patients, were short-circuited in the case of the infirmaries. This may explain why beds in poor law infirmaries were often used for emergency admissions of non-poor patients as well.[74] These were often patients in advanced stages of tuberculosis, where successful treatment was highly unlikely. It is not surprising that the infirmaries did not, as a general rule, offer any systematic treatment. They lacked financial resources, personnel and the necessary accommodation; even allowing for regional disparities, most poor law infirmaries were providing care for the terminally ill rather than any attempt at therapeutic treatment.

> It is only fair to remark that the Poor Law Institution is as a rule the 'last ditch' of the T.B. sufferer, and it is open to question if modern lines of Sanatorium treatment would in fact be of much benefit to him. He comes in as a rule to die and not to be cured.[75]

These tuberculosis wards in poor law infirmaries suffered from an incredible institutional mortality, often loosing 30–50 per cent of their patients over the course of a year.[76] As such, poor law infirmaries remained one of the more important places where patients went shortly before death.[77] However, similar to their overall contribution to tuberculosis care, the number of tuberculosis cases dying there started to decline after 1911 from 22 per cent of all male tuberculosis deaths in 1912 to 14 per cent in 1920, while hospitals saw a rise in male tuberculosis deaths from 8 per cent in 1912 to 19 per cent in 1920.[78] However, the simplified admission procedures made sure that in addition to the advanced cases, many other patients arrived with the hope of being transferred to a proper sanatorium later on. While the infirmary could be accessed after a day's worth of waiting, the number of days to wait before getting into a sanatorium stood at about thirty.[79] Using a poor law infirmary as a gateway to a treatment facility was therefore a real option.

Comments on the health status of individual patients and other details mentioned by the reporting doctors of the LCC may help to exemplify these two fundamentally different functions of poor law infirmaries. One group of patients consisted of terminally ill cases, whose deaths were more or less imminent. The report mentions a twenty-seven-year-old, single woman from London. She was transferred to the Islington Infirmary by the local tuberculosis officer. After receiving residential treatment in the Great Northern Hospital, the officer decided that sanatorium treatment was no longer going to be helpful, instead she was sent to the infirmary.[80] Another case, a thirty-eight-year-old man from London, was initially diagnosed as pneumonia. He had spent some time in the West London Hospital, and was then looked after by the local tuberculosis dispensary. There, the tuberculosis officer decided to transfer him into the Kensington Infirmary acknowledging that his disease was already too advanced for sanatorium treatment to have any beneficial effect.[81] And finally there was a sixty-one-year-old male patient in the Woolwich Infirmary who suffered from advanced tuberculosis; for him a treatment cycle in a sanatorium was deemed to be completely out of the question.[82]

The second group of patients consisted of relatively early cases where either applications for admission into a sanatorium had already been made, or were at least seriously considered. A seventeen-year-old man was temporarily admitted into St. George's Infirmary, where he expected an imminent decision on a promising application to go to Grosvenor Sanatorium.[83] A different type of patient was a twenty-three-year-old woman staying temporarily at Islington Infirmary. The medical superintendent of this infirmary had recommended an application for sanatorium treatment; however, the patient declined because she preferred to stay with relatives at the coast. All she wanted from her stay in the infirmary was to recover her ability to travel to her relatives.[84] This case is interesting because it points to informed decision-making on the part of the patient as well as to the fact that poor law institutions had become part of an institutional setup and had lost much of their stigmatising effect. Finally, there was a forty-five-year-old man hoping to be getting out of Islington Infirmary soon. He was extremely keen on getting back into a sanatorium having been a patient at Godalming Sanatorium before. He had left that sanatorium because family problems required his presence at home.[85]

These individual case stories confirm that poor law infirmaries fulfilled two distinct functions by serving as care centres for terminal cases as well as operating as waiting areas for patients suitable or hoping for a sanatorium bed. This dual functionality was mainly based on the flexible structures of these usually large institutions. Their favourable attributes included low waiting times, the simple admission procedures and the opportunity to get help with an application for sanatorium treatment. At the same time they offered care for hopeless cases, again helped by the surprising flexibility of a poor law institution, even though they mostly lacked the facilities to provide proper treatment. Thus quite often the institutional career of a tuberculosis case must have started and ended in poor law infirmaries.

Yet another perspective on a patient's institutional career is available through a biographical perspective that examines sanatorium treatment in an individual's disease history.[86] Clearly, this whole issue is very difficult to address due to problems with available sources. But a unique collection including admission records and follow-up information concerning patients of the Brompton Hospital Sanatorium in Frimley allows the study of patients after discharge from the sanatorium.[87] The question is thus: can admission and follow-up records reveal a more complete story about the place that the sanatorium treatment had in the biography of tuberculosis victims? At what point was the treatment in the disease history? what were its immediate results? And do these histories reveal anything about repeated contact with medical institutions? It is worthwhile noting that the purpose of collecting the follow-up information in the first place was to be able to ascertain the effects of sanatorium treatment.[88] These studies confirmed that about 50 per cent of the discharged patients died within five years. However, the Frimley material also allowed the researchers to look at several factors influencing the survival rates. With the interest on survival rather than on ability to work, the British sanatoriums usually offered longer treatment than the German sanatoriums. The Frimley studies showed that the length of treatment had indeed quite a direct influence on the survival figures, which was seen as reassurance to allow sojourns of four or more months, longer than in most working-class sanatoriums in Britain and on the continent.

But Frimley was an elite working-class institution in more ways than one, where patients were treated under fairly exceptional circumstances.[89] A qualitative analysis of the follow-up registers offers an interesting new perspective on patient survival. First and foremost, the follow-up register is a document of death and disappearance. While Linda Bryder, who discovered and secured the sources during a visit to Frimley, estimated that follow-up stories for 90 per cent of the patients are available, more recent calculations show that no more than 60 per cent of the discharged patients subsequently had an entry in the records. Those missing 40 per cent had either disappeared or died too soon after discharge to find their ways into the books. No less remarkable is the fact that several patients for which there are entries in the follow-up notes were discharged as being cured or as being much better only to die within a couple of days.[90] A considerable number of patients, however, lived on and had repeated contacts with other medical and social institutions. It seems that the follow-up studies confirm what Frimley doctors had always suspected, namely that the first two years of afterlife were crucial for the long-term prospect of survival.

Probably a bit of an extreme case, albeit very interesting in terms of an institutional career, is the story of Julia.[91] After the first of two treatment cycles at Frimley, Julia was initially helped by a charity to find work outside of the sanatorium; however, after World War I she came back and was accepted as a servant into the staff of the sanatorium. A few years later, she resurfaced in the Lady Almoner office of Frimley, the follow-up record keeper of the sanatorium, to ask for further treatment. Her second round of treatment was followed by a stay in the Pinewood Sanatorium of the Metropolitan Asylums Board in 1922. Shortly thereafter, she was accepted as a member of staff at Frimley again, but was soon let go after staying out a night without permission. Again several years later, another charitable society sent notice to Frimley that Julia had been admitted to a London hospital for several operations after she had had an illegal abortion. Continuous 'stalking by a man' led to a relocation to Liver-pool, organised by several charitable organisations, which was fol-lowed by a stay in West Ham infirmary back in London and an operation at St. Bartholomew's around 1930. Afterwards, Julia finally seems to have found relative happiness and stopped reporting to Frimley.

There are other examples of patients staying in an almost life-long contact with medical institutions, often in relation to chest surgery. Several life-histories of patients treated at Frimley record complications as a consequence of the treatment usually received at the Brompton Hospital. The sanatorium at Frimley was discreetly transformed from a therapeutic institution to a convalescent centre. Often, whether or not this functional change happened depended on a sanatorium's willingness to build up the infrastructure for chest sur-gery itself. Where there was a referring specialist hospital, as in the case of Frimley, this was of course a foregone conclusion. Elsie, a patient at Frimley in 1924, struggled against the disease for twelve years and through four or five major operations before finally loosing the battle.[92] Her story is filled with hope, despair, and regular contact with medical institutions for advice and repeat operations. The typical operation of the time, the artificial pneumothorax, was relatively easy and aimed at collapsing one of the lungs. The problem for the patients, apart from the direct physical pain, which must have been quite severe, was that A.P. made regular visits to doctors necessary to keep the lung collapsed. With surgery and its methods becoming refined over time, more complicated operations such as thoracoplastic surgery were performed. These aimed at permanently keeping one of the lungs or at least the affected part of it collapsed by using a range of metals to replace chest bones. The physical effects of these operations were tough and the survival rates not very impressive so they were usually presented as medicine's last resort for very advanced cases. However, this aspect of the history of tuberculosis still partly remains in the dark. What is known is that Britain was relatively reluctant to implement chest surgery.[93] In Germany however, already in the mid- 1920s, chest surgery was extremely popular as many sanatoriums had built up their infrastructure. Based on a survey from all German sanatoriums for adult patients it can be shown that the necessary infrastructure for chest surgery was available in 173 of 178 institutions by 1930.[94] Again somewhat of an exception in the UK, Frimley developed into a convalescent home for discharged surgery patients from Brompton Hospital as the emphasis on labour therapy had long started to fade.

The Frimley follow-up register confirms this change in tuberculosis treatment as patients wrote letter after letter in which they mentioned the consequences of invasive treatment. One such patient was Rose, a sixteen-year-old girl arriving at Brompton in 1925 with a fairly advanced tuberculosis. Her father had died in service during the war while her mother succumbed in London to tuberculosis. Having been in the hospital, Rose was transferred to Frimley after it was determined that there were no tubercle bacilli left in her sputum. She stayed for 130 days and was discharged as 'improved' in July. The Lady Almoner wanted to recruit Rose to work in the sanatorium, but since Rose was not very popular among her fellow patients and the staff, she preferred to work somewhere else. However, the discharging doctor confirmed that Rose was not fit for work. That said, she stayed with an aunt in Essex for a while and seemed to have recovered well enough for a doctor to confirm her to be fit for work. Early in 1926 she took up a position in a sanatorium, but was soon let go for being 'too free to the men'. This brought her back to a private position, with Lady Baines, where she was working very hard and stayed until her wedding in 1928. 'Glands of the neck' developed into a serious problem and had to be removed by help of an operation in the Brompton hospital. In 1929 she came back to the out-patient department and subsequently to the Lady Almoner. Her husband had recently been made redundant and the family was suffering from serious financial problems due to a recent house purchase. In 1930 she brought a newborn child to be examined in Frimley and the Lady Almoner described both as 'very miserable looking'. Rose had slimmed more than was good for her and was coughing heavily. Doctors urgently recommended another round of treatment at the sanatorium, but Rose rejected the idea saying that she could not abandon her jobless husband and her weak child. Even without the treatment she seemed to recover well enough from her deplorable condition. She wrote a 'cheerful letter' to the sanatorium, felt healthy and gave birth to her second child. In 1933, she was again admitted to the Brompton Hospital to receive tuberculosis treatment, where she stayed for four months. After this treatment, Rose stayed relatively healthy as her reports now came in more seldom. A tuberculosis officer recommended her in 1942 to undergo chest surgery. It is unclear where Rose received such treatment, however, and contacts with Brompton and Frimley broke down until the mid-1950s when Rose's daughter helped to reinstate the communication. A new marriage after her first husband had died did not bring much luck. The second husband had already died from cancer. Rose was now working as a cleaner in Exeter, where a doctor yet again advised her to undergo major chest surgery in 1957! Rose declined and stated that she preferred to be left in peace and certainly did not intend to be examined again or undergo any further treatment. Rose obviously had had enough and decided to ignore medical advice after more than thirty years of regular interaction with institutions, doctors and dispensary personnel.

Conclusion

The analysis of the institutional career of tuberculosis reveals several interesting issues which are of broader concern to the historiography of medical institutions. From the point of view of the patients, these institutions contributed to a wider medical experience as a life-long process. In order to understand modern medical culture, it is absolutely essential to study the repeated interaction of patients and doctors, inmates and institutions, social policy and hospital funding. This perspective offers a lot of potential for future research as the agency of patients has to be studied in relation to admission applications, decisions for early discharge and refusal of treatment. The expectation that patients developed tuberculosis, received one round of treatment, and later on died, is just not a realistic representation of the history and needs to be revised. Conservative sanatorium treatment in whatever form may have helped a patient to recover briefly, but was ultimately doomed as a therapeutic answer to the tuberculosis problem not least because it produced a conflict between its emphasis on life style and ultimately living-standards which contrasted so dramatically with the working-class patients' experience of life after the sanatorium. The introduction of chest surgery, however, changed the playing field from the point of view of the patients. Not only did it hurt to undergo chest surgery with no clear prospect of success in the longer term, it also brought about a much more invasive treatment. For patients, it was often not easy to discern between long-term disease symptoms, and problems that were caused by the intervention. Often the consequences of the treatment rather than the disease itself became the focus of repeated medical attention. In fact, recent studies show that late complications of thoracoplastic surgery may currently be contributing to the renewed dissemination of tuberculosis.[95]

Chest surgery led to a non-compliant patient in a new sense, one that refused surgery-based treatment out of consideration of quality of life after the intervention.

From the point of view of the history of the institutions themselves, the institutional career refers to two separate processes. These are related to the 'ageing' of institutions in the sense of loosing an aura of modernity as they started to loose a certain element of fashion over the course of time. Classic open-air treatment was a spectacular and new treatment regime during the late nineteenth century; it became standardised for the doctors, and no less part of the patients' routine during the early twentieth century. And finally it had its last stand subsequently with doctors trying to convince the public (and the patients) that rest treatment was actually the ideal moral and medical background to educate the patients in a hygienic life style. This aspect of the story is not so much about a clear-cut superiority of the new therapies over sanatorium treatment, but about a changing attitude to the same treatment over time by patients, doctors, and the general public. At the forefront of tuberculosis treatment after World War I, a sanatorium without the relevant equipment for chest surgery soon found itself rather left behind. This leads to the second element of an institutional career, the competition between institutions. Tuberculosis institutions competed with each other not only via the available treatment, but also through their location in the case of open-air sanatoriums, the social structure of their patients, survival ratios and other factors influencing the choice of patients and funding bodies. The way an institution was supplied with financial resources by the agency responsible for maintaining it also played a fundamental role. Between Germany and England, between social integration through hygienic education and labour-therapy in the tradition of poor law institutions, there was an incredible range of different regimes, intentions and ways to finance cure. At the end of the day the framework of an institutional career of tuberculosis serves to bring together seemingly distinct elements of the history of medical treatment. It allows us to study monetary issues of cost and control together with implications for patients and their dependants. And ultimately, it helps to bring back an element of agency to the study of patients' experience.

Notes

1   L. Bryder, *Below the Magic Mountain: A Social History of Tuberculosis in Twentieth-Century Britain* (Oxford 1988); F. Condrau, *Lungenheilanstalt und Patientenschicksal: Sozialgeschichte der Tuberkulose in Deutschland und England im späten 19. und frühen 20. Jahrhundert*, Kritische Studien zur Geschichtswissenschaft, 137 (Göttingen, 2000). All translations from German in this article are the author's.

2   In order to grapple with the *transnational* context of sanatorium treatment one has to go back to contemporary writers, i.e. F.R. Walters, *Sanatoria for Consumptives in Various Parts of the World (France, Germany, Norway, Russia, Switzerland, the United States, and the British Possessions): A Critical and*

Detailed Description together with an Exposition of the Open-Air or Hygienic Treatment of Phthisis (London, 1899, 1913).

3 The definition of an early case was a hotly debated problem at the time. See L. Teleky, 'Die Bekämpfung der Tuberkulose', in A. Gottstein et al. (eds), *Handbuch der sozialen Hygiene und Gesundheitsfürsorge* (Berlin, 1926), 3, pp.207–341.

4 A. Grotjahn, 'Die Krisis in der Lungenheilstättenbewegung', *Medizinische Reform*, 15 (1907), pp.219–23.

5 See a concise account by one of the pioneers of German sanatorium treatment, P. Dettweiler, 'Einige Bemerkungen zur sogenannten Ruhe- und Luftliegekur bei Schwindsüchtigen', *Zeitschrift für Tuberkulose und Heilstättenwesen*, 1 (1900), pp.96–100, 180–7.

6 The history of chest surgery for tuberculosis remains to be written. See one of the German pioneers for an early account, L. Brauer, 'Der therapeutische Pneumothorax', *Deutsche Medizinische Wochenschrift*, 17 (1906), pp.652–7; a more elaborate discussion can be found in F. Condrau, 'Behandlung ohne Heilung: zur sozialen Konstruktion des Behandlungserfolgs bei Tuberkulose im frühen 20. Jahrhundert', *Medizin, Gesellschaft und Geschichte*, 19 (2000), pp.71–93.

7 M. Paterson, 'Graduated Labour in Pulmonary Tuberculosis', *The Lancet*, 86.1 (1908), pp.216–20.

8 Labour was soon regarded as a appropriate way of spending time and getting physical exercise for working-class patients. See L.G. Cox, 'The Present Position of Institutional Treatment', *British Journal of Tuberculosis*, 19 (1925), pp.27–36.

9 A.H. Murken, 'Heilanstalten für Tuberkulöse: zur Geschichte der Lungensanatorien und ihrer Therapiekonzeption im 19. Jahrhundert', in W. Göpfert and H.-H. Otten (eds), *Metanoeite: Wandelt euch durch neues Denken. Festschrift für Professor Hans Schadewaldt zur Vollendung des 60. Lebensjahres* (Düsseldorf 1983), pp.107–24; A.H. Murken, 'Vom Heilpalast zum Sanatorium des Volkes', *Die Waage*, 21 (1982), pp.64–72.

10 Q. Miller, *Le Sanatorium: Architecture d'un isolement sublime* (Lausanne, 1992); M. Campbell, 'What Tuberculosis did for Modernism: The Influence of a Curative Environment on Modernist Design and Architecture', *Medical History*, 49 (2005), pp.463–88.

11 A. Adams and T. Schlich, 'Design for Control: Surgery, Science, and Space at the Royal Victoria Hospital, Montreal, 1893–1956', *Medical History*, 50 (2006), pp.303–24.

12 E.g. B.-I. Puranen, *Tuberkulos: en sjukdoms förekomst och dess orsaker, Sverige 1750–1980*, Umea Studies in Economic History, 7 (Umea, 1984); Bryder, *Magic Mountain*; M. Worboys, 'The Sanatorium Treatment for Consumption in Britain, 1890–1914', in J.V. Pickstone (ed.), *Medical Innovations in Historical Perspective* (New York, 1992), pp.47–71; G. Göckenjan, *Kurieren*

und Staat machen: Gesundheit und Medizin in der bürgerlichen Welt (Frankfurt a.M., 1985).

13 See the extremely helpful analysis of V. Pohland, *Das Sanatorium als literarischer Ort: Medizinische Institution und Krankheit als Medien der Gesellschaftskritik und Existenzanalyse* (Frankfurt a. M., 1984); for the French perspective see I. Grellet and C. Kruse, *Histoires de la tuberculose: les fièvres de l'âme, 1800–1940* (Paris, 1983); P. Guillaume, *Du désespoir au salut: les tuberculeux aux 19e et 20e siècles* (Paris, 1986).

14 Worboys, *Sanatorium.*

15 Condrau, *Lungenheilanstalt.*

16 See, as a very useful contribution on the ineffectiveness of treatment, T. Gorsboth and B. Wagner, 'Die Unmöglichkeit der Therapie am Beispiel der Tuberkulose', *Kursbuch*, 94 (1988), pp.123–46.

17 See for an overview of the poor law medical services R.G. Hodgkinson, *The Origins of the National Health Service. The Medical Services of the New Poor Law, 1834–71* (London, 1967); A. Powell, *The Metropolitan Asylums Board and its Work, 1867–1930* (London, 1930).

18 F. Tennstedt, *Sozialgeschichte der Sozialpolitik in Deutschland: vom 18. Jahrhundert bis zum Ersten Weltkrieg* (Göttingen, 1981), p.95.

19 J. Frerich and M. Frey, *Handbuch der Geschichte der Sozialpolitik in Deutschland*, vol. 1: *Von der vorindustriellen Zeit bis zum Ende des Dritten Reiches* (Munich, 1993); F. Tennstedt, *Vom Proleten zum Industriearbeiter: Arbeiterbewegung und Sozialpolitik in Deutschland 1800 bis 1914* (Cologne, 1983).

20 A. Labisch, *Homo Hygienicus: Gesundheit und Medizin in der Neuzeit* (Frankfurt a. M., 1992), pp.170–80.

21 See U. Frevert, *Krankheit als politisches Problem 1770–1880: soziale Unterschichten in Preussen zwischen medizinischer Polizei und staatlicher Sozialversicherung*, Kritische Studien zur Geschichtswissenschaft, 62 (Göttingen, 1984), pp.60–9; S.F. Eser, *Verwaltet und verwahrt: Armenpolitik und Arme in Augsburg, vom Ende der reichsstädtischen Zeit bis zum Ersten Weltkrieg*, Historische Forschungen der Historischen Kommission der Akademie der Wissenschaften und der Literatur, 20 (Sigmaringen, 1996), pp.115–24; R. Spree, 'Krankenhausentwicklung und Sozialpolitik in Deutschland während des 19. Jahrhunderts', *Historische Zeitschrift*, 260 (1995), pp.75–106.

22 F. Driver, *Power and Pauperism: The Workhouse System, 1834–84*, Cambridge Studies in Historical Geography, 19 (Cambridge, 1993), p.64.

23 A. Newsholme, 'The Causes of the Past Decline of Tuberculosis and the Light thrown by History on Preventive Measures for the Immediate Future', *Supplement to the Transactions of the 6th International Congress on Tuberculosis in Washington 1908* (Philadelphia, 1908), pp.80–109.

24 See A. Hardy, *The Epidemic Streets: Infectious Disease and the Rise of Preventive Medicine 1856–1900* (Oxford, 1993); J.V. Pickstone, *Medicine and Indus-*

trial Society: A History of Hospital Development in Manchester and its Region, 1752–1946* (Manchester, 1985).

25 *Report on the Accommodation for Tuberculosis in Poor Law Infirmaries of London*, 2.11.1922: The National Archive (TNA), Poor Law Hospitals, Treatment of Tuberculous Persons, 1922–3, MH 55:145.

26 'Tuberculosis Patients Under the Poor Law', *British Medical Journal* (hereafter *BMJ*) (1898), pp.1891ff.

27 'The Treatment of Tuberculosis in Hospitals and Infirmaries', *BMJ* (1902), pp.1542–5, 1599–1602, 1658–62.

28 F.S Togood, 'Tuberculosis and Metropolitan Pauperism', *British Journal of Tuberculosis*, 2 (1907), pp.166–77.

29 *Annual Report of the Metropolitan Asylums Board*, 1900, p.I.

30 J.D. Macfie, 'The Future of Sanatorium Benefit', *British Journal of Tuberculosis*, 5 (1911), pp.267ff.; J.D. Macfie, 'Ten Years' Experience of Sanatorium Benefit', *Tubercle*, 4 (1922/1923), pp.496–500; Departmental Committee on Tuberculosis, *Final Report of the Departmental Committee on Tuberculosis*, 2 vols (HMSO Cd. 6641/6654, London 1913).

31 R. Porter, 'Hospitals and Surgery', in R. Porter (ed.), *Cambridge Illustrated History of Medicine* (Cambridge 2001), pp.202–45.

32 A. Labisch and R. Spree, 'Die Kommunalisierung des Krankenhauswesens in Deutschland während des 19. und frühen 20. Jahrhunderts', in J. Wysocki (ed.), *Kommunalisierung im Spannungsfeld von Regulierung und Deregulierung im 19. und 20. Jahrhundert*, Schriften des Vereins für Socialpolitik, Neue Folge, 240 (Berlin, 1995), pp.7–48.

33 *Statistisches Jahrbuch für das Deutsche Reich*, 26 (1915), p.448; R. Spree, 'Quantitative Aspekte der Entwicklung des Krankenhauswesens im 19. und 20. Jahrhundert: "Ein Bild innerer und äußerer Verhältnisse"', in A. Labisch and R. Spree (eds), *'Einem jeden Kranken in einem Hospitale sein eigenes Bett': Zur Sozialgeschichte des Allgemeinen Krankenhauses in Deutschland im 19. Jahrhundert* (Frankfurt a. M., 1996), p.74.

34 L. Granshaw, '"Fame and Fortune by Means of Brick and Mortar": The Medical Profession and Specialist Hospitals in Britain, 1800–1948', in L. Granshaw and R. Porter (eds), *The Hospital in History* (London, 1989), pp.199–220.

35 H. Rosin, 'Die englischen Schwindsuchthospitäler und ihre Bedeutung für die deutsche Schwindsuchtpflege', *Deutsche Vierteljahresschrift für öffentliche Gesundheitspflege*, 24 (1892), pp.252–76.

36 'Treatment', *BMJ* (1902), pp.1542, 1599, 1658.

37 R. Pinker, *English Hospital Statistics 1861–1938* (London, 1966), p.114.

38 On finances of voluntary hospitals see S. Cherry, 'Accountability, Entitlement, and Control Issues and Voluntary Hospital Funding, 1860–1939', *Social History of Medicine* 9 (1996), pp.215–34.

39 F.B. Smith, *The Retreat of Tuberculosis* (London and New York, 1988), p.64.

40 *Report of the Tuberculin Treatment, Sub-Committee, Brompton Hospital, in National Heart and Lung Institute, Imperial College, London (NHLI)* (1891).

41 Bryder, *Magic Mountain*, pp.176ff.

42 H. Timbrell Bulstrode, *On Sanatoria for Consumptives and Certain Other Aspects of Tuberculosis Question, Supplement to the Report of the Medical Officer for 1905-06 to the 35th Annual Report of the Local Government Report* (reprinted, with omissions and additions from HMSO Cd. 3657, London, 1908).

43 I. Langerbeins, *Lungenheilanstalten in Deutschland von 1854–1945* (Cologne, 1979), p.8.

44 F. Condrau, 'Lungenheilstätten im internationalen Vergleich: zur Sozialge-schich-te der Tuberkulose im 19. und frühen 20. Jahrhundert', *Historia Hospitalium*, 19 (1993–4), pp.220–34.

45 M.S. Paterson, *Auto-Inoculation in Pulmonary Tuberculosis* (London, 1911).

46 M.S. Paterson, 'Graduated Labour in Pulmonary Tuberculosis', *The Lancet* 86 (1908.1), pp.216–20.

47 A. Labisch and R. Spree, 'Neuere Entwicklungen und aktuelle Trends in der Sozialgeschichte der Medizin in Deutschland: Rückschau und Ausblick', *Vierteljahrschrift für Sozial- und Wirtschaftsgeschichte*, 84 (1997), pp.171–210, 305–21.

48 E. Rumpf, 'Prophylaxe oder Therapie der Lungentuberkulose?', *Zeitschrift für Tuberkulose*, 11 (1907), p.31.

49 E. von Leyden, 'Die Wirksamkeit der Heilstätten für Lungenkranke', in idem, *Populäre Aufsätze und Vorträge* (Berlin, 1907), p.71.

50 O. Roepke, 'Tuberkulose und Heilstätte', *Beiträge zur Klinik der Tuberkulose*, 3 (1904), pp.9–18.

51 E. von Leyden, 'Ueber Specialkrankenhäuser', *Arbeiten aus der ersten medizinischen Klinik zu Berlin*, 2 (1891), p.27.

52 A. Grotjahn, 'Die Lungenheilstättenbewegung im Lichte der Sozialen Hygiene', *Zeitschrift für Soziale Medizin*, 2 (1907), pp.196–233.

53 F. Wehmer, 'Rückblick auf Brehmers Lebensarbeit', *Beiträge zur Klinik der Tuberkulose*, 31 (1914), pp.457–79.

54 F. Köhler, *Grundzüge der Behandlung der Lungentuberkulose* (Leipzig, 1927), p.4.

55 Condrau, 'Behandlung'.

56 R. Spree, 'Zu den Veränderungen der Volksgesundheit zwischen 1870 und 1913 und ihren Determinanten in Deutschland (vor allem in Preußen)', in W. Conze and U. Engelhardt (eds), *Arbeiterexistenz im 19. Jahrhundert: Lebensstandard und Lebensgestaltung deutscher Arbeiter und Handwerker* (Stuttgart, 1981), pp.235–92.

57 For methodological considerations see R. Porter, 'The Patient's View: Doing Medical History from Below', *Theory and Society*, 14 (1985), pp.175–98; B. Luckin, 'Towards a Social History of Institutionalization', *Social History*, 8 (1983), pp.87–94.

58   A very helpful study on the problems of historical diagnosis is J. Brügelmann, *Der Blick des Arztes auf die Krankheit im Alltag 1779–1850: Medizinische Topographien als Quelle für die Sozialgeschichte des Gesundheitswesens* (Berlin, 1982).

59   *Die vorbeugende Krankenpflege und die Invalidenfürsorge der Landesversicherungsanstalt der Hansestädte nebst Beschreibung und Plänen der von ihr für die Versicherten errichteten Anstalten*, Heilstätten, Genesungsheime, Invalidenheim (Lübeck, 1904).

60   H. Gebhardt, 'Ausbreitung der Tuberkulose unter der versicherungspflichtigen Bevölkerung', in G. Pannwitz (ed.), *Bericht über den Kongress zur Bekämpfung der Tuberkulose als Volkskrankheit* (Berlin, 1899), pp.80–92.

61   For some of the diagnostic problems see J. Lachmund, *Der Abgehorchte Körper: zur historischen Soziologie der medizinischen Untersuchung* (Opladen, 1997); B. Pasveer, *Shadows of Knowledge: Making a Representing Practice in Medicine. X-Ray Pictures and Pulmonary Tuberculosis, 1890–1930* (Amsterdam, 1992).

62   See for the German classification of stages of tuberculosis L. Teleky, *Bekämpfung: Sechzig Jahre Landesversicherungsanstalt Hansestadt Hamburg 1891–1951* (Hamburg, 1951), pp.214–17.

63   On measuring survival after treatment in a German sanatorium see G. Liebermeister, 'Die Sicherung des Kurerfolges bei der Tuberkulose vom ärztlichen Standpunkt aus', *Zeitschrift für Tuberkulose*, 42 (1925), pp.531–6; F. Köhler, 'Die Dauererfolge der Behandlung Lungentuberkulöser in den Deutschen Heilstätten', *Tuberculosis*, 7 (1908), pp.243–58; H. Weicker, *Tuberkulose–Heilstätten–Dauererfolge* (Leipzig, 1903); Dr. Friedrich, *Die Erfolge der Freiluftbehandlung bei Lungenschwindsucht*, Arbeiten aus dem Kaiserlichen Gesundheitsamte, 18 (Berlin, 1901).

64   Thomas himself was advised to stay in the sanatorium for treatment as well, but wisely chose to flee the scene. On the Manns' connection to Davos, see C. Virchow, *Medizinhistorisches um den 'Zauberberg': 'Das gläserne Angebinde' und ein pneumologisches Nachspiel*, Augsburger Universitätsreden 26 (Augsburg, 1995); T. Sprecher (ed.), *Das Zauberberg-Symposium 1994 in Davos*, Thomas-Mann-Studien, 11 (Frankfurt a. M., 1995).

65   P.Q. Edwards and L.B. Edwards, 'The Story of the Tuberculin Test from an Epidemiologic Viewpoint', *American Review of Respiratory Diseases*, 81 (1960), pp.1–47; G.W. Comstock et al., 'The Prognosis of a Positive Tuberculin Reaction in Childhood and Adolescence', *American Journal of Epidemiology* 99 (1974), pp.131–8.

66   G.W. Comstock, 'Tuberculosis: A Bridge to Chronic Disease Epidemiology', *American Journal of Epidemiology*, 124 (1986), pp.1–16; Informationsdienst des Bayerischen Statistischen Landesamtes, *Die Tuberkulose in Bayern 1954* (Munich, 1955), p.14.

67   M.W.T. Bromme, *Lebensgeschichte eines modernen Fabrikarbeiters, hrsg. und eingeleitet von Paul Göhre* (Jena, 1905).

68   Teleky, *Bekämpfung: Sechzig Jahre Landesversicherungsanstalt Hansestadt Hamburg 1891–1951* (Hamburg, 1951), p.23.

69   C. Hamel, *Deutsche Heilstätten für Lungenkranke. Geschichtliche und statistische Mitteilungen*, 6 vols (Tuberkulose-Arbeiten aus dem Kaiserlichen Gesundheitsamte, vols 2–14, 1904–1918); Gebhard, 'Ausbreitung'.

70   W. von Leube, 'Spezialkrankenhaus für Tuberkulöse in den vorgeschriebenen Stadien der Erkrankung: Tuberkulosekrankenhäuser (Heimstätten "Invalidenheime") – Krankenhauspflege', in *Der Stand der Tuberkulose-Bekämpfung in Deutschland. Denkschrift dem Internationalen Tuberkulose-Kongress in Paris 1905* (Berlin, 1905), pp.252–61; *Die vorbeugende Krankenpflege und die Invalidenfürsorge der Landesversicherungsanstalt der Hansestädte [...]*.

71   Spree, *Krankenhausentwicklung*.

72   *Report on the Accomodation for Tuberculosis in Poor Law Infirmaries of London, 2.11.1922* (TNA, Poor Law Hospitals, Treatment of Tuberculous Persons, 1922–3, MH 55:145).

73   For the number of beds for tuberculosis, see *On the State of the Public Health. Annual Report of the Chief Medical Officer of the Ministry of Health for the Year 1922* (London, 1923), p.88.

74   Most notably, this included the admission of paying patients to poor law infirmaries.

75   Mr. Francis, commentary of the Report on the Accomodation for Tuberculosis (TNA, MH 55:145).

76   In 1922 Camberwell Infirmary lost 45% of all tuberculosis patients. For more details, see *Annual Report of Camberwell Infirmary, 1922, Report on the Accomodation for Tuberculosis* (TNA, MH 55:145).

77   *Tuberculosis Notification of Poor Law Cases, Regulations, 1908* (TNA, MH 55: 523).

78   GRO, *Decennial Supplements of the Annual Reports of the Registrar General's Office* (1921), p.99. Women appear to have died outside of institutions more often than men.

79   *Report on an Inquiry into the Use of Poor Law Infirmaries for the Treatment of Tuberculosis, March 1923* (TNA, MH 55:145).

80   Admission 15.8.1922, in *Report on an Inquiry* (TNA, MH 55:145).

81   Admission 17.1.1923.

82   Admission 28.11.1922.

83   Admission 5.2.1923.

84   Admission 9.1.1923; discharge of this patient was imminent.

85   Admission 25.11.1922.

86   This perspective owes a lot to demographic studies of hospital afterlife. A. Brändström, 'Cured or Killed? Life-Histories for Nineteenth Century Swedish Hospital Patients', in A. Brändström and L.-G. Tedebrand (eds),

Health and Social Change: Disease, Health and Public Care in the Sundsvall District 1750–1950 (Umea, 1993), pp.25–54.

87   Brompton Hospital Sanatorium (BHS), Frimley: Clinical Records, 1906–31; BHS, Frimley: Patients Follow-Up Records, 1906–59, formerly at the Wellcome Unit for the History of Medicine, Oxford. Unfortunately, it has been difficult to track the location of the patient related sources as the trail ends in the Wellcome Library for the History of Medicine, the Surrey County Record Office and the National Heart and Lung Institute at the Imperial College, London.

88   P.H. Horton-Smith et al. (eds), 'The Expectation of Survival in Pulmonary Tuberculosis: An Analysis of 8766 Cases Treated at the Brompton Hospital Sanatorium Frimley', *Brompton Hospital Reports*, 4 (1935); *An Inquiry into the After-Histories of Patients Treated at the Brompton Hospital Sanatorium at Frimley, during the Years 1905–14*, Medical Research Council, Special Report Series, 85 (London, 1924).

89   A more elaborate discussion of Frimley's status as an elite institution can be found in Condrau, *Lungenheilanstalt*, pp.135–40; see also F. Condrau, 'Die Patienten von Lungenheilanstalten 1890–1930. Deutschland und England im Vergleich', in A. Labisch and R. Spree (eds), *Von der Armenfürsorge zur kommunalen Dienstleistung. Finanzwirtschaft und Patienten Allgemeiner Krankenhäuser in Deutschland während des 19. und frühen 20. Jahrhunderts* (Frankfurt a.M., 2001), pp.427–48.

90   An example is Charles: Frimley patient # 5982.

91   Frimley patient # 3816, 1914; this case has been cited in J.R. Bignall, *Frimley: The Biography of a Sanatorium* (London, 1979), pp.93–5.

92   Frimley patient # 7698.

93   Bryder, *Mountain*.

94   Compiled using *Verzeichnis der deutschen Einrichtungen für Tuberkulöse*, Deutschen Zentralkomitee für Tuberkulose (Berlin, 1930).

95   E. Kniehl et al., 'Rupture of Therapeutic Oleothorax Leading to Paraffin Oil Aspiration and Dissemination of Tuberculosis: A Fatal Late Complication of Tuberculosis Therapy in the 1940s', *Wiener Klinische Wochenschrift*, 110 (1998), pp.725–8.

Part Five: The Demographic Impact

Alysa Levene

Chapter 15: Saving the Innocents: Nursing Foundlings in Florence and London in the Eighteenth Century

The eighteenth century was a period of great expansion in institutional provision for abandoned infants, or 'foundlings' in Europe. While some countries such as Italy, Spain and Portugal had systematically provided care for foundlings within hospitals since the medieval era, other countries, including England and Germany, were slower to follow suit. In these latter countries, the growth of foundling hospitals was prompted when eighteenth-century Enlightenment imperatives to take responsibility for the underprivileged fused with innovative charitable projects and concerns to increase national populations.[1] At the same time there was massive growth in the scale of infant abandonment in Europe, and foundling hospitals, both new and long-established, found themselves under an increasing burden to care for growing numbers of charges whilst continuing to balance their financial books. This chapter considers one of the most critical aspects of the care of foundling infants, but also one of the most expensive: how they were nursed. It will examine how far two European foundling hospitals, the Spedale degli Innocenti of Florence, and the London Foundling Hospital, were able to respond to the need to find nurses for large numbers of babies, and how they attempted to overcome shortages through policy changes.

As hinted at already, the two hospitals had quite different pedigrees. The Innocenti was the longest-running foundling home in continuous operation by the eighteenth century, and is also one of the best documented. It was opened in January 1445 under the joint impetus of the silk guild (one of the city's *arti maggiori* or major guilds), and the commune of Florence. Until the closure in 1875 of the famous *ruota*, or wheel, which facilitated anonymous abandonment, the hospital admitted all infants offered to it, be they illegitimate offspring of women who needed to hide their 'shame'; the legitimate children of couples in financial difficulties, or who had already reached their optimal family size; and in the early period at least, the offspring of slaves (sometimes sired by their masters). Admissions to the hospital remained fairly constant between the mid-sixteenth and the early eighteenth centuries, with approximately 500 infants entering every year. From the 1720s however, the pan-European explosion in child abandonment is reflected in continuously rising admissions, which had reached approximately 1200 per year by 1800.[2]

The London Foundling Hospital, in contrast, did not receive its foundation by Royal Charter until 1739, and admitted its first infants in 1741. Like other contemporaneous London charities, it was organised on a joint-stock basis, and was funded by subscribers and charitable donations.[3] Admissions were small-scale and selective: babies had to be initially under two months, and free of contagious disease. Admissions rarely exceeded 200 per year. High demand for places, however, prompted the hospital's governors to petition Parliament for financial support, which resulted in a state-funded 'General Reception' of all babies offered between 1756 and 1760. The age limit was raised to one year, and the screening for health was removed. Admissions soared: over 4,000 babies per year were abandoned at the hospital, and over 15,000 in total were admitted during the period of the General Reception. In 1760, the funding was withdrawn because of high costs, high mortality among the foundlings, and perceived 'abuses' such as putative fathers and parish officials sending babies to the hospital against the mother's will to escape the burden of supporting them.[4] After 1760, admissions were again small-scale and explicitly restricted to London-born illegitimate children, and mothers were asked to petition the hospital with their history before being admitted to a ballot for admission.

Although the two hospitals had different histories and catered for different levels of demand, there was a common aim to raise infants by placing them with external wet nurses in surrounding rural areas as soon as possible after admission. Babies would be cared for by these foster mothers until they were returned to the foundling hospitals for training and education: at 18 months at the Innocenti, and at five years at the London hospital. This preference for wet nursing in a family environment rather than raising infants on paps and broths in the hospital was given medical backing in the eighteenth century by doctors newly interested in childcare. The London hospital, for example, sought the opinion of the Royal College of Physicians, and of influential doctors such as Sir Hans Sloane on the best method of rearing infants, while the Innocenti asked the well-known Florentine doctor Antonio Cocchi for his advice.[5] In most cases, wet nursing was preferred to dry where possible, although Cocchi in particular noted that the type of women who were willing to nurse for the hospital might not necessarily be well-suited to doing it well. In such cases, dry nursing might be preferred, as long as a proper method (such as that he went on to outline) was followed. Other medical treatise-writers were also increasingly advocating the benefits of breast milk for infants in this period, reinforcing the wisdom of the hospitals' policies.[6] Wet nursing was not cheap, however, and at the Innocenti in particular, the cumulative cost was sometimes prohibitive, especially as financial support from the silk guild waned up to its abolition in 1770. In fact, despite the general preference for breast-feeding among eighteenth-century doctors, those involved in running foundling homes frequently questioned whether it was practical or necessary. The London hospital did make a brief experiment of both wet- and dry-nursing before deciding unequivocally in favour of breast-feeding wherever possible, and experiments were also carried out in parts of France.[7] Although such trials almost always found that artificial feeding brought higher risks of death, the costs of wet nursing, and the necessity to rely on uneducated women, kept the question alive.[8]

Clearly, the experience of wet nursing was affected by both demand- and supply-side factors. The hospitals needed to recruit a sufficient number of nurses, but to do so, the wage had to be more lucrative than a woman's earnings from agriculture or other employments. It had to be sufficiently low, however, that the hospitals were not bankrupted to keep their children alive. When women were not forthcoming to nurse the foundlings, the hospitals needed either alternatives or incentives. These conflicts and balances are illustrated in this chapter via selected entry cohorts to the two hospitals. The supply of nurses in different years is examined, along with the different approaches the institutions took to maintaining a balance of effective feeding methods, and the impact they had on mortality levels. These approaches generally involved changes in nursing wage levels, more active recruitment of women, and trials of different feeding methods. The discussion will indicate how successful the hospitals were in managing staff levels, and how their policies impacted on the likelihood that a foundling would be successfully placed with a foster nurse.

Sources and Samples

The entry cohorts at the Innocenti were selected because of their relationship with the nursing regime. The value of cohort study as a methodological approach was established for the Innocenti records both by Carlo Corsini, and by Paolo Viazzo, Maria Bortolotto and Andrea Zanotto. The work produced by these scholars has illuminated aspects of the hospital's regime, and its relationship with surrounding areas.[9] One of Viazzo et al.'s key findings for the current study was that the hospital frequently had problems recruiting sufficient numbers of nurses. Most notably, they found that it directly tried to influence the supply in 1779 by raising wages. In order to keep the costs down, however, the nursing period was shortened from 18 to 12 months. The change in policy did produce lower rates of infant mortality, and a higher rate of wet nursing in the short term, but early weaning and return to the hospital resulted in lower survival rates among one to two year olds. Mortality rates were 229 per thousand in the second year of life in the 1777 cohort, but a massive 632 per thousand in the 1782 cohort, with a concentration between 15 and 16 months.[10] In 1786, the nursing period was brought back to 18 months with a resulting fall in second-year mortality, although what happened to wage levels remains unclear. Viazzo et al. investigated the impact of the 1779 wage raise by focusing on entry cohorts on either side: 1777 and 1782. They found a smaller overall proportion of infants being placed with wet nurses in the former year, and with a longer average wait in the hospital before a nurse was found. This examination of entry cohorts thus placed a strong emphasis on the nursing system and its mechanics and incentives as an important factor governing survival chances. Dr Viazzo has kindly made available the data for the 'poor' year of 1777 (consisting of 814 children) for this comparative study.

A second Innocenti cohort was selected to shed light on how at other times the hospital tried to manage a policy of artificial feeding rather than wage manipulation. The advice of the previously mentioned Antonio Cocchi on artificial feeding was sought by the Innocenti's *Spedalingo*, Francesco Rucellai, in 1744.[11] Scattered evidence suggests that a small-scale trial of artificial feeding was made following Cocchi's comments, but its impact and background are unknown. The entry cohort of 1744 (560 children) was thus selected for further investigation, and also to shed more light generally on a little-studied decade of the hospital's history. The 1740s seem to have been another period of poor financial health for the hospital, but at this time the possibility of artificial feeding was pursued rather than a rise in nursing wages.

For the London hospital, a sampling technique was used to examine the cohort who entered the institution up to the end of the General Reception (1741-60). The sample consists of the first ten per cent of entrants in each month (1650 children) and is designed to be representative of all entrants to the hospital in this period. After 1760, the admissions process and stipulations on type of child meant that the population of foundlings was quite different in composition. In all cases, individual-level data on nursing were extracted from admissions books and other entry documents.[12]

Experiences of Nursing

The data on babies admitted in the three cohorts allow us to examine the likelihood that foundlings would be placed with external wet nurses, how rapidly they were placed, and whether this varied by season. We will see that the two hospitals operated at different levels of efficiency with regard to their nursing systems, and that the success of the system in finding enough nurses varied from cohort to cohort at the Innocenti.

Fig. 15.1 illustrates the proportion of foundlings in the three cohorts who were sent to an external nurse, and how long they had to wait for a placement. The graph indicates that the 1744 cohort at the Innocenti did better than that of 1777 in terms both of the likelihood a baby would be placed at all, and the speed with which a nurse was found. The London hospital sample, however, did better on both fronts. There, 85 per cent of children in the sample were placed with a wet nurse, and over three quarters of the intake had been found a nurse within a week of abandonment. Indeed, 26 per cent were sent out on the day that they were received into the hospital. This indicates that the hospital had a highly efficient system of nursing, with an effective recruitment policy, and a reservoir of women waiting at the hospital for babies, even at times of high demand like the General Reception.[13] At the Innocenti in 1744, the overall proportion of nursing placements was also high: 77 per cent, but only 36 per cent of entrants had been found a nurse within a week, and a tiny 0.2 per cent were sent out on the day they came in to the hospital. The recruitment of nurses in 1744 was thus reasonably good, although the system was slow to find the maximum number of children an ongoing supply of breast milk. The cohort is comparable to Viazzo et al.'s of 1782, after the 1779 nursing reforms, when 79.8 per cent of children were found a nurse, and 98 per cent of these were placed within two months of entry.[14] In 1777, however, the nursing system was running far less optimally: comparatively few children were placed with a nurse, and there was a substantial interval between entry to the hospital and placement. Only 41 per cent of those entering in this year were eventually found a

Figure 15.1
Speed of placement with external wet nurses, London Foundling Hospital (1741–60) and Spedale degli Innocenti (1744 and 1777)

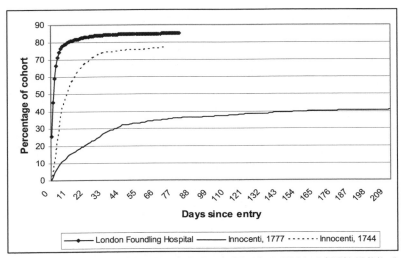

Source: London Foundling Hospital, General Register LMA, A/FH/A09/2/1–5;
Innocenti, *Balie e bambini*, AOIF Serie XVI, 1744 and 1777

nurse, 10 per cent went out within a week, and 0.3 per cent on the day of arrival. The average wait for those who went to a nurse was 35.1 days, compared with 10.8 days in 1744.

A comparison with the mortality rates of the cohorts illustrates how critical it was to find wet nurses promptly. The London hospital sample had an infant mortality rate of 630.5 per thousand live births, which was already at least double that seen among contemporary London infants, and perhaps three to four times that in the English provinces.[15] At the Innocenti, however, the 1777 cohort had an infant mortality rate of 835.2 per thousand. A lack of data on age at entry precludes the calculation of a comparable rate for 1744. Statistical analysis suggests that the efficiency of the nursing system played an important role in setting the level of mortality in different years.[16] No children in any of the cohorts survived to leave the hospital without having been placed with a nurse at all, although some of those admitted in 1777 were still alive to be placed up to seven months after entry, indicating a reasonable ability to keep children alive in the hospital.[17] This topic will be discussed further below. It is clear, however, that the survival prospects of infant foundlings were severely compromised where wet-nursing was restricted.

The calculation of an average wait time before going to nurse masks the fact that there were seasonal variations. It is likely that an attractive enough nursing wage would deter women from taking up work in other seasonal sectors such as agriculture when it became

Figure 15.2
Seasonal wait for external nursing placement, London Foundling Hospital (1741–60), and Spedale degli Innocenti (1744 and 1777)

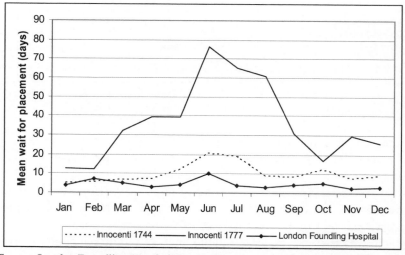

Source: London Foundling Hospital General Registers and Inspections Books, 1741–64 (LMA, A/FH/A10/001/001/01-02); Innocenti *Balie e bambini*

available. The pattern of placement times over the year is thus further revealing as to how the system of nursing worked. Fig. 15.2 shows the patterns from the cohort data, illustrating a common model at the two hospitals. In all three cohorts, babies had to wait for longer in the hospital for a nurse to be found over the summer months, although it was a more marked pattern at the Innocenti than at the London hospital, and more so there in 1777 than in 1744. This may partly relate to the respective opportunities for female labour in agriculture in the two locations, but the difference in scale between the two Innocenti cohorts suggests that it was mainly a function of the nursing wage. In 1777 in particular, nursing for the foundling hospital was clearly a less worthwhile occupation for women during the summer, and the length of time infants had to wait for a nurse lengthened dramatically. This was especially unfortunate for the foundlings' survival prospects, since this was a season notoriously dangerous for the risks of death from gastric disease. These risks were exacerbated if infants were being fed on dry food, since high temperatures raise the risk of bacterial contamination of food and vessels.[18] The seasonal pattern is not related to the index of admissions, which consistently show a peak in the winter at both hospitals.[19]

Hospital policy may also have played a role in the speed with which infants were placed with external wet nurses. Although the evidence suggests that hospital officers aimed to place their charges with external nurses as soon as possible, they may have felt that some infants would benefit from a strengthening stay in the hospital first. Others may have been too sick to travel, or carried a disease which might be transmitted to a nurse. Data from the London hospital show that an increasing proportion of infants entered in a poor state of health over the course of the General Reception, and had to be sent to one of the hospital's infirmaries. A growing percentage of these babies did not survive to be placed with a wet nurse.[20] Diseases such as congenital syphilis were also a worry for hospital officers, since they could be transmitted to nurses via breast-feeding.[21] This danger would clearly be a disincentive for women to put themselves forward as nurses. Factors such as ill-health, therefore, might also affect the proportion of infants placed with nurses, and this might vary according to policy in a particular year. Overall, however, the data examined here show that wet nursing was the norm.

Nursing Shortages and Hospital Policy

Increasing wages for nurses was almost certainly the most effective way of recruiting more women to work for foundling hospitals. Given the financial constraints most hospitals were operating under, however, this was rarely possible, and officials instead had to turn to other policies to attract enough women. As noted above, we know that the Innocenti's *Spedalingo* considered the option of artificial feeding in 1744, and that the London hospital also briefly trialled this method of nursing. Other options included increasing the number of nurses inside the hospital (either from necessity or in an attempt to maintain a more closely supervised system of mixed breast- and dry-feeding),[22] or recruiting women more actively outside the hospital. Of these, using artificial foods was perhaps the most obvious course of action when nurses were in short supply, since it reduced the hospital's reliance on external staff. It was, however, extremely difficult to carry out successfully, and the care with which Antonio Cocchi prepared his plan for artificial feeding indicates how seriously contemporaries took the issue.

Cocchi was one of the foremost intellectual figures in mid-eighteenth-century Florence, a practitioner at the Santa Maria Nuova hospital, and a strong advocate of simplicity and modernisation in medical practice generally.[23] After considering the mechanics of infants' digestion, he decided that artificial feeding could confidently be used at the Innocenti for babies over 30 days, and from birth if the child was healthy. The method might also be used for children who were prematurely returned from nurse. However, he made a series of stipulations on the conditions which should be observed: a well-lit and furnished room must be used, with one cradle for two infants rather than four as before; the supervisor (ideally an ex-foundling) and employees must be diligent and faithful in feeding, clothing and washing the infants; and the food must consist of fresh cow's milk, mixed with pure, heated water in a clean carafe, with supplements of bread paps lightly boiled in water or milk. On weaning, an egg might be introduced into the pap, and at five months, meat broth might be added. Records should be kept of every child in order that the system might be monitored and improved.[24]

In his recommendations for clean and hygienic conditions, Cocchi was undoubtedly astute, since vessels used for feeding are easily contaminated, and the keeping of many infants cramped together in unsanitary conditions assisted the spread of contagion. The food prescribed also avoided some of the worst deficiencies of dry-nursing, although it lacked the antibodies and precise protein and mineral composition of breast milk. Its milk basis staved off the worst dangers of rickets and scurvy, and contained fat, which is essential for an infant's diet. McClure points out that the paps used for dry-nursed children at the London Foundling Hospital (for example, for those who were sick) did not always contain milk, which would have dramatically reduced their nutritive value.[25]

Despite these provisos, however, it seems that the Innocenti did not embark on a policy of more widespread dry nursing. The data from 1744 have shown that wet nursing was still the norm, and that in fact, placements with external nurses were relatively rapid. A previously uncited archival source, however, indicates that a small-scale experiment into artificial feeding did take place in 1745, but that it was deemed a total failure. A report by one Francesco Cerusico records a meeting which took place on 18 August 1745, where a memorial was read out against the *Spedalingo*, Rucellai, charging him with an attempt 'di fare allattare i piccoli bambini con il Latte di Vaccha, e che di sedici ne morirono quindici' ('to raise small children on cow's milk, and that of 16 so fed, 15 had died').[26] The one survivor had been removed from the experiment. Apparently Rucellai had indeed taken Cocchi's recommendation of artificial feeding to heart, perhaps in an attempt to cut down the expenses of wet nursing. The disapproval which is clear from this brief account was still felt in the 1760s, however, when the *Commissario*, Neri Badia noted that the care necessary for such a scheme of artificial feeding was impossible to obtain from the people who offered themselves for the job.[27] Clearly, artificial feeding was not felt to be a lasting or effective substitute for wet nursing.

An alternative – though related – policy on nursing, was to recruit more women to serve inside the hospital rather than in their own homes. This again meant that the system could be more closely supervised by hospital officials, and if combined with a system of mixed breast- and artificial-feeding, could reduce the numbers of women needed. It was noted above that infants admitted to the Innocenti in 1744 rarely survived for long inside the hospital compared with those in 1777, and it may have been these babies which Rucellai envisaged being fed by hand to keep them alive. This was again a topic which seems to have been more actively considered at the Innocenti than at the London hospital, which did not deviate from its policy on universal external wet nursing after its early years.

A register of internal nurses for the Innocenti reveals its pattern of recruitment.[28] In 1777 there was a marked seasonal pattern, with more nurses being employed in March, August/September and November. In the 1740s the main nursing peak was in May, with the late summer and autumn highs less marked. It is quite possible that this does not represent a deliberate policy of higher levels of recruitment at certain times of the year, but rather reflects the times when women were more likely to offer themselves as nurses. Over the course of 1775 however, the phrase 'si potese alle solite condizioni di servire nell'estate futura' (she was told of the usual conditions of serving for the next summer) becomes common in the register entries. This suggests that the Innocenti officials were trying to increase the number of internal nurses over the summer months. The average period of employment as an internal nurse was short, however. Between 1740 and 1743 it was 6.8 months, although by the mid 1770s it had risen to 9.1 months, possibly as a result of the requirement to work through the summer.[29] Recruitment levels had also risen, from an average of 32 new nurses per year in the early 1740s, to 54.3 by the mid-1770s (although admissions were also rising). Certainly, in May 1776 the *Commissario* was writing to parish priests, asking them to send women to the Innocenti to work as nurses.[30] The women were asked to wean their own child, unless it had recently died. Of the 217 women entering the Innocenti as internal nurses between 1774 and 1777, 12.4 per cent had lost their own child, and 78.8 had sent their child either to the Innocenti, or to another foundling home. This is suggestive of an informal system whereby women who abandoned babies then worked for the hospital as a nurse, although such a scheme

was not formally in operation at the Innocenti until 1791. This phenomenon, taken in conjunction with the appeal to priests, suggests that
the hospital was attempting to recruit more internal nurses as well as
external by the time of the 1777 Innocenti cohort.

Several censuses of staff and children in the Innocenti illustrate
that the situation varied considerably from year to year. In December
1742, for example, the year of Rucellai's appointment, there were 37
'*allatanti*' infants (nurslings), inside the house, with 24 nurses and six
soprabbalie (head nurses), or 1.5 infants to each of the regular nurses.
There were also approximately 30 other young children in the house,
who may have been cared for by some of these nurses. Another survey
was made on 30 June 1746, at which time there were 22 suckling
infants to 12 nurses, plus six head nurses, or 1.8 each. There were a
further 23 other young children also present. Cocchi noted that in
1744 there were 12 nurses in the house, with more than 36 infants
being nursed, rising as high as 77 in summer. This represented a minimum of 3 infants to one nurse. For his hand rearing regime Cocchi
advocated no more than 5 infants for 2 nurses.[31] The 1740s do thus
appear to have been a time of relatively high reliance on internal
nurses, although at times the ratio of babies to nurses could have supported near-exclusive breast-feeding. At the end of the eighteenth
century and beginning of the nineteenth, the Innocenti was again
relying on a large number of internal nurses. Between 1801 and 1805
there were never fewer than 50 nurses inside the hospital, rising to a
maximum of 70 in summer. The ratio of nurses to children never rose
above one to three.[32]

In the mid-1760s, however, surveys show that the ratio of babies
to nurses was relatively low. In 1767, there were 15 nurslings to 10
nurses (1.5 per nurse), and in 1768, 13 infants to 12 nurses (1.1 per
nurse).[33] We should note that the situation may have varied considerably according to the season in which the census was taken. Viazzo et
al. examined staff levels around the time of the 1779 nursing reforms,
finding that prior to this, the number of nurslings in the house varied
from 30 in winter to around 125 in summer, with approximately 50
nurses for them in the summer months (1.5 per nurse). After the
reform the numbers of infants staying in the hospital fell until the
1780s.[34] Clearly, internal staffing levels varied considerably, no doubt

related both to seasonal patterns of admissions, and to alternative female employments. The stipulation on internal nurses serving over the summer, however, suggests an attempt to control for shortages of external nurses.

While artificial feeding seems not to have been followed to any great extent at either hospital, therefore, internal nursing at the Innocenti was sometimes particularly promoted. On the whole, however, the latter policy seems to have been pursued as a means to keep infants alive until an external placement could be found for them. An account of 1745 detailing admissions and deaths under Rucellai and his predecessor specifically notes that a preference for external nurses in the countryside was 'il vero metodo per far vivere i Lattanti' (the right way to keep nurslings alive).[35] With this commitment in mind, the best policy for the hospitals to pursue was the more intensive recruitment of external nurses. It has already been noted that the Innocenti appealed to priests in rural locations to send women to act as nurses. The London hospital seems to have been particularly effective in their attempts, using an extensive network of local inspectors.

In this respect, the London Foundling Hospital benefited from the fact that there was relatively little competition for wet nurses in England, certainly compared with the situation in Tuscany.[36] Private nursing was not a particularly active phenomenon, and poor law officials started to use the practice intensively only after a law of 1767 made it mandatory for London parishes.[37] The hospital also had a wide range of contacts in rural areas because of the spheres of influence of its high-society supporters.[38] They were able to recommend suitable local people to act as unpaid inspectors, and they in turn were in an ideal position to search out women who could act as nurses. Although the hospital governors did sometimes note that there were difficulties getting enough nurses, individual inspectors seem to have few problems in finding potential employees, and some successfully placed several hundreds of infants in one locality during the General Reception.[39] The Innocenti, however, lacked this network of inspectors, and were also working in a more saturated market. The number of other foundling hospitals in the region, coupled with an active private market for nurses, made it much harder to seek out new nurses.

Conclusion

Both the London Foundling Hospital and the Spedale degli Innocenti remained basically committed to the health benefits of external wet-nursing for young foundlings. Cohort data have shown that their success rates in recruiting enough women to ensure most infants could be placed in foster families varied, however. The London hospital was able to place a large majority of foundlings with external nurses very rapidly, almost certainly because of its network of inspectors, and the lack of competition on any large scale. The Innocenti had a more varied record, with relatively high success rates in 1744 and 1782, but a much poorer record in 1777. Nonetheless, the hospital in Florence pursued alternatives to external wet nursing in 1744 as well as the 1770s, when the improvement in nurses' salaries did attract more women to work for the institution. The success of the nursing policy was clearly related to the survival outcomes of the foundling infants, with the Innocenti having a particularly horrifying mortality rate in 1777 (although the work of Viazzo et al. has shown that a longer feeding period in that year than in 1782 kept second-year mortality down). At the London hospital, mortality rates, though still extremely high, were lower than at the Innocenti, at least partly because of the higher chance that foundlings would be found nurses quickly.

In the 1740s, it was artificial feeding which attracted attention, although records do not specify whether this was an attempt to improve survival chances for the infants, or whether it was part of an attempt to cut costs. Although a positive report was received from an eminent Florentine doctor, however, the attempt was unsuccessful. The negative impact of artificial feeding seems to have been absorbed to the extent that it was not trialled again even in the straitened circumstances of the 1770s. At times, the Innocenti also attempted to recruit more women to work as nurses inside the hospital. Their success rate seemed to improve when women using the hospital were asked to serve over the summer months; an arrangement which later became formalised, and which was used at other foundling hospitals as well (although not in London). The busy nursing market in Tuscany seems to have prevented the Innocenti from effectively implementing a policy of more active recruitment of external nurses. The London hospital did pursue this aim, and backed up by a sufficiently attractive wage, had high enough success rates that they did not need to revisit the artificial feeding debate in any lasting way. For most of the century, of course, the London hospital had to deal with only relatively small numbers of foundlings, but the scale of their operations during the General Reception indicates how enormous a task it was to find enough nurses to promote family fostering at eighteenth-century foundling hospitals.

Notes

1   O. Ulbricht, 'The Debate about Foundling Hospitals in Enlightenment Germany: Infanticide, Illegitimacy and Infant Mortality Rates', *Central European History*, 18 (1985), pp.211–56; D. Andrew, *Philanthropy and Police: London Charity in the Eighteenth Century* (New Jersey, 1989), pp.54–7. It should be noted that the English Poor Laws had long supported abandoned babies outside the foundling hospital model.

2   P.P. Viazzo, M. Bortolotto and A. Zanotto, 'Five Centuries of Foundling History in Florence', in C. Panter-Brick and M.T. Smith (eds), *Abandoned Children* (Cambridge, 2000), pp.75–6. The reasons for this explosion in infant abandonment are unclear, although it parallels the rise in illegitimate births in the same period. G. Da Molin (*Nati e abbandonati: aspetti demografici e sociali dell'infanzia abbandonata in Italia nell'età moderna* (Bari, 1993), p.178) suggests that it was a result of a change in popular attitudes away from earlier ecclesiastical directives towards marriage, accompanied by demographic pressure, and a rise in the age of marriage. Pregnancy may thus have occurred more frequently outside marriage, while an increasing number of legitimate infants were being abandoned in response to poor economic conditions. The increasing number of foundling hospitals may also have encouraged the practice. M. Livi Bacci (*The Population of Europe: A History*, English translation, Oxford, 2000, pp.150–1) sees the eighteenth-century rise in abandonment in Europe as a response to 'the higher cost – absolute or relative – of offspring'. Abandonment was therefore the pre-birth-control-era's response to family limitation, although he recognises that other factors were also important.

3   See Andrew, *Philanthropy and Police*, pp.46–9.

4   R. McClure, *Coram's Children: the London Foundling Hospital in the Eighteenth Century* (New Haven, 1981), pp.97–101.

5   For example, see London Foundling Hospital General Committee Minutes, 20 Aug. 1740, London Metropolitan Archive (hereafter LMA), A/FH/K02/001, although at this stage, artificial feeding was recommended. On 1 October 1744, the General Committee recorded their resolve to breast-feed as many infants as possible. S. Contardi (ed.), *Antonio Cocchi: scritti scelti* (Florence, 1998); M.M. Goggioli (ed.), *Antonio Cocchi: relazione dello Spedale di S. M. Nuova di Firenze* (Florence, 2000).

6   For example, M. Underwood, *A Treatise on the Diseases of Children, with General Directions for the Management of Infants from the Birth*, 2 vols (London, 1789); J. Nelson, *An Essay on the Government of Children* (London, 1756); W. Moss, *An Essay on the Management, Nursing and Diseases of Children from the Birth* (Egham, 1794); W. Buchan, *Domestic Medicine, or a Treatise on the Prevention and Cure of Diseases by Regimen and Simple Medicines* (London, 1769).

7   M-F. Marel, 'À quoi servent les enfants trouvés? Les médecins et le problème de l'abandon dans la France du XVIIIè siècle', in *Enfance abandonée et société en Europe XIVe–XXe siècle*, Collection de l'école française de Rome (Rome, 1991), pp.840–50; G. Cappelletto, 'Gli affidamenti a balia dei bambini abbandonati in una comunità del territorio veronese nel settecento', in *Enfance abandonnée*, p.327. Artificial feeding was also practised within natal families in some parts of Europe, although it was generally accompanied by high mortality. See, for example, U-B. Lithell, 'Breast-feeding Habits and their Relation to Infant Mortality and Marital Fertility', *Journal of Family History*, 6 (1981), p.183; J. Dupâquier, *La population française aux XVIIe et XVIIIe siècles* (Paris, 1979), pp.51–8; J.E. Knodel, *Demographic Behaviour in the Past: A Study of Fourteen German Village Populations* (Cambridge, 1988), Appendix F, pp.542–8; A. Brändström, 'The Impact of Female Labour Conditions on Infant Mortality: A Case Study of the Parishes of Nedertorneå and Jokkmokk, 1800–96', *Social History of Medicine*, 1.3 (1988), pp.329–58.

8   Cocchi also put forward some benefits to infants of artificial feeding, for example, that it saved them the hard work of suckling, and protected them against the risks of contagion passed from the nurse.

9   C. Corsini, 'Materiali per lo studio della famiglia in Toscana nel secoli XVII–XIX: gli esposti', *Quaderni Storici*, 33 (1976), pp.998–1052; idem, 'Breastfeeding, Fertility and Infant Mortality: Lessons from the Archive of the Florence Spedale degli Innocenti', in *Historical Perspectives on Breastfeeding*, published by order of UNICEF and the Istituto degli Innocenti (Florence, 1991), pp.63–83; P.P. Viazzo, M. Bortolotto and A. Zanotto, 'Continuity, Change and Chances: A Long-Term Perspective on Child Abandonment in Florence, 1445–1995', conference paper at 'Nobody's Children: Anthropological and Historical Perspectives on Child Abandonment and the Lives of Children without Fam-

ilies' (Durham, 1995), p.22; Viazzo, Bortolotto and Zanotto, 'Medicina, economia e etica: l'allattamento dei trovatelli a Firenze fra tradizione e innovazione (1740–1840)', *Bollettino di Demografia Storica*, 30/31 (1999), pp.147–59.

10   Viazzo *et al.*, 'Medicina, economia e etica', pp.155–6.

11   Archive of the Spedale degli Innocenti of Florence (hereafter AOIF), Affari Generali, LXXVI, 76, No. 9.

12   London Foundling Hospital General Registers, 1741–60 (LMA, A/FH/A09/2/1–5) and billet books, 1741–60 (LMA, A/FH/A09/001); Innocenti *Balie e bambini* (AOIF, *Serie* XVI, No. 105–6), 1–173.

13   For more detail on the nursing system at the London Foundling Hospital see A. Levene, *Childcare, Health and Mortality at the London Foundling Hospital, 1741–1800: 'Left to the Mercy of the World'* (Manchester, 2007), ch. 5.

14   Viazzo et al., 'Five Centuries', p.84.

15   See A. Levene, 'The Estimation of Mortality at the London Foundling Hospital, 1741–99', *Population Studies*, 59.1 (2005), pp.89–99.

16   Levene, 'Health and Survival Chances', pp.224–65; *eadem*, 'The Survival Prospects of European Foundlings in the Eighteenth Century: The London Foundling Hospital and the Spedale degli Innocenti of Florence', *Popolazione e Storia* (forthcoming).

17   Viazzo *et al.* ('Five Centuries', p.84) also note 'the foundling home's ability to keep infants alive for long periods in the hospital' in 1777.

18   A nineteenth-century commentator and medical officer at the Innocenti noted that even breast-fed infants were affected: many were returned in summer emaciated and in a poor state of health. F. Bruni, *Storia dell' I.E.R. spedale di S. Maria degl'Innocenti di Firenze e di molti altri pii stabilimenti*, 2 vols (Florence, 1819), 1, p.111.

19   A. Levene, 'Health and Survival Chances at the London Foundling Hospital and the Spedale degli Innocenti of Florence, 1741–99' (unpublished PhD thesis, University of Cambridge, 2002), pp.116–18.

20   Levene, *Childcare, Health and Mortality*, ch. 5.

21   D. Kertzer, 'Syphilis, Foundlings and Wetnurses in Nineteenth-Century Italy', *Journal of Social History*, 32.3 (1999), pp.589–602.

22   Given the still-popular belief that children imbibed their nurses' personal qualities with their milk, the avoidance of potentially unsuitable women was also desirable on this front.

23   Contardi, *Antonio Cocchi*; Goggioli, *Antonio Cocchi*.

24   AOIF, Affari Generali, LXXVI, 76, No. 9.

25   McClure, *Coram's Children*, p.195.

26   AOIF, Affari Generali, LXII, 74, No. 68.

27   AOIF, Affari Generali, LXXVI, 76, No. 9.

28   AOIF, Balie di casa, Affari Generali, *Serie* XI, Nos 2 and 3.

29   This is comparable to the foundling hospital at Perugia between 1700 and 1709, where the average stay of an internal wetnurse was eight months, with most nurses caring for fewer than ten children in total (L. Tittarelli, 'Le *balie di casa* e le *balie di fuori* nell'ospedale di S Maria della Misericordia di Perugia nel primo decennio del XVIII secolo', in *Enfance abandonée*, p.1144).

30   AOIF, *Serie* XXVI, No. 1, Malatti di nostri fanciulli e medicinali. 'Istruzione per i sigg. Parochi e avvertimenti per i bali.'

31   AOIF, Statistiche XLIV, No. 2, 1742, 1746; Affari Generali LXXVI, 76, No. 9.

32   M. Bortolotto and P.P. Viazzo, 'Assistenza agli esposti e declino della mortalità infantile allo Spedale degli Innocenti di Firenze nella prima metà dell'ottocento', *Bollettino di Demografia Storica*, 24–5 (1996), p.30.

33   AOIF, Affari Generali, LXXVI, 76, No. 61.

34   Viazzo *et al.*, 'Medicina, economia e etica', p.157.

35   AOIF, Affari Generali LXII, 72, No 27.

36   C. Klapisch-Zuber, *Women, Family and Ritual in Renaissance Italy*, English translation (Chicago, 1985); G.D. Sussman, *Selling Mothers' Milk: the Wet-Nursing Business in France, 1715–1914* (Illinois, 1982).

37   This was a consequence of 'Hanway's Act', following many of the principals followed at the London Foundling Hospital. See D.M. George, *London Life In the Eighteenth Century* (Harmondsworth, 1925), pp.58–9.

38   McClure, *Coram's Children*, pp.28–30.

39   Levene, *Childcare, Health and Mortality*, ch. 5.

Diego Ramiro Fariñas

Chapter 16: Mortality in Hospitals and Mortality in the City in Nineteenth- and Twentieth-Century Spain: The Effect on the Measurement of Urban Mortality Rates of the Mortality of Outsiders in Urban Health Institutions

Introduction

One of the most important challenges faced by historical demographers is to identify the causes behind the decline of mortality which has occurred since the later nineteenth century.[1] This is one of the most important lacunae which inhibit a full comprehension of the demographic evolution of populations. It is ironic that although we know in ever greater detail *how* this process took place, we still do not know *why*. In the absence of such knowledge we cannot explain how most of the developed countries have reached such a high expectancy of life at birth, mostly due to the decline in mortality. Nor can we contribute effectively to the scientific and popular debate of health-related issues which is attracting increased attention.

We know that in the long process of mortality decline in Spain, for example, life expectancy at birth has increased from around 29.8 years in the mid-nineteenth century to 79.67 years in 2002, with the probability of dying before reaching age 5 falling from a common level of over 450 per thousand during most of the nineteenth century, to slightly more than 5 per thousand in 2002. These are not just numbers but the realities of radical changes affecting the everyday life of the generations born during the past two centuries. In the mid-nineteenth century, half of all those born would die before the age of five. By contrast, virtually all babies today will reach adulthood, commence work and (if they so desire) marry and procreate. The mortality transition thus impacts on many other social and economic factors.

Within the transition process, there are two key periods to which, in my opinion, historical demographers need to direct more attention. One of these periods runs from the 1840s to the 1880s. This is the period when, in most European countries, there was a crucial change in demographic rates. Early childhood mortality ($_4q_1$) and infant mortality rate (q_0) began to decline, initiating simultaneously a continuous and sustained rise in life expectancy. However, despite constituting one of the most important demographic events in the history of humanity, and an open and vivid debate concerning the causes of that decline, at the beginning of the twenty-first century we still do not know why humans started to survive in larger numbers.

Figure 16.1
Infant Mortality Rate (q_0) in Urban and Rural Spain, 1900–33

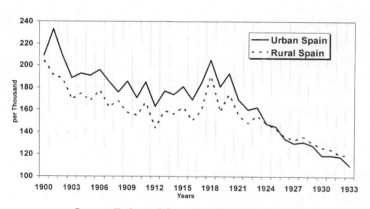

Source: Estimated from Vital Statistics for 1900–33

The second critical period is the first third of the twentieth century (see Figs 16.1 and 16.2). During this period a number of basic changes occurred which in combination had a profound impact on demography. In the first place, early childhood mortality, which in Spain usually exceeded infant mortality, declined steadily and more

Figure 16.2
Early Childhood Mortality ($_4q_1$) in Urban and Rural Spain, 1900–33

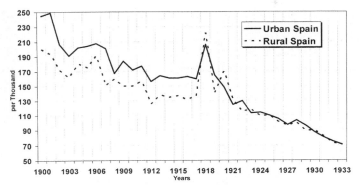

Source: Estimated from Vital Statistics for 1900 to 1933

quickly than infant mortality to fall to a level below the infant mortality rate. In the second place, there is the magnitude of the improvement in mortality. Both infant and early childhood mortality declined dramatically between 1900 and 1930, by 40 per cent in the case of infant mortality and by 60 per cent for child mortality. And finally, there was the crucial change in the experience of urban populations. On one hand, the natural growth rate in urban areas ceased to be negative, a common situation throughout the greater part of the nineteenth century, and became positive. The positive natural growth rate in conjunction with the constant arrival of migrants in the cities increased their populations very quickly. On the other hand, the rates of infant and early childhood mortality in the cities declined faster than those in the rural areas, with the result that by the 1920s childhood mortality in the rural areas exceeded that in urban areas. It is this last aspect, the differences between the level of urban and rural mortality, on which I am going to focus in the present analysis, by offering a new perspective on urban mortality and the process of the urbanisation and modernisation of European societies.

Sources and Methods

For this study and for the estimation of the various indicators of mortality, data on births and deaths were taken from vital statistics (*Movimiento Natural de la Población*) and data relating to population from Censuses, together with estimates on infant and child mortality (q_0 and $_4q_1$) published in the *Anuario Estadístico de España* (Statistical Yearbook of Spain) for the national level between 1990 and 1997. Data used in the last part of this article, in which information on an individual level has been recorded, have been directly obtained from the Civil Registers of each municipality.

The structure and contents of the official publications, used for the first part of this study, has led to some problems in their use. For example, census data and those from the vital statistics normally offer information by provinces and their capitals. When other information is available for urban areas different from provincial capitals, the information relates to municipalities over a specific size (normally over 10,000 or 20,000 inhabitants), a scale that normally changes across sources and time. Furthermore, only certain demographic variables are available (normally only total deaths and births). In practical terms it is, therefore, impossible to achieve a clear distinction between rural and urban areas from the sources utilised. However, it is possible to reach an approximation of this differentiation if one distinguishes the figures for the provincial capitals (as representative of the urban areas) from those for the remaining municipalities (as representing the rural areas).

Obviously, the use of this criterion has the disadvantage that it treats a number of urban areas as if they are rural. For example, in 1860, seven provincial capitals had a population of less than 10,000 inhabitants. Even in 1900, one provincial capital was still below 10,000 inhabitants. On the other hand, in 1860, two towns, which were not capitals, exceeded 50,000 inhabitants and nineteen, 20,000 inhabitants. One hundred years later, six non-capitals cities exceeded 100,000 inhabitants and twenty-four exceeded 50,000. At an intermediate date, 1900, three non-capital towns exceeded 50,000 inhabitants and twenty-six, 20,000 inhabitants. However, since there are no other available means of assessing mortality estimates that differentiate between urban and rural populations, we have to accept this method of disaggregation that gives us the nearest possible approximation to reliable results. Thus, in order to obtain the data for the rest of the municipalities (rural areas), the figures for the provincial capitals (urban areas) have been subtracted from those for the overall figures for the provinces. Nevertheless, it is necessary to bear in mind that the distinctions are imprecise and therefore it is important to take the appropriate precautions in interpreting the statistics. Another problem which affects the analysis is that for the same spatial units (provinces and capitals), it is not always possible to obtain data disaggregated by single years of age. At the same time, changes in the classifications cause great difficulty in elaborating a homogeneous and continuous series of demographic indicators.

In many cases, it has been necessary to adopt corrective measures to overcome such problems with the data. Two fundamental problems were encountered in the course of this study. The first relates to the absence of data on deaths in the first day of life, which stems from the custom of categorising such children as stillbirths. The need to take account of this sub-category has been argued by various authors.[2] Clearly, this has important implications in terms of measurement and for the interpretation of the infant mortality transition in Spain. The second problem stems from differences in the age classifications in the data collected in the vital statistics which make it difficult accurately to calculate the Early Childhood Mortality Rate ($_4q_1$), hereafter ECMR.

These different characteristics of the official statistics had an enormous impact on the groundwork for this study and, naturally, on the methods used. Thus, in the analysis of the structure of mortality in Spain, several key indicators were used: the probability of dying in the first year of life (q_0) and ECMR, the probability of dying in adulthood ($_{40}q_{20}$) and some estimations of life expectancy at several ages (e_0, e_{20}, e_{60}). The data used to calculate the childhood mortality estimates at national level (q_0 and $_4q_1$) for the years 1900 to 1997 were taken directly from vital statistics and the Statistical Yearbooks of Spain.[3]

In the calculation of q_0 it was necessary to introduce an adjustment in order to deal with the problem caused by the legal concept of live birth.[4] For administrative effects only live births are considered 'if the foetus born has a human figure and has lived twenty-four hours out of the mother', considering all others as 'abortive creatures' and not including them in births or deaths of infants. To try to correct this deficiency, mortality has been estimated for the first day of life using correcting measures.[5] For the estimation of ECMR ($_4q_1$) it has been necessary to follow different methods according to the documentation available.

For the second part of this study, information on an individual level, and only for the period 1877–8, has been recollected from the Civil Registers of two Central Spanish cities: Toledo (ca. 23,000 inhabitants in 1900) and Salamanca (ca. 25,000 inhabitants in 1900). A bigger sample of twenty Toledan rural municipalities (between c. 1,500 to c. 8,500 inhabitants in 1900), with information on mortality by age in single years, and months during the first year of life will be used for the same time period.[6] The first of these databases includes information on mortality by age, sex, birthplace and place of death in addition to other information. The population of the sample of urban and rural municipalities from Toledo represents slightly more than 26 per cent of the total population of that province. Estimations of mortality indicators have been done using the procedures established in the first part of this work.

Urban Mortality and Migration: The Effect of the Arrival of Migrants on Urban Institutional Mortality

It is well-known that the level of urban mortality was higher than that of rural mortality until well into the twentieth century. Weber wrote 'it is almost everywhere true that people die more rapidly in cities than in rural districts'.[7] Indeed, ever since Malthus characterised the phenomenon now known as the 'urban graveyard effect', the study of urban mortality has attracted the interest of many scholars. The Spanish case is no different. In Fig. 16.3 I have plotted in the form of a scatter diagram the probability of dying before reaching age five and the probability of dying in adulthood ($_{40}q_{20}$). Two time series are specified, one covering rural areas and the other urban ones. The principal difference between urban and rural areas becomes evident in adulthood, while childhood mortality that was initially higher in urban areas had reached very similar levels in urban and rural areas by the 1920s. However, this does not mean that we need to focus only on adult mortality to explain all the differences between urban and rural mortality. Some examples will demonstrate that adult mortality it is not the only key factor that can explain such patterns.

The terrible image of the cities was nourished, to a large extent, by two of their principal features: acting as a pole of attraction for the working-age population and their role as administrative centres. The first occasioned a continuous inflow of the rural population fleeing from the country, where the same employment opportunities did not exist as were to be found in the cities. Migration, 'not drop by drop, but in cascade',[8] increased the population density of the cities, which was already higher than that found in the countryside. This served to promote the diffusion of diseases in a city environment that was typically dirty and unhealthy and offered poor housing, often constructed near swampy areas. This increase in the diffusion of diseases was engendered by increased direct personal contact resulting from crowding, and through the increased contamination of water and food.

As administrative centres, the cities had to sustain, aside from other institutions, hospitals, prisons, retirement homes and foundling hospitals, with their pernicious effects on mortality. The impact on urban mortality was accentuated because sections of the institutional population were not usually resident in the cities but in the contiguous rural areas. Moreover, the cities also served as religious and military administrative centres, bringing further inhabitants to the cities.[9]

On the other hand, fertility and nuptiality were lower in the cities, resulting in lower natural urban growth rates than in the rural areas. Growth rates were usually negative. Nevertheless, the cities still grew in population. This phenomenon, known as the 'natural decrease problem', has inclined some authors to assert that the 'city populations

Diego Ramiro Fariñas

Figure 16.3
Change in Mortality of Children (5q0) and Adults (40q20) in Urban and Rural Spain, 1904–33

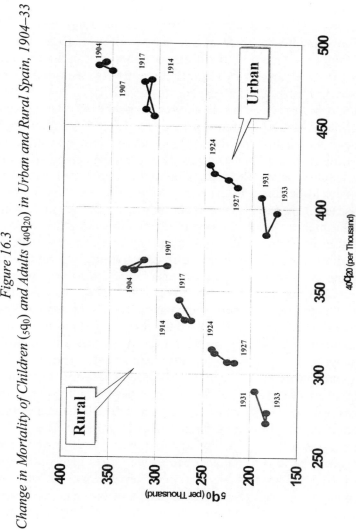

Source: Estimated from Census of Population for 1900, 1910, 1920 and 1930 and
Vital Statistics for 1904–7, 1914–17, 1924–7 and 1931–3

were only sustained due to migration'.[10] The ideas held by the advocates of the 'urban natural decrease' model and the advocates of the 'urban migration' model have made the study of the conditions of urban life a key subject in demography. In this respect, the effect of migration and its interaction with mortality are the key elements in the process.

An important unresolved issue is whether living conditions in the cities were really that bad and whether due allowance in the measurement of mortality has been accorded to the fact that the cities were the administrative centres and poles of attraction for migrants. When Sharlin developed his 'urban migration' model, he considered that the arrival of migrants in the cities changed the balance between births and deaths, since the migrants, according to his theory, inflated the number of deaths, while contributing far less to the number of births than did the permanent residents.[11] In terms of mortality, the obvious impact would be an increase in the number of deaths of persons of working age. It is important now to pause in the argument. By presenting a simple theoretical exercise which focuses on the effect of the arrival of migrants on the level of mortality, one can determine the different kinds of possibilities that could influence estimates of the level of mortality in urban areas. Assume, for the sake of argument, that the mortality of the locally born population of the city constitutes the normal level of mortality, that is to say, if a person is born in a city and then dies there, this will represent the base level of mortality. If an individual is born in the city and then decides to migrate and dies outside the city walls, the result will be that the level of mortality recorded for the city will be lower because that death will not be registered in the city registration system. Conversely, if an outsider arrives in the city and dies, this would increase the level of mortality recorded for the city. If an outsider comes to the city and then decides to migrate again, the effect could be either to leave the measured level of mortality unchanged, or, should that outsider have been registered in the census, to lower the calculated level of general mortality in the city (as the population assumed to be at risk of death will be increased without any comparable increase in the number of deaths). I am going to focus below on the third of these possibilities, those outsiders who arrived in the city and died.

Let us now take this simple theoretical analysis a stage further by introducing the further proposition that there is a registration system covering all the inhabitants of the city. The characteristics of the mortality of outsiders in the city in such a situation are set out in Fig. 16.4. I have included several different scenarios. One could be that the level and age structure of mortality of outsiders exactly matches that

Figure 16.4
A Simple Model of the Effect of the Mortality of Outsiders on the General Mortality Level of the City

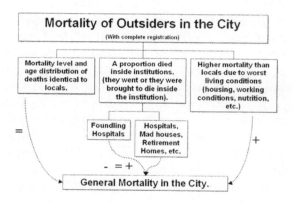

of the locally born inhabitants. Another includes those persons who died in institutions (foundling hospitals, hospitals, asylums for the insane, retirement homes, etc) following voluntary or involuntary incarceration. A third could be that outsiders experienced higher mortality than the locally born inhabitants due to exposure to poorer living conditions (housing, working conditions, nutrition...). How might these different possibilities affect the general mortality of the city? The first would not change the general mortality level. The third, which is widely accepted by historical demographers as representing the reality of conditions experienced by migrants to the city, would increase mortality levels in the city. The second scenario involving the mortality of outsiders in institutions could reduce mortality levels, if the institutions were effective and had mortality rates lower than those of the general population of the city. However, it would not change the mortality level if the conditions inside and outside the institutions were the same; and it could increase the level of mortality if the conditions were worse inside the institution than they were outside it. I will now focus on this last hypothesis. Moreover, the impact on the measured level of mortality could even be heightened should the registration system be incomplete, that is to say, that deaths of outsiders were registered but that the outsiders were not registered in the census.

It is important to point out that little attention in the debate has so far been given to the influence on the level of urban mortality of the geographical distribution of health and welfare agencies. By the middle of the nineteenth century, in countries such as Spain, most of the health institutions were located in the principal cities, and not until much later were such facilities expanded to smaller cities or towns. The rural population residing in the vicinity of the city and demanding health care needed to travel to the city's health institutions to receive attention. A proportion of those temporary migrants died in the city, increasing the number of deaths in the cities. By the end of the nineteenth century, around 4 per cent of total deaths in Spain took place in health or charitable institutions – such as foundlings hospitals, hospices, madhouses, maternity hospitals, hospitals, asylums – a total of almost 90,000 deaths.[12] However, this was not equally distributed between urban and rural areas. In urban Spain, on average, between 17 and 19 per cent of total deaths occurred inside the walls of health or charity institutions. In some provincial capitals more than one third of their total deaths took place in institutions (three of them in 1886–8, Gerona, León and Huesca). In ten provincial capitals in 1900 (Gerona, Toledo, Salamanca, Zamora, León, Huesca, Pamplona, Palencia, Córdoba and Burgos) this was around 30 per cent. In cities like Gerona and Toledo, almost 40 per cent of deaths occurred inside institutions. By 1888, in thirty-three out of forty-nine cities and forty of forty-nine in 1900 more than 15 per cent of their deaths took place in health and charity institutions. This is not surprising if we consider that Spain had at that time a very centralised health and charitable network system.[13]

The deaths of these temporary migrants, in the Spanish case, were normally not registered in the places of origin but instead were registered in the localities where they had died. At the same time, these outsiders were not always registered in the census. That means that such migrants contributed deaths to the total of urban deaths, while they did not appear in the registered population that was used as the total population at risk of dying. One such example, with similar consequences, is given by Revenga. In 1904, in his work *Mortality in Spain*, he attributed to the laws of 7 July 1888 and 30 June 1892 (which determined the tax rates to be applied for a consumption tax based on the size of the population of each settlement) the possibility of errors in the calculation of the total population of some urban settlements, with the consequent overestimation of the rate of mortality. With reference to the experience of several Spanish cities with around 12,000 inhabitants, he wrote 'the extraordinary fact is, that in many of the towns which have a level of mortality much higher than the provincial average, the number of inhabitants approaches one of the size categories fixed by those laws [...]' and that 'if the figure shown for the population of Spain has been under-estimated, as we maintain, the level of mortality is over-estimated'.[14] Both English and Spanish data indicate the scale of the problem. In seven London hospitals during the last third of the nineteenth century, 12 per cent of deaths were of persons normally resident outside the city.[15] In an earlier period (1774–81) almost 75 per cent of all patients at Westminster General Dispensary in London were born outside London.[16]

The effect that foundling hospitals had on overall urban mortality levels has also received little attention. Such institutions were usually located in provincial capitals, and collected abandoned children from the entire province. Although it is true that in some cases the orphans in foundling hospitals were sent to rural areas to be raised, the majority of them died during their first days or weeks in the orphanages, before they could be sent to the countryside. The high probabilities of dying in this type of institution, characterised by Stone (1966) as 'highly effective infanticide agencies', certainly inflated the level of childhood mortality in the cities.

By 1900, in urban areas in Spain, 7 per cent of their children's deaths took place inside health and charity institutions.[17] The smallest provincial capitals, under 20,000 inhabitants, had on average 14 per cent, cities between 20,000 and 100,000 inhabitants had 9 per cent, and cities with over 100,000 inhabitants and Madrid, 4 and 7 per cent respectively of their children's deaths took place in institutions. Rural areas had an almost insignificant 0.2 per cent. However, this overall picture hides some very important contrasts. On the one hand, in cities such as Zamora, Salamanca and Toledo, more than one quarter of their child deaths took place in institutions. On the other hand, cities such as Ávila, Huelva or Málaga had almost no mortality in institutions at these ages. By 1877–8, more than 10 per cent of all deaths registered in the city of Toledo, took place inside the walls of the Foundling Hospital, and the deaths of foundlings represented, in the period 1925 to 1930, one fifth of all deaths of children under the age of five.

Certainly our understanding of the pattern and level of urban mortality would be transformed should it prove possible to distinguish the mortality in the hospitals from other types of city mortality. It would also help if we could calculate the numbers of deaths of outsiders which were registered as deaths but for which there is no reference to that person either in the city census or in the birth registers.

The focus of many of the studies dealing with urban–rural differences on mortality has been the search for factors involved in the appearance of the so-called urban supra-mortality or 'urban penalty'.[18] In this search, some have considered the effect of migration and mortality in institutions on the measurement of the level of urban mortality. That is the case, for example, of Robert Lee who has studied Bremen[19] and Graham Mooney et al. who have examined the case of London[20] Others, like Reher, or Pérez Moreda, Ramiro, and Sanz,[21] focused their analysis on the explanation of the differences between urban and rural childhood mortality. But despite their important contributions, some of these studies have been limited by the availability of data, or by the limitations imposed by published statistics. Moreover, some of them concentrated their analysis on the working age population, avoiding the analysis of mortality at other ages and, also, when mobility has been considered, such as in Mooney's study of London, intra-city movements were the focus of attention while migrants arriving from outside the city were ignored.

Many important questions affecting our understanding of the impact of urbanisation thus remain unanswered. For example, it is still unclear to what extent the presence of heath facilities in the cities influenced urban mortality either directly (higher mortality in such institutions than in the general population) or indirectly (acting as poles of attraction for migrants from outside the cities). We need to establish whether urban mortality was so high partly as a result of the influence of an administrative effect whereby deaths were recorded in the place of occurrence and not in the place of origin of the deceased. The migration of a very small proportion of the population from the countryside to the city, some to live and work, others just to use their health facilities, with the unfortunate among them dying inside them, could have had a major impact on urban mortality. We need to determine whether the age distribution of deaths of outsiders in the city was of any importance for the estimation of life expectancy at birth. We also need to look at the significance of the fact that the higher mortality was concentrated in specific age groups, for example, through the forced migration of children to the foundling hospital, rather than distributed evenly across all age groups. When account is taken of these influences, the mortality of those inhabitants who had been born in the city may not have been so bad as it is usually depicted. Finally, we need to explore further the paradox that cities grew because of migration even though this migration increased levels of urban mortality.

Discussion: An Indirect Test of the Influence of Outsiders on the Level of Urban Mortality

Addressing all the issues raised above will require the accurate measurement of the impact on the level of urban mortality of the deaths of migrants, the re-allocation of those deaths to the home areas of the migrants, and the re-estimation of mortality in urban environments. Only a considerable research effort on these lines will yield a revised image of the reality of urban and rural mortality during the course of modernisation. One indirect approach, once it has been established, as regards whose deaths are those of outsiders and where the deaths had occurred, would be to deduct the deaths of migrants from the totals of registered deaths.[22] Another would be adding to the population recorded in the census an equivalent number of inhabitants as implied by the deaths of outsiders. In this case we would effectively be assuming that none of the outsiders were ever registered in the census, though this must be improbable. A less drastic solution would be to make the same sort of correction but limit it to those deaths of outsiders which occurred in institutions. In the case of the foundling hospital, for example, most of the children who arrived from outside the city died in a few days and before they could be registered.

Figure 16.5
Percentage of Deaths by Birthplace and Place of Death in Toledo,
1877–8

Place of Death	Locals	Outsiders	Total	% Outsiders
Outside Institutions	83	50	66	39
Foundling Hospitals	8	13	11	63
Hospitals (without Foundling Hospitals)	9	37	23	81
Number of Cases = 1423	100	100	100	51

Source: Civil Registers from Sample Localities

The first step, then, is to estimate the proportion of mortality attributable to the deaths of outsiders to the city. In this case I am going to use as an example the city of Toledo in 1877–8, a medium-sized city, with around 20,000 inhabitants at the time. In this city (see Fig. 16.5), 17 per cent of the inhabitants born in the city died inside an institution. For those born outside the city, the percentage who died in an institution was much higher (50 per cent). One third of all deaths in Toledo during these two years occurred in institutions. Of those deaths inside hospitals[23] 81 per cent were of outsiders, as were 63 per cent of the deaths in the foundling hospitals. Of all deaths in Toledo, 51 per cent were those of outsiders. If we consider only children, by 1877–8,

Toledo and Salamanca had 42 and 20 per cent, respectively, of their children's deaths taking place in institutions (see Fig. 16.6). For those born outside the city, the percentage who died in an institution was much higher (70 and 41 per cent). Of these deaths inside the institutions, 42 per cent in Toledo and 30 per cent in Salamanca were migrants. Of all children's deaths in Toledo and Salamanca, 25 and 14 per cent, respectively, corresponded to outsiders.

Figure 16.6
Percentage of Deaths of Children by Birthplace and Place of Death:
Toledo and Salamanca, 1877–8

	Place of Death	Locals	Outsiders	Total	% Outsiders
Toledo	Outside Institutions	68	30	58	13
	Inside Institutions	32	70	42	42
	Cases = 565	100	100	100	25
Salamanca	Place of Death	Locals	Outsiders	Total	% Outsiders
	Outside Institutions	84	59	80	10
	Inside Institutions	16	41	20	30
	Cases = 565	100	100	100	14

Source: Civil Registers from Sample Localities

The structure of mortality by age and birthplace also shows important differences.[24] For example for children, while individuals native born in Toledo and Salamanca had a mainly homogenous mortality structure, going from high percentages in the first year to a small percentage in the fifth year of life, migrants, suffered a higher concentration of deaths in the first year of life and also, in relative terms, in the fifth one. This structural pattern by age seems to be closely related with childhood mortality patterns of permanent residents in the city who died at home, on the one hand, and on the other hand, foreigners who arrived to the cities and died in a health or charitable institution. However, around 70 per cent of all children's deaths of migrants to health institutions (movers in search of health attention) died during the first year of life, while native born individuals dying in their own homes (permanents) corresponded to around 4 per cent. By the second year of life, almost all mortality of foreigners in institutions had already taken place, with more than 90 per cent of all deaths happening during the first year. This different structural childhood mortality by age and the concentration of deaths in certain age ranges, namely infant mortality, had important implications for overall urban mortality, which experienced an inflation of mortality in very specific age groups affecting other estimations such as life expectancy.

Let us move to the second stage of the argument. This involves the estimation of the general level of mortality in the city. We therefore calculated a life table for Toledo for 1877, using the census which was carried out in that year in conjunction with data from the civil register from 1877 and 1878 for deaths and from 1875–8 for births, the latter in order to avoid using census data to estimate infant and early childhood mortality (q_0 and $_4q_1$). Since in the civil registers there is not only information on age, sex and cause of death, but also data on birthplace and place of death – that is to say, if the individual died at home, in a hospital or in a foundling hospital – it is possible to estimate urban mortality without introducing the distortion of including the deaths of the residents of institutions and of those who had not been born in the city. It is also possible to establish which institutions had the most impact on the registered level of urban mortality and in some cases to compare the age and cause of deaths patterns of the institutionalised and non-institutionalised population.

In Fig. 16.7, I have included some estimates of mortality (e_0, e_{20}, e_{60}, q_0, $_4q_1$, $_{40}q_{20}$) for the City of Toledo, using the census data for 1877 and data from the civil register. In addition, I have included comparable estimates of mortality for a sample of Toledan villages, a sample which represents around 4 to 5 per cent of all the rural population of the province.[25] As can be seen, the differences between the urban area and the rural areas approximate those discussed above. Life expectancy in the city of Toledo was five years lower than in the rural areas and the city experienced higher child and adult mortality.

However, the registered level of mortality of the city is modified dramatically if we re-estimate the level of mortality to take into account the effect of the deaths of outsiders. If we deduct from the general mortality of the city those deaths of outsiders who died in the

Figure 16.7
The Effect of Deaths of Outsiders inside Institutions on Life Expectancy and Probabilities of Dying at Different Ages in the City of Toledo, 1877–8

	e_0	e_{20}	e_{60}	q_0	$_4q_1$	$_{40}q_{20}$
Without Foundling H	29.9	–	–	195	259	–
With Foundling H	27.0	–	–	238	295	–
Without Hospitals	28.7	40.8	14.6	–	–	430
With Hospitals	25.9	35.5	10.4	–	–	534
With both	27.1	35.5	10.4	238	295	534
Without Both	33.3	40.8	14.6	195	259	430
Total	25.8	35.3	10.1	250	316	536
Rural Sample	*31.2*	*40.0*	*12.7*	*256*	*255*	*422*

Source: Civil Registers from Sample Institutions

foundling hospital, the registered life expectancy at birth increases by more than 4 years, and the suggested level of infant mortality declines by more than fifty points, falling below that found in the rural areas, while the level of childhood mortality becomes the same as that in rural areas. If instead of deducting those deaths we included them in the denominator, that is to say, we add them to the total of persons recorded by the census in appropriate age groups, the estimate of life expectancy in the city increases by 1.2 years. If, in a further calculation, we exclude those deaths of outsiders which took place in hospitals, the estimate of life expectancy at birth in the city increases by three years, and the level of adult mortality becomes equivalent to that of the rural areas. Excluding the deaths of outsiders in both types of institutions, foundling and other hospitals, from the calculation of general mortality in the city of Toledo, produces estimates of life expectancy at birth that are more than two years higher in urban than in rural areas.

It is more complicated to measure the effect of the second scenario which involves the mortality of outsiders in institutions and which states that mortality levels could be reduced, if the institutions were effective and had mortality rates lower than those of the general population of the city. It would not change the mortality level if the conditions inside and outside the institutions were the same (despite the fact that there is a probable under-registration of moving population in the city census); and it could increase the mortality level if the conditions were worse inside the institution than they were outside it. To be able to carry out a test with this scenario it is necessary to have information on mortality by birthplace, place of death and age and the same level of detail for the population at risk. Sadly this information is not available for all age ranges and with this level of detail, and it is only possible to have this information if access to individual level data on deaths, births and census population is granted, which normally is not easily accessible or can be non-existent. However, and only for Salamanca, we have been able to estimate infant mortality inside and outside the foundling hospital, and the proportion by which the city Infant Mortality Rate (IMR) increased due to the presence of the foundling hospital.[26] IMR in Salamanca was 233 per thousand by 1877–8; in the Salamanca's foundling hospital it was 484 per thousand, meaning that half of the children did not survive to the following year, while IMR in the city without the births and deaths in the foundling hospital was 171 per thousand. This means that IMR increases by almost 25 per cent if deaths and births from the foundling hospital are taken into consideration. The reduction of sixty-two points in the IMR makes an urban area such as Salamanca healthier during the first year of life than most surrounding rural areas. The effect at other ages is more reduced. We must remember that deaths of foundlings are mostly concentrated in the first year of life.

Given such results it would be unwise, therefore, to continue to argue that living conditions in the city were worse than those in rural areas. Admittedly, this is only one case study, possibly an extreme one, and it is necessary to measure the impact of the mortality of migrants on the estimates of the level of mortality in the city in a more direct way.

This simple example must nevertheless force us to reassess whether mortality in the cities was in reality as high as it is often represented. In turn we need to reconsider many of our ideas about the process of urbanisation and modernisation, in which the cities, until now, have always played the role of terrifying human slaughterhouses, a role that I think did not reflect the reality. Rather I would argue that the cities suffered because of their success as dynamic centres and for that reason, poles of attraction for migrants.

Notes

1   This work constitutes one element of the projects 'Demographic Modernization and the Decline of Mortality in Urban and Rural Spain: 1860–1960', financed by the Ministry of Science and Technology (BSO2000–0673), carried out at the University Complutense of Madrid, 'Mortality and Migration during the First Third of the Twentieth Century: Spain in an International Comparison', financed by the Ministry of Science and Technology (BSO2002–01521), and 'Mortality in Institutions and Urban Demography: Madrid in an International Comparative Perspective', funded by the Ministry of Education and Science (SEJ2005–06334), carried out at the Spanish Council for Scientific Research. I would also like to thank those present at the ESTER seminar on 'Health, Medicine and Society' which took place at the University of Liverpool in 1997 and where the basic ideas of this contribution were presented, the Cambridge Group for the History of Population and Social Structure seminar, and the 'Población, Espacio y Sociedad' of the Facultad de Ciencias Políticas y Sociología of Madrid seminar, for their helpful comments and suggestions.

2   M. Pascua, *La mortalidad infantil en España* (Madrid, 1934); A. Arbelo Curbelo, 'Necesidad demográfico sanitaria de rectificar el concepto legal de nacido vivo', *Revista Internacional de Sociología*, 9 (1951) (36), pp.393–405; A. Arbelo Curbelo, *La mortalidad de la infancia en España, 1901–50* (Madrid, 1962), and R. Gómez Redondo, *La mortalidad infantil española en el siglo XX* (Madrid: CIS, Siglo XXI, 1992) and more recently D. Ramiro, 'La evolución de la mortalidad en la infancia en la España interior, 1785–1960' (unpublished PhD dissertation, University Complutense of Madrid, 1998), and A. Sanz Gimeno, *La mortalidad de la infancia en Madrid. Cambios demográfico-sanitarios en los siglos XIX y XX* (Madrid, 1999).

3   D. Ramiro Fariñas and A. Sanz Gimeno, 'Childhood Mortality in Central Spain, 1790–1960: Changes in the Course of Demographic Modernisation', *Continuity and Change*, 15.2 (2000), pp.235–67.

4   F. Dopico and D.Reher, *El declive de la mortalidad en España, 1860–1930*, Monográfias 1 (Zaragoza, 1998).

5   See Ramiro and Sanz, 'Childhood Mortality'.

6   Detailed information regarding this sample of Toledan rural municipalities can be found in Ramiro, 'La evolución de la mortalidad en la infancia', and Ramiro and Sanz, 'Childhood Mortality'.

7   A.F. Weber, *The Growth of Cities in the Nineteenth Century: A Study in Statistics* (New York, 1899), p.343

8   S. Aznar, *Despoblación y colonización* (Madrid, 1930), pp.28–9.

9   See for example D. Ramiro, 'Urban and rural mortality in Central Spain: 1858–1960', ESTER seminar on 'Health, Medicine and Society', Liverpool, 7–11 September 1997, or D. Ramiro, 'Urban and Rural Mortality in Central Spain during the Nineteenth and Twentieth Century', BSPS Annual Conference, 1999, University College, Dublin, 6–8 September, in which a theoretical framework, based on a case study, is used to analyse the effects of mobility and mortality in institutions on mortality in urban areas.

10 E.A. Wrigley, *Historia y población: Introducción a la demografía histórica*, (Barcelona, 1990), p.98.

11 A good illustration of this debate can be found in: A. Sharlin, 'Natural Decrease in Early Modern Cities: A Reconsideration', *Past and Present*, 79 (1978), pp.126–38; R. Finlay, 'Natural Decrease in Early Modern Cities', *Past and Present*, 92 (1981), pp.169–74; A. Sharlin, 'A Rejoinder', *Past and Present*, 92 (1981), pp.175–80; N. Keyfitz, 'Do Cities Grow by Natural Increase or by Migration?', *Geographical Analysis*, 12.2 (1980), pp.143–56; A. van de Woude, 'Population Developments in the Northern Netherlands (1500–1800) and the Validity of the "Urban Graveyard Effect"', *Annales de Demographie Historique* (1982), pp.55–75; R.I. Woods, 'What Would One Need to Know to Solve the "Natural Decrease in Early Modern Cities" Problem?', in R. Lawton, *The Rise and Fall of Great Cities* (London, 1989), pp.80–95; E.A. Hammel and C. Mason, 'My Brother's Keeper: Modelling Kinship Links in Early Urbanization', in D. Reher and R.S. Schofield (eds), *Old and New Methods in Historical Demography* (Oxford, 1993), pp.318–42; C. Galley, 'A Model of Early Modern Urban Demography', *Economic History Review*, 48.3 (1995), pp.448–69, and R. Lee, 'Urban Labour Markets, In-Migration, and Demographic Growth: Bremen, 1815–1914', *Journal of Interdisciplinary History*, 30.3 (1999), pp.437–73.

12 Between 1879 to 1882, 94.9 per cent of all deaths took place at home, 4.2 in health and charity institutions, 0.1 in correctional centres and prisons, 0.2 in the street and 0.6 in open fields (*Movimiento Natural de la Población*, 1886–92, p.34).

13 P. Carasa Soto, *El sistema hospitalario español en el siglo XIX: De la asistencia benéfica al modelo sanitario actual* (Valladolid, 1985).

14 R. Revenga, *La muerte en España, estudio estadístico sobre la mortalidad* (Madrid, 1904), p.15.

15 G. Mooney et al., 'Patient Pathways: Solving the Problem of Institutional Mortality in London during the Later Nineteenth Century', *Social History of Medicine*, 12.2 (1999), p.247.

16 J. Landers, *Death and the Metropolis: Studies in the Demographic History of London, 1670–1830* (Cambridge, 1993), p.47.

416   *Diego Ramiro Fariñas*

17   This estimation is the percentage of children under 5 years old dying in
     institutions over the total of deaths of children under 5 years old.
18   See for example G. Kearns, 'The Urban Penalty and the Population History of
     England', in A. Brändström and L.G. Tedebrand (eds), *Society, Health and
     Population during the Demographic Transition* (Stockholm, 1988), pp.213–36;
     G. Kearns, 'Le handicap urbain et le declin de la mortalité en Angleterre et au
     Pays de Galles, 1851–1900', *Annales de Demographie Historique* (1993),
     pp.75–105; or more recently Lee, 'Urban labour markets'; Mooney et al.,
     'Patient Pathways'; D. Ramiro and A. Sanz, 'Structural Changes in Childhood
     Mortality in Spain, 1860–1990', *International Journal of Population Geog-
     raphy*, 6 (2000), pp.61–82; D.S. Reher, 'In Search of the "Urban Penalty": Ex-
     ploring Urban and Rural Mortality Patterns in Spain during the Demographic
     Transition', *International Journal of Population Geography*, 7 (2001), pp.105–
     27; M. Haines, 'The Urban Mortality Transition in the United States, 1800–
     1940', *Annales de Demographie Historique* (2001), pp.33–64.
19   Lee, 'Urban Labour Markets', pp.437–73.
20   Mooney et al., 'Patient Pathways', pp.227–69.
21   In the case of Reher, 'In Search of the "Urban Penalty"', and V. Pérez Moreda,
     D. Ramiro Fariñas and A. Sanz Gimeno, 'Dying in the City: Urban Mortality in
     Spain in the Middle of the Health Transition, 1900–1931', in E. Sonnino (ed.),
     Living in the City (14th–20th Centuries) (Rome, 2004), the analysis of childhood
     mortality is one component of an overall analysis of mortality by age groups.
22   The best way in which this problem could be solved is by searching in the
     census for those individuals recorded in the civil registers, thereby making it
     possible to estimate more directly the degree of under-registration of migrants
     in the census.
23   Hospitals include all institutions apart from the foundling hospitals.
24   The structure of mortality in this case refers to how deaths are distributed
     according to age. Total deaths under five years old = 100.
25   Rural means in this case municipalities with fewer than 10,000 inhabitants
26   In Salamanca, births recorded those children who were registered as foundlings,
     therefore allowing the estimation of IMR inside the foundling hospital by
     dividing children dying during the first year of life by births in the foundling
     hospital. The rest of the city IMR has been estimated by removing from births
     and deaths those children from the foundling hospital. It is possible that some of
     the foundlings who died in institutions were registered as births outside the
     foundling hospital, and that effect would reduce the differences between institu-
     tional and non-institutional mortality, therefore reducing the effect of foundling
     mortality over overall urban mortality. However, this is a very difficult problem
     to disentangle.

List of Contributors

ANNMARIE ADAMS, School of Architecture, McGill University

STEVE CHERRY, School of History, University of East Anglia

FLURIN CONDRAU, Centre for the History of Science, Technology and Medicine, University of Manchester

MARINA GARBELLOTTI, Centre for Italo-German Historical Studies, University of Trento

LOUISE GRAY, Wellcome Trust Centre for the History of Medicine at University College London

ERIC GRUBER VON ARNI, Independent Scholar

JOHN HENDERSON, School of History, Classics and Archaeology, Birkbeck University of London

PEREGRINE HORDEN, Department of History, Royal Holloway University of London

ALYSA LEVENE, School of Arts and Humanities, Oxford Brookes University

SERGIO ONGER, Department of Social Studies, University of Brescia

ALESSANDRO PASTORE, Faculty of Arts and Philosophy, University of Verona

DIEGO RAMIRO FARIÑAS, Institute of Economics and Geography, Spanish Council for Scientific Research, Madrid

CAROLE RAWCLIFFE, School of History, University of East Anglia

KEVIN C. ROBBINS, Department of History, Indiana University Purdue University Indianapolis

MAX SATCHELL, Department of Geography, University of Cambridge

MATTHEW THOMAS SNEIDER, Department of History, University of Massachusetts-Dartmouth

CHRISTINE STEVENSON, Courtauld Institute of Art, University of London

ANDREA TANNER, Great Ormond Street Hospital for Children, London, and School of Social Science, Kingston University

Index